Mastering The Boards and Clinical Examinations In Internal Medicine

CARDIOLOGY

A.B.R. Thomson

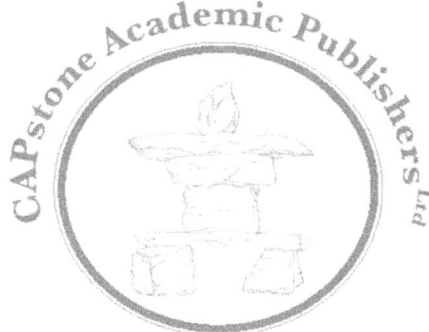

CAPstone (Canadian Academic Publishers Ltd) is a not-for-profit company dedicated to the use of the power of education for the betterment of all persons everywhere.

"The Democratization of Knowledge"
Peace through Medicine

 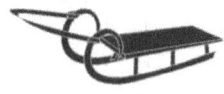

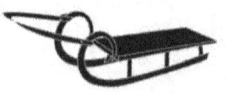

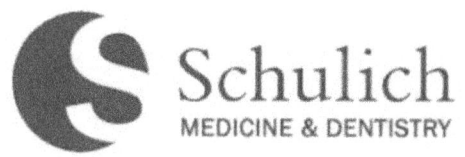 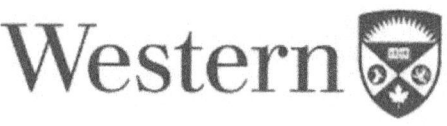

THE WESTERN WAY

Medical drawings by S. Lee and E. Howell

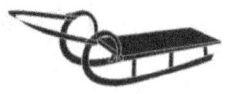

Mastering the Boards: Cardiology   A.B.R. Thomson

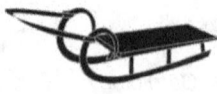

Mastering the Boards: Cardiology   A.B.R. Thomson

TABLE OF CONTENTS

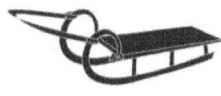

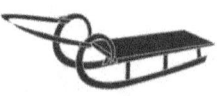

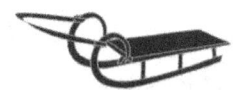

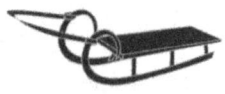

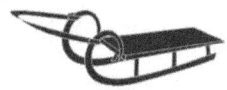

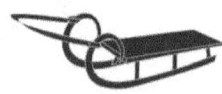

DISCLAIMER

The primary purpose of this publication is education. The author, editor and publisher acknowledge that the development of new material opens to way for possible errors – what is correct today might not be the standard of care tomorrow. Readers are advised to ensure that the doses of drugs which they use are in compliance with their country's product information, and that the use of any therapeutic agent, be it a pharmaceutical or a technology, should be guided by local guidelines. There is often a wide diversity of professional opinion, and guidelines from one country are not always congruent with another.

The author, editor and publisher do not guarantee the safety, reliability, accuracy, completeness or usefulness of this material.

They disclaimer any and all liability for damage and claims that may result from the use of information, publications, technologies, products, and for series provided in this publication.

We have made every attempt to trace the holders of copyright for material reproduced in this book. If by some oversight we have omitted a copyright holder, please contact us.

Thank you

A. B. R. Thomson

 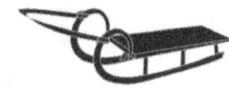

MASTERING THE BOARDS AND THE CANMED OBJECTIVES

Medical expert
The discussion of complex cases provides the participants with an opportunity to comment on additional focused history and physical examination. They would provide a complete and organized assessment. Participants are encouraged to identify key features, and they develop an approach to problem-solving.

The case discussions, as well as the discussion of cases around a diagnostic imaging, pathological or endoscopic base provides the means for the candidate to establish an appropriate management plan based on the best available evidence to clinical practice. Throughout, an attempt is made to develop strategies for diagnosis and development of clinical reasoning skills.

Communicator
The participants demonstrate their ability to communicate their knowledge, clinical findings, and management plan in a respectful, concise and interactive manner. When the participants play the role of examiners, they demonstrate their ability to listen actively and effectively, to ask questions in an open-ended manner, and to provide constructive, helpful feedback in a professional and non-intimidating manner.

Collaborator
The participants use the "you have a green consult card" technique of answering questions as fast as they are able, and then to interact with another health professional participant to move forward the discussion and problem solving. This helps the participants to build upon what they have already learned about the importance of collegial interaction.

Manager
The participants are provided with assignments in advance of the three day GI Practice Review. There is much work for them to complete before as well as afterwards, so they learn to manage their time effectively, and to complete the assigned tasks proficiently and on time. They learn to work in teams to achieve answers from small group participation, and then to share this with other small group participants through effective delegation of work. Some of the material they must access demands that they use information technology effectively to access information that will help to facilitate the delineation of adequately broad differential diagnoses, as well as rational and cost effective management plans.

Health advocate
In the answering of the questions and case discussions, the participants are required to consider the risks, benefits, and costs and impacts of investigations and therapeutic alliances upon the patient and their loved ones.

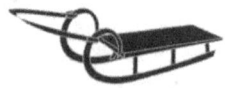

Scholar
By committing to the pre- and post-study requirements, plus the intense three day active learning Practice Review with colleagues is a demonstration of commitment to personal education. Through the interactive nature of the discussions and the use of the "green consult card", they reinforce their previous learning of the importance of collaborating and helping one another to learn.

Professional
The participants are coached how to interact verbally in a professional setting, being straightforward, clear and helpful. They learn to be honest when they cannot answer questions, make a diagnosis, or advance a management plan. They learn how to deal with aggressive or demotivated colleagues, how to deal with knowledge deficits, how to speculate on a missing knowledge byte by using first principals and deductive reasoning. In a safe and supportive setting they learn to seek and accept advice, to acknowledge awareness of personal limitations, and to give and take 360^0 feedback.

Knowledge
The basic science aspects of gastroenterology are considered in adequate detail to understand the mechanisms of disease, and the basis of investigations and treatment. In this way, the participants respect the importance of an adequate foundation in basic sciences, the basics of the design of clinical research studies to provide an evidence-based approach, the designing of clinical research studies to provide an evidence-based approach, the relevance of their management plans being patient-focused, and the need to add "compassionate" to the Three C's of Medical Practice: competent, caring and compassionate.

"They may forget what you said, but they will never forget how you made them feel."

Carl W. Buechner, on teaching.

"With competence, care for the patient. With compassion, care about the person."

Alan B. R. Thomson, on being a physician.

 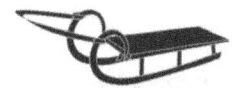

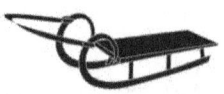

DEDICATION

To Harold and Mary Fran,

And

John and Ellen Hill

 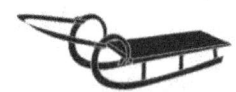

PROLOGUE

HREs, better known as, High Risk Examinations. After what is often two decades of study, sacrifice, long hours, dedication, ambition and drive, we who have chosen Internal Medicine, and possibly through this a subspecialty, have a HRE, the [Boards] Royal College Examinations. We have been evaluated almost daily by the sadly subjective preceptor based assessments, and now we face the fierce, competitive, winner-take-all objective testing through multiple choice questions (MCQs), and for some the equally challenging OSCE, the objective standardized clinical examination. Well we know that in the real life of providing competent, caring and compassionate care as physicians, as internists, that a patient is neither a MCQ or an OSCE. These examinations are to be passed, a process with which we may not necessarily agree. Yet this is the game in which we have thus far invested over half of our youthful lives. So let us know the rules, follow the rules, work with the rules, and succeed. So that we may move on to do what we have been trained to do, do what we may long to do, care for our patients.

The process by which we study for clinical examinations is so is different than for the MCQs: not trivia, but an approach to the big picture, with thoughtful and reasoned deduction towards a diagnosis. Not looking for the answer before us, but understanding the subtle aspects of the directed history and focused physical examination, yielding an informed series of hypotheses, a differential diagnosis to direct investigations of the highly sophisticated laboratory and imaging procedures now available to those who can wait, or pay.

This book provides clinically relevant questions of the process of taking a history and performing a physical examination, with sections on Useful background, and where available, evidence-based performance characteristics of the rendering of our clinical skills. Just for fun are included "So you want to be a such-and-such specialist!" to remind us that one if the greatest strengths we can possess to survive in these times, is to smile and even to laugh at ourselves.

Sincerely,

[signature]

Emeritus Distinguished University Professor, U of A
Adjunct Professor, Western University

ACKNOWLEDGEMENTS

Patience and patients go hand in hand. So also does the interlocking of young and old, love and justice, equality and fairness. No author can have thoughts transformed into words, no teacher can make ideas become behaviour and wisdom and art, without those special people who turn our minds to the practical - of getting the job done!

Thank you, Naiyana and Duen for translating those terrible scribbles, called my handwriting, into the still magical legibility of the electronic age. Thank you, Sarah, and Becky for your creativity and hard work.

My most sincere and heartfelt thanks go to the excellent persons at JP Consulting, and CapStone Academic Publishers. Jessica, you are brilliant, dedicated and caring. Thank you.

When Rebecca, Maxwell, Megan Grace, Henry Felix, Toby and Grady ask about their Grandad, I will depend on James and Anne, Matthew and Allison, Jessica and Matt, and Benjamin to be understanding and kind. For what I was trying to say and to do was to make my professional life focused on the three C's - competence, caring, and compassion - and to make my very private personal life dedicated to family - to you all.

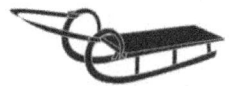

ARE YOU PREPARING FOR EXAMS IN GASTROENTEROLOGY AND HEPATOLOGY?

See the full range of examination preparation and review publications from CAPstone on Amazon.com

Gastroenterology and Hepatology

First Principles of Gastroenterology and Hepatology in Adults and Children - Volume I – Gastroenterology (ISBN: 978-1494345624)

First Principles of Gastroenterology and Hepatology in Adults and Children - Volume II - Hepatology and Paediatrics (ISBN: 978-1494345501)

Medical Mini Review Series in Gastroenterology and Hepatology: Efficient Refresher for the Busy Clinical Gastroenterologist (ISBN: 978-1502472199)

Medical Mini Review Series in Gastroenterology and Hepatology: Efficient Refresher for the Busy Clinical Gastroenterologist (ISBN: 978-1502472199)

Guideline-Based Management in Gastroenterology (ISBN: 978-1515078623)

Guideline-Based Management in Hepatology (ISBN: 978-1502928078)

Practice Review in Gastroenterology (ISBN: 978-1500855321)

Practice Review in Hepatopancreatobiliary Diseases and Nutrition (ISBN: 978-1500855734)

Endoscopy and Diagnostic Imaging - Part I: Skin, Nail and Mouth Changes in GI Disease; Esophagus; Stomach; Small intestine; Pancreas (ISBN: 978-1477400579)

Endoscopy and Diagnostic Imaging - Part II: Colon and Hepatobiliary (ISBN: 978-1477400654)

Scientific Basis for Clinical Practice in Gastroenterology and Hepatology (ISBN: 978-1475226645)

The Physiology and Pathophysiology of Gastrointestinal and Hepatopancreaticobiliary Disorders: Preparing for Professional Competence. (ISBN: 978-1500298265)

General Internal Medicine

Achieving Excellence in the OSCE - Part One: Cardiology to Nephrology (ISBN: 978-1475283037)

Achieving Excellence in the OSCE - Part Two: Neurology to Rheumatolgy (ISBN: 978-1475276978)

Mastering the Boards and Clinical Examinations in Internal Medicine, Part I: Cardiology, Endocrinology, Gastroenterology, Hepatology and Nephrology (ISBN: 978-1461024842)

Mastering The Boards and Clinical Examinations In Internal Medicine, part II: Neurology, Respirology and Rheumatology (ISBN: 978-1478392736)

Bits and Bytes: Surviving Morning Rounds (ISBN: 978-1478295365)

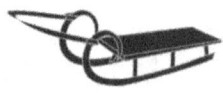

Mastering the Boards: Cardiology   A.B.R. Thomson

CARDIOLOGY

 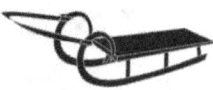

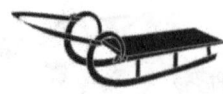

GENERAL INTRODUCTION

Useful background: the "O to W" of any history"

O= **O**nset and duration
P = **P**rovoking and alleviation factors
Q = **Q**uality of pain (e. g. "Is the pain sharp or dull? Is it throbbing?")
R = **R**adiation of pain
S = **S**everity (on a scale from 1 to 10)
T = **T**iming and progression (e. g. Is the pain constant or intermittent?")
U = "How does it affect '**U**' in your daily life?"
V = déjà **V**u? (e.g. "Has it happened before?"
W = '**W**hat do you think is causing it?"

Source: Filate W, et al. *The Medical Society, Faculty of Medicine, University of Toronto* 2005, page 7.

Sensitivity   PID   present in disease
Specificity   NIH   negative in health

PLR = sensitivity/ 1-sensitivity
NLR = 1-sensitivity/specificity

Accuracy of the history and physical exam
  o One study in general medical clinic found that 55% of patients had been assigned correct diagnosis at the end of the history, and that number rose to 73% by the end of the physical examination.

Source: Sackett DL, et al. *JAMA* 1992; 267: 2650-265; and Filate W, et *The Medical Society, Faculty of Medicine, University of Toronto* 2005, page 5.

• Take a directed history for disease of the cardiovascular system.

➢ Cardiovascular symptoms
  o Chest pain
  o Dyspnea – exertion, paroxysmal nocturnal dyspnea (PND), orthopnea
  o Cough
  o Palpitations
  o Ankle swelling
  o Intermittent claudication

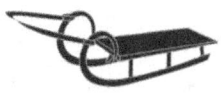

- ➤ Associated symptoms
  - ○ Left side heart failure (L-HF)
    - - Fatigue
    - - SOB, SOBOE orthopnea
    - - Cough, hemoptysis
    - - Baseline exercise in tolerance
    - - Cyanosis
    - - Cool extremities
    - - Palpations
    - - Nausea, vomiting
  - ○ Right side heart failure (R-HF)
    - - Edema of ankles, sacrum
    - - Tender hepatomegaly
    - - Determine New York class of HF
  - ○ Syncope
  - ○ Fatigue
  - ○ Weight gain
- ➤ Functional status (New York Heart Association Classification, Angina/ dyspnea activity on activity and relationship to exercise)
  - ○ Class I – intense
  - ○ Class II – ordinary
  - ○ Class III – less than ordinary
  - ○ Class IV – at rest
- ➤ Associated conditions/risk factors
  - ○ Hypertension
  - ○ Hyperlipidemia
  - ○ Hyperhomocysteinemia
  - ○ Obesity
  - ○ Diabetes
  - ○ Physical inactivity
  - ○ Smoking
  - ○ Causes of L/R- HF
  - ○ Family history
  - ○ Personal past history of CAD, PVD, rheumatic fever, cardiac murmur, cardiac surgery, cardiac events, medications
  - ○ Risk factors for CAD

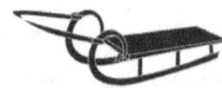

Abbreviations: CAD, coronary artery disease; HF, heart failure; L-CHF, left side heart failure; PND, paroxysmal nocturnal dysphea; PVD, peripheral vascular disease; R-HF, right side heart failure; SOB, shortness of breath; SOBOE, shortness of breath on exertion

Adapted from: Talley N.J, et al. *Maclennan & Petty Pty Limited* 2003, page 27.

- Perform a focused inspection of the patient for cardiac disease.

➢ Body appearance
  - Frightened, struggling, diaphoretic, tachypneic – pulmonary edema
  - Anasarca of congestive heart failure
  - Tall stature, long extremities, and sparse subcutaneous fat of Marfan syndrome. Patients are prone to mitral valve prolapse and aortic dilatation and dissection.
  - Tall stature and long extremities of Klinefelter syndrome. Patients may have atrial or ventricular septal defects, patent ductus arteriosus, and even tetralogy of Fallot.
  - Long extremities, kyphoscoliosis, and pectus carinatum of homocystinuria. Patients often present with thrombosis of medium-sized arteries.
  - Tall stature and thick extremities of acromegaly (associated with hypertension, cardiomyopathy, and conduction defects).
  - Short stature, webbed neck, low hairline, small chin, wide-set nipples, and sexual infantilism of Turner syndrome (associated with coarctation of the aorta and valvular pulmonic stenosis).
  - Dwarfism and polydactyly of Ellis-van Creveld syndrome (associated with atrial septal defects and common atrium).
  - Morbid obesity and somnolence of obstructive sleep apnea (associated with hypoventilation, pulmonary hypertension, and cor pulmonale)
  - Truncal obseity, thin extremities, moon face, and buffalo hump and hypertensive patients with Cushing syndrome.
  - Mesomorphic, overweight, balding, hairy, and tense middle-aged patient prone to coronary artery disease.
  - Hammer toes and pes cavus of Friedreich ataxia (associated with hypertrophic cardiomyopathy, angia, and sick sinus syndrome).

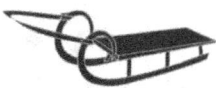

- o Waddling gait, lumbar lordosis, and calf pseudohypertrophy of Duchenne muscular dystrophy (associated with hypertrophic cardiomyopathy and pseudoinfarction pattern of EKG).
- o Straight back of ankylosing spondylitis (associated with aortic regurgitation and complete heart block).
- o Ataxic gait of tertiary syphilis (associated with aortic aneurysm and regurgitation).
- o Preferential sqatting of patients with tetralogy of Fallot.
- o Levine's sign (clenched fist over the chest of patients with acute myocardial infarction).

> Face
- o Hypertelorism, pigmented moles, and webbed neck of Turner syndrome.
- o Premature aging of Werner syndrome and progeria (associated with premature coronary artery and systemic atherosclerotic disease).
- o Gargoylism of Hurler syndrome (associated with mitral and/or aortic disease).
- o Round and chubby face of congenital valvular pulmonic stenosis
- o Elfin face (small chin, malformed teeth, wide-set eyes, patulous lips, baggy cheeks, blunt and upturned nose) of congenital stenosis of the pulmonary arteries and supravalvular aortic stenosis (often associated with hypercalcemia and mental retardation).
- o Epicanthic fold, protruding tongue, small ears, short nose, and flat bridge of Down syndrome (associated with endocardial cushion defects)
- o Saddle-shaped nose of polychondritis (associated with aortic aneurysm)
- o Drooping eyelids, expressionless face, receding hairline, and cataracts of Stenierts disease (myotonia dystrophica, associated with conduction disorders and mitral valve prolapse).
- o Dry and brittle hair, loss of lateral eyebrows, puffy eyelids, apathetic face, protruding tongue, and thick, sallow skin of patients with myxedema (with peridcardial and coronary artery disease).
- o Tightening of skin and mouth, scattered telangiectasisias, and hyper/hypopigmentation of scleroderma (with pulmonary hypertension, pericarditis and myocarditis).
- o Flushed cheeks and cyanotic lips of mitral stenosis (arcocyanosis).

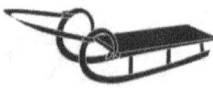

- o Paroxysmal facial and neck flushing of patients with carcinoid syndrome (with pulmonic stenosis and tricuspid stenosis/regurgitation).
- o Deafness and cataracts of rubella syndrome (associated with patent ductus arteriosus or stenosis of the pulmonary artery).
- o Short palpebral fissures, small upper lip, and hypoplastic mandible of fetal alcohol syndrome (associated with atrial or ventricular septal defects).
- o Unilateral lower facial weakness of infants with cardiofacial syndrome, which is encountered in 5-10% of infants with congenital heart disease (usually ventricular septal defect) and often is noticeable only during crying.
- o Pulsatility of the earlobes in patients with tricuspid regurgitation.
- o Macroglossia of Down syndrome, myxedema and amyloidosis (which is associated with restrictive cardiomyopathy and congestive heart failure).

> Eyes
  - o Lid lag, stare, and exophthalmos of hyperthyroidism (associated with supraventricular tachyarrhythias, angina, and high-output failure)
  - o Stare and proptosis of increased central venous pressure.
  - o Xanthelasmas of hyperproteinemia and coronary artery disease.
  - o Blue sclerae of osteogenesis imperfecta (associated with aortic regurgitation).
  - o Icteric sclerae of cardiac cirrhosis.
  - o Enlarged lacrimal glands of sarcoidosis (associated with restrictive cardiomyopathy, conduction defects, and possibly, cor pulmonale).
  - o Dislocated lens of Marfan syndrome.
  - o Conjunctival petechiae of endocarditis.
  - o Conjunctivitis of Reiter disease (associated with pericarditis, aortic regurgitation, and prolongation of the P-R interval).
  - o Fissuring of the iris (coloboma) of total anomalous pulmonary venous return.
  - o Retinal changes of hypertension and diabetes (associated with coronary artery disease and congestive heart failure).
  - o Roth spots of bacterial endocarditis.

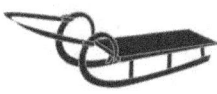

- ➤ Skin
  - o Jaundice of hepatic congestion.
  - o Cyanosis of right-to-left shunt.
  - o Pallor of anemia and high-output failure.
  - o Bronzing of hemochromatosis (associated with restrictive cardiomyopathy).
  - o Telangiectasias of Rendu-Osler-Weber syndrome (at times associated with pulmonary arteriovenous fistulas).
  - o Neurofibromas, café-au-lait spots, and axillary freckles (Crowe's sign) of Von Recklinghausen's disease (associated with pheochromocytomas).
  - o Symmetric vitiligo (especially of distal extremities) of hyperthyroidism.
  - o Butterfly rash of lupus erythematosus (associated with endo-, myo-, and pericarditis).
  - o Eyelid with purplish discoloaration of dermatomyositis (associated with cariomyopathy, heart block, and pericarditis).
  - o Skin nodules and macules of sarcoidosis (associated with cariomyopathy and heart black).
  - o Xanthomas of dyslipidemia.
  - o Hyperextensible skin and joints of Ehlers-Danlos syndrome (associated with mitral valve prolapse).
  - o Coarse and sallow skin of hyperthyroidism.
  - o Skin nodules 9sebaceous adenomas), shagreen patches and periungual fibromas of tuberous sclerosis (associated with rhabdomyomas of the heart and arrhythmias).

- ➤ Extremities
  - o Cyanosis and clubbing of central mixing (as in right-to-left shunts, pulmonary arteriovenous fistulas, and drainage of the inferior vena cave into the left atrium).
  - o Differential cyanosis and clubbing of patent ductus arteriosus with pulmonary hypertension (the reversed shunt limits cyanosis and clubbing to the feet and spares the hands).
  - o Reversed differential dyanosis and clubbing of transposition (aorta originating from the right ventricle): hands are cyanotic and clubbed, but feet are normal.
  - o Sudden pallor, pain, and coldness of peripheral embolization.

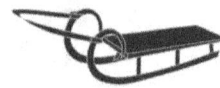

- o Osler's nodes (swollen, tender, raised, pea-sized lesions of fingerpads, palms, and soles) and Janeway lesions (small, nontender, erythematous or hemorrhagic lesions of palms of soles) seen in bacterial endocarditis.
- o Clubbing and subungual splinter hemorrhages of bacterial endocarditis.
- o Tightly tapered and contracted fingers of scleroderma, with ischemic ulcers and hypoplastic nails (often associated with pulmonary hyertension, myocardial disease, pericarditis, and valvulopathy).
- o Raynaud's phenomenon of scleroderma
- o Arachnodactyly and hyperextensible joints of Marfan syndrome (associated with aortic disease and regurgitation).
- o Hyperextensible joints of osteogenesis imperfecta (associated with aortic regurgitation).
- o Simian line of Down syndrome (associated with ostium primum defects).
- o Ulnar deviation of rheumatoid arthritis (associated with pericardial, valvular, or myocardial disease).
- o Nicotine stains of hcain smokers (clue to underlying coronary artery disease).
- o Leg edema of congestive heart failure.
- o Mainline track lines of intravenous drug abuses (presenting with tricuspid regurgitation, septic embli, and endocarditis).
- o Liver pals (erythema of thenar and hypothenar eminence) of chronic hepatic congestion.

- ➤ Thorax and Abdomen
  - o Thoracic bulges of venticular or atrial septal defects.
  - o Systolic and rarely diastolic murmurs of pectus carinatum, pectus excavatum, and straight back syndrome.
  - o Pectus carinatum, pectus excavatum, and kyphoscoliosis of Marfan syndrome.
  - o Barrel chest of emphysema (often associated with cor pulmonale).
  - o Loss of thoracic kyphosis or straight back syndrome (associated with mitral valve prolapse)
  - o Cor pulmonale of severe kyphoscoliosis
  - o Right upper quadrant pulsation of tricuspid regurgitation.
  - o Bulging flanks (ascites) of right-sided or biventricular heart failure.

Printed with permission: Mangione S. *Hanley & Belfus* 2000, pages 176-9.

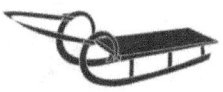

- Perform a focused physical examination for disease of the heart and cardiovascular system.

➢ Inspection
  o General appearance
    - Scleral icterus
    - Mitral facies (rosy cheeks with blue tinge from pulmonary hypertension [PHT] and low cardiac output [MS])
    - Palour
    - Wasting
    - Oxygen mask
    - Marfan syndrome (MS) (aortic and mitral regurgitation)
    - Down syndrome (DS) (congenital heart disease)
    - Turner syndrome (TS) (coarctation of the aorta)

  o Mouth
    - High arched palate (MS)
    - Diseased teeth
    - Tongue, lips – central cyanosis, petechiae

  o Hands, feet
    - Clubbing
    - Splinter hemorrhages in nail beds
    - Osler nodes (Raised, red, tender nodules on the pulps of the fingers or toes, or on the thenar or hypothenar eminences)
    - Janeway lesions (Raised, red, non-tender nodules on the pulps of the fingers or on the palms)
    - Short, broad hands (DS)
      ▪ Single palmar crease (DS)
      ▪ Incurving fifth finger (DS)
      ▪ Hyperflexible joints (DS)
        - Lymphedema (TS)
        - Short 4th metacarpal bone (TS)
        - Increased carrying angle of elbow (TS)
      ▪ Aracanydactyly (spider fingers) (MS)
      ▪ Periocular xanthemalasma

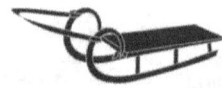

- o Neck
  - Carotid arteries
  - Jugular venous pressure (JVP) elevated
  - Webbing, low hairline, redundant skin folds on back of neck (TS)

- o Chest
  - Funnel shaped chest
  - Widely spaced nipples

- o Vital signs
  - PR, BP, RR, % O_2 saturation
  - Colour – white, blue, grey
  - Distress
  - Chest incisions, pacemakers
  - Signs of peripheral vascular disease
  - Fundic vessel abnormalities (hypertension, diabetes)

- o Palpation
  - PMI (apex beat)
  - Thrills and heaves
  - Reduced peripheral pulses

- o Percussion
  - Cardiomegaly (pulmonary edema)
  - Pleural effusion

- o Auscultation
  - Supine and upright, 5 areas, bell and diaphragm for S1/S2
  - L. lateral decubitus bell for S3/S4
  - Base of heart, lean forward, bell for diastolic murmur
  - Auscultate carotids (axilla)

➤ Signs of left side heart failure (L-HF)
  - o Dyspnea, cough, hemoptysis
  - o Basal crepitations
  - o Cyanosis
  - o Hypotension
  - o Cold extremities
  - o Fever, sweating

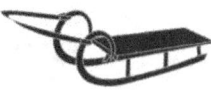

- ➢ Signs of right side heart failure (R-HF)
  - ○ ↑ JVP
  - ○ Hepatojugular reflux
  - ○ Tender hepatomegaly
  - ○ Pulsatile murmur
  - ○ Hepatic bruit

- ➢ Signs of other causes of HF
  - ○ Hypertension
  - ○ Vascular disease
  - ○ Endocarditis
  - ○ Constrictive pericarditis
  - ○ Arrythmia
  - ○ Anemia
  - ○ Hyperhtyroidism, pheochromocytoma
  - ○ Pregnancy
  - ○ Heat stroke
  - ○ Non compliance with other medications
  - ○ PE, AE-COPD, pneumonia
  - ○ High salt diet (salt shaker at bedside)
  - ○ Acute/chronic renal failure
  - ○ Nephrotic syndrome

- ➢ MAYO precipitating factors in heart failure
  - ○ Diet (excessive sodium or fluid intake, alcohol)
  - ○ Non-compliance with medication or inadequate dosing
  - ○ Sodium retaining medications (NSAIDs)
  - ○ Infection (bacterial or viral)
  - ○ Myocardial ischemia or infarction
  - ○ Arrhythmia (atrial fibrillation, bradycardia)
  - ○ Breathing disorders of sleep
  - ○ Worsening renal function
  - ○ Anemia
  - ○ Metabolic (hyperthyroidism, hypothyroidism)
  - ○ Pulmonary embolus

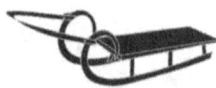

- Perform a focused physical examination of the cardiovascular system for 5 syndromes suggested from the inspection of a person's **body appearance**.

Syndromes	Cardiac abnormalities
o Acromegaly	– Hypertension – Cardiomegaly – Conduction defects
o Ankylosing spondylitis	– AR (aortic regurgitation) – CHB (complete heart block)
o Cushing	– Hypertension
o Duchenne muscular dystrophy	– HOCM (hypertrophic obstructive cardiomyopathy – Pseudoinfarction pattern on ECG
o Ellis-van Creveld	– ASD – Common atrium
o Friedreich ataxia	– HOCM – Angina – SSS (sick sinus syndrome)
o Homocysteinuria	– Thrombosus, medium-sized arteries
o Klinefelter	– ASD (atrial septal defect) – VSD (ventricular septal defect) – PDA (patent ductus arteriosus) – T of F (tetralogy of Fallot)
o Marfan	– MVP (mitral valve prolapsed) – Aortic dilation & dissection
o Pickwick	– Cor pulmonale – PHT (pulmonary hypertension) – Hypoventilation
o Tetralogy of Fallot	– Preference for the squatting position
o Turner	– Coarctation of aorta – VPS (valvular pulmonary stenosis)

Adapted from: Mangione S. *Hanley & Belfus* 2000, page 177.

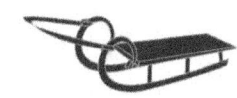

- Give how long does it take to enjoy the health benefits of stopping smoking.
    - Benefits begin immediately
    - After myocardial infarction
        - OR (odds ratio) of death in these stopping vs. not stopping is 0.54
        - In 3 yr, MR (mortality of non-smokers with previous smokers becomes equivalent)

Useful terms:

- Bigeminal pulse
    - Irregular rhythm, alternating strong and weak beats, due to premature contraction opeing aortic valve, premature contraction not opening aortic valve, 3:2 heartblock

- Buerger test for PVD
    - Elevate legs 45° → pallor; lower legs 90° → cyanosis

- Campbell sign
    - Trachea descends with inspiration; seen in acute respiratory distress, COPD, or other causes of severe airway obstruction

- Hamman sign
    - Mediastional crunch, timed with systolic and diastolic components of heart beat, due to mediasintal air, such as with a pneumothorax

- Kussmaul respiration
    - ↑ Rate and depth of breathing is caused by anion-gab metabolic acidosis (MAKE UPL):
        - Methanol
        - ASA
        - Ketoacidosis
        - Ethylete glycol
        - Uremia
        - Paraldehyde
        - Lactic acidosis

- Kussmaul sign
    - ↑ JVP on inspiration, in RV failure when JVP is ↑ (on inspiration, JVP normally falls). On inspiration, normally BP ↓, PR↑

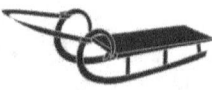

- ○ Pulsus alternans — Regular rhythm, alternative strong and weak beats

- ○ Pulsus paradoxus — Systolic blood pressure > 10-12 mmHg with inspiration (common is cardiac tamponade [98% prevalence] and acute asthma [< 50% prevalence])

- ○ Sinus arrhythmia — Normal ↓ PR on expiration

Abbreviations: BP, blood pressure; COPD, chronic obstructive pulmonary disease; JVP, jugular venous pressure; PR, pulse rate; PVD, peripheral vascular disease; RV, right ventricle

Source: Hauser SC, et al. *Mayo Clinic Gastroenterology and Hepatology Board Review.* 3rd Review. pages 598 and 600.

Tidbits

- ○ Albuminuria, any amount of albuminuria, is an independent risk factor for CV (cardiovascular) event

- ○ These CV event associated with renal disease include hospitalizations for HF (heart failure), and ↑ all-cause mortality (as well as CV events themselves, such as MI [myocardial infection])

- ○ It is not clear if this ↑ risk (5-30x ↑ risk!) is due just to the usual CV risk factors, e.g.

  - \> age

  - HBP (hypertension)

  - DM (diabetes mellitus)

  - Dyslipidemia

  - Smoking

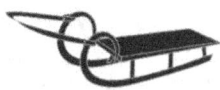

HYPERTENSION

- Give a classification of the subtypes of hypertension.

	mmHg		Rx
	SBP	DBP	
o Normal	< 120	< 80	No
o Prehypertension	120-139	80-89	Only for target organ damage (TOD)
o Isolated systolic hypertension (HBP)	> 140	< 80	Non Rx → Rx
o Stage I (HBP)	140-159	90-99	Rx to BP to, < 140 / 90 in DM/CKD, < 130/80
o Stage II	> 160	> 100	When > 20/10 above target-usually needs 2 Rx > 200/120, symptoms, TOD: hospitalize, and urgent Rx
o Hypertensive crisis - Urgencies	> 120		Rx within hours if - Optic disk edema - End organ complications - Perioperative hypertension
- Emergencies	> 210	> 130	Accelerated hypertension - Blurred vision - Headaches - Focal neurological symptoms - Immediate Rx 20%-25% ↓ BP
- Malignant			- As above, plus - Papilledema

- Give examples of end-organ damage (ESD) from hypertension.

  - CNS
    - Intracranial bleeding
    - Encephalopathy
    - CVA (stroke)
    - Seizures
    - Coma

  - Heart
    - Acute myocardial infarction
    - Instable angina
    - L-HF (left-sided congestive heart failure)
    - Aortic dissection

  - Lung
    - Pulmonary edema

  - Kidney
    - Acute renal failure

  - Pregnancy
    - Eclampsia

About 90% of the patients with hypertension have no known cause

- Give causes of secondary hypertension.

  - CVS
    - Coarctation of the aorta

  - Lung
    - Obstructive sleep apnea

  - Kidney
    - Renovascular disease
    - Renal parenchymal disease

  - Endocrine
    - Obesity
    - Cushing syndrome
    - Hyperaldosteronism (1°)
    - Pleochromocytoma
    - Genetic causes of salt retention (adrenal-renal axis)

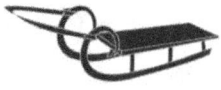

- Give the reversible /modifiable conditions which may be corrected to improve the management and control of the primary as well as secondary hypertension.

  - Oral intake
    - ↑ intake of
      - Salt
      - Alcohol
      - Caffeine
      - Calories (↑ BMI)
    - ↓ intake of
      - Fresh fruits
      - Vegetables
      - K^+ (potassium)
  - ↓ physical exercise
  - Possible, stress (mental / emotional)
  - Drug / toxins
  - During use
    - NSAIDs
    - Cyclosporin
    - Corticosteroids
    - Anti-depressants
    - Thyroid hormones
    - Erythropoietin
    - Cocaine
    - Amphetamines
  - During withdrawal
    - Opioid analgesics
    - β-blockers
    - α2-agonists (central)
    - Alcohol

SO YOU WANT TO BE A CARDIOLOGIST!

When a hypertensive patient suddenly stops their anti-hypertensive therapy a undergo withdrawal from alcohol, cocaine, opioid analgesics, central α2-agonists, β-blockers, they may develop rebound hypertension. This rebound hypertension is heated with sodium nitroprusside, nitroglycerin, or phentolamine.

- Give the reason why rebound hypertension is not treated with β-blockers
  - Using a β-blocker with intrinsic activity (ISA; such as carteolol or acebutolol), has the risk of unopposed α-adrenergic activity, developing worsening hypertension.

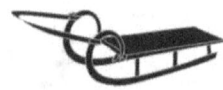

> Comments
>> o Treatment with first-line anti-hypertensive drugs such as diuretics and calcium channel blockers (CCB) were shown in the ALLHAT study to ↓ cardio- and cerebrovascular morbidity and mortality rates. Beta-blockers (BB) and angiotensin-converting enzyme (ACE) inhibitors are also 1st-line.
>> o Patients not responsive to a diuretic alone, or stage 2 hypertension (SBP > 160, DBP > 100 mmHg) will require a diuretic plus another 1st-line drug.
>> o When to change within a drug class
>>> - When adverse effects occur from the index drug
>>> - If a drug within one class fails to ↓ BP, then using another drug within that class does not usually work well

---

Care caution for hypertension
> o In the patient on an ACE inhibitor or ARB, do these drugs have to be stopped if there is a ↑ concentration of serum creatinine (Cr)?
>> - Stop ACE inhibitor or ARB therapy only if Cr > 33% of baseline in stage 1 uncomplicated hypertension.
> o In the stage 1 uncomplicated hypertensive patient with renal disease, in whom lifestyle modification has failed, which class of diuretic is used.
>> - Use a loop diuretic, since thiazides are not effective when GFR < 30 mL/min per 1.73 m^2

- For blood pressure > 180 / 120 mmHg, give the end organ damage you would seek in the situation of possible **hypertensive emergency**.

o Eye	– Retinal hemorrhages
	– Papilledema
o CNS	– Altered LOC (level of consciousness)
	– CVA (focal neurological deficits)
o CVS	– Myocardial infarction
	– Aortic dissection
o Renal	– AKI (acute kidney injury)

Remember

> Even women with well controlled hypertension have an increased risk of pre-eclampsia

> There is an increased risk for a woman to develop pre-eclampsia if she has been a sufferer of migraine headaches

---

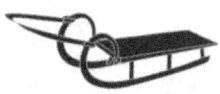

Mastering the Boards: Cardiology   A.B.R. Thomson

THERAPEUTICS

Diuretics

- Site of action of diuretics

Class	Site of action	Target
o Thiazides	– Distal convoluted tubules	▪ Thiazide-sensitive Na/Cl cotransporter
o Furosemide	– Thick ascending loop of Henle	▪ Na/ K/2Cl cotransporter
o Spironolactone	– Anti-aldosterone	
o Amiloride, triamterone	– Distal nephrone	▪ Na+ channel ▪ Na+ absorption / K+ secretion

K+ sparing diuretics such as spironolactone and amiloride are relatively weak diuretics, and are often combined with a thiazide or loop diuretic.

- Give the reason why a patient with L-sided heart failure will be given a thiazide or furosemide plus spironolactone.

    - In the setting of L-HF, spironolactone may ↑ myocardial function, independent if its diuretic effect.

- Give common adverse effects (AEs) of diuretics.

AEs	Thiazides	Loop	K-sparing spironolactone	Triamterene
o 1° electrolytes				
- ↓ Na	+			
- K	↓	↓	↑	↑
o 2° electrolytes				
- ↓ Mg	+	+		
- Ca	↑	↓		

 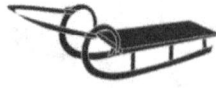

AEs	Thiazides	Loop	K-sparing spironolactone	Triamterene
o Symptoms				
- Weakness	+			
- Muscle cramps	+			
- Impotence	+			
- Gynecomastia			+	-
- Ototoxicity		+		
o Metabolic				
- ↑ blood sugar	+			
- ↑ uric acid	+			
- ↑ LDL / TG	+	-	-	-
o Renal stones	+			+
o Pancreatitis	+			+

CLINICAL PROBLEM SOLVING: DIURETICS

A patient on thiazide or loop diuretics develops hypokalemia. In addition to lowering the dose or recommending or K+ supplement, what pharmacotherapy remains an option.
- o Add a K+ sparing agent, or
- o Switch to a K+ sparing agent

The patient is given aldactone plus a thiazide, and the combination corrects the hypokalemia, but develops painful gynecomastia. Apart from stopping this aldosterone antagonist, give the other option
- o Triampterine is also a K+ sparing diuretic, but it does not cause gynecomastia, so a switch within this class of drug is reasonable (spironolactone → triampterine)
- o The gynecomastia resolves, but the patient develops hyperglycemia and dyslipidemia (↑ LDL, ↑ TG). Apart from lowering the dietary intake of lipids or using a statin / clofibrate, give the useful change in diuretic.

A loop diuretic does not cause hyperglycemia or dyslipidemia, so again a switch within class would be helpful (thiazide → loop diuretic)

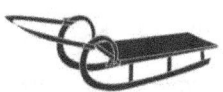

β-adrenergic antagonists (aka "β-blockers" [BB])

- o BB ↓ risk of
    - CVA (cerebrovascular accident)
    - MI (myocardial infarction)
    - HF (heart failure)

- o Action
    - Competitive inhibition of effect of catecholamines or β-receptors
        - ↓ HR (heart rate)
        - ↓ CO (cardiac output)
        - ↓ PV (plasma volume)
    - ↓ renin
        - Reset baroreceptor
    - CNS-mediated antihypertensive effect
    - ↑ prostaglandin release → vasodilation
    - ↑ density of β receptors

- Type of β-blockers, and their adverse effects (AEs)
    - o β1 blockers (cardioselective at low dose)
    - o β1 plus β2 blocking effects
        - Non-selective
        - Give the caution to patients with
            - Reactive airway disease
            - Diabetes mellitus (DM)
            - Peripheral vascular disease (AVD)
    - o Isolated sympathomimetic activity (ISM)
    - o α- and β-antagonist properties

➢ Adverse effects (AEs) of β-blockers

- o CV
    - AV (atrioventricular) block   +
    - HF (heart failure)   +
    - First-dose effect   +
    ↓ HDL, ↑ TG
    Abrupt withdrawal
    Hypertension
    Angina

- o CNS
    - Syncope   +
    - Orthostatic hypertension   +
    - Dizziness headaches   +

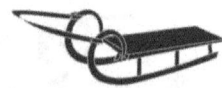

- ○ MSK
  - - Raynaud phenomenon +
  - - Impotence +
  - - Insomnia +
  - - Depression +
  - - Nasal congestion +

- • Unique AEs of BBs
  - ○ Nebivolol
    - - ↑ vasodilation

  - ○ Propanolol (non-selective)
    - - Nasal congestion
    - - Insomnia
    - - Depression

  - ○ Labetalol (α and β antagonist)
    - - Hepatitis
    - - ANA-positive, lupus-like syndrome
    - - Tremors
    - - Postural hypotension
  - ○ Selective α1 adrenergic antagonist
    - - First dose effect (> BP ↓ with first dose)

  - ○ Doxazosin (α-adrenergic antagonist)
    - - ↑ risk of HF, CVA, CAD

  - ○ Blood lipid changes
    - - ↓ total cholesterol
      - ▪ Centrally acting adrenergic agents (guanabenz guanfacine)
    - - ↓ HDL, ↑ TG
      - ▪ β1 plus β2
        - Non-selective
    - - ↑ HDL
      - ▪ Pindolol
        - ISA (intrinsic sympathomimetic action)
    - - Little effect
      - ▪ Labetelol, carvedilol (α and β antagonist)
      - ▪ Prazosin, terazosin, doxazosin (selective α1 adrenergic antagonists)

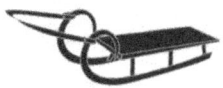

Adrenergic agents

➢ Adverse Effects (AEs)

- Centrally acting (clonidine)
    - ○ CNS   -   Drowsiness
    - ○ Mouth   -   Dry
    - ○ CV   -   Bradycardia
        -     -   Postural hypotension
        -     -   HF (heart failure)
        -     -   Acute withdrawal syndrome (AWS)
            - ▪ Sweating
            - ▪ ↑ BP
            - ▪ ↑ HR
    - ○ Endocrine   -   Gynecomastia
        -     -   Impotence

- Methyldopa
    - ○ Blood   -   Hemolytic anemia
    - ○ Liver   -   Hepatitis, autoimmune-like
    - ○ MSK   -   ANA-positive, lupus-like syndrome

*precipitation of heart failure in persons with ↓ LV function

- Guanabenz, guanafacine

Postural hypotension, severe → ↓ CO (cardiac output)
                                   ↓ peripheral resistance
                             ↑ venous pooling

- Guanethidine
    - ○ Impotence
    - ○ Diarrhea

- Reserpine
    - ○ Depression
    - ○ Nasal stiffness
    - ○ Sedation

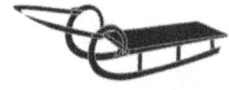

Calcium Channel Blockers (CCBs)

Types		NI / NC	Hepatic metabolism
o Diphenylalkylamines	- Verapamil	+	+
o Benzodiazepines	- Diltiazem	+	+
o Dihydropyridines (DHP)	- Nifedipine	+/-	+
o Second generation more vasoselective, longer acting	- Amlodipine - Glelodipine - Nicardipine		+

CLINICAL ALERTS

- Give the explanation for the extra caution to be considered when prescribing a diphenylalkylamine or benzothiazepine calcium channel blocker in the patient with a cardiac conduction abnormality.

  Diphyalkylamine CCB such as verapamil or benzodiazepine CCB such as diltiazam have negative cardiac inotropic and negative chromotropic effects so may ↑ HF (heart failure) in a patient who has ↓ LV function and a cardiac conduction abnormality.

- Give the reason why the short-acting dihydropyridine CCBs are not used to treat hypertension.

  The short-acting dihydropyridine CCBs (such as nifedipine), cause ↓ risk of cardiac ischemic events)

- Give the reason why none of the CCBs should be given shortly after a myocardial infarction (MI).

  o CCBs given shortly after a myocardial infarction causes ↑ mortality rate, especially in unstable patient with heart failure.

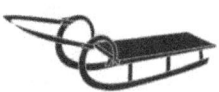

- Give the precaution which must be respected in the use IV nicardipine

  o The calcium channel blocker nicardipine is potentially toxic to the vessel into which it is being injected
  o IV nicardipine must be given into a central venous line
  o IV nicardipine has been given IV, the site of administration must be changed q 12 h

---

A TRICK QUESTION

The CCB nifedipine has a rapid onset within 30 min when given sublingually and causes only minor facial flushing and postural hypotension.

- Give the reason why sublingual nifedipine is not recommended for the acute management of hypertension.

  o In the setting, nifedipine is associated with ↑ risk of
    - MI (myocardial infarction)
    - CVA (stroke)

Inhibitors of renin-angiotensin system

- Angiotensin converting enzymes (ACE) inhibitors

ACE inhibitors are ↓ risk of MI, CVA, and death in patients with hypertension in the setting of HF (heart failure) or ↓ EF (left-ventricle ejection fraction), as well as in those without HF or ↓ EF

- Give metabolic adverse effects of first line therapy for hypertension which may be partially corrected by ACE inhibitors or ARBs.

  o ↑ blood glucose (hyperglycemia)
  o ↓ K+ (hypokalemia)*
  o ↑ cholesterol (hypercholesterolemia)
  o ↑ uric acid (hyperuricemia)

* Except in chronic renal failure, when ACE inhibitor in presence of ↓ GFR may ↑ serum K+.

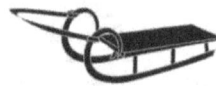

➢ Adverse effects (AEs) of ACE inhibitors and ARBs

AEs	ACE Inhibitors	ACE-I with sulfhydryl group (captopril)	ARBs
o Angioneurotic edema	+	+	
o Chronic dry cough	+	+	
o Hypotension	+	+	
o Taste disturbance		+	
o ↓ WBC (leucopenia)		+	
o Glomerulopathy		+	
o Allergy			+
o Rash			

o ARBs are useful who cannot tolerate the AEs of the ACE inhibitors

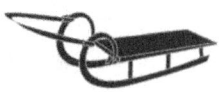

```
SO YOU WANT TO BE A CARDIOLOGIST!

• Give an example of a high renin state, which is associated with sudden or
  severe hypertension which is particularly well treated with an ACE
  inhibitor.

    o Scleroderma renal crisis and renovascular hypertension are rare
      causes of hypertension and responds well to an ACE inhibitor
```

Parenteral Anti-hypertensive Drugs

- o Diuretics, beta-blockers, CCB, ACE inhibitors are available in
  intravenous (IV) forms for use when a rapid decline in blood
  pressure is desired, and the direct-acting vasodilators are
  especially potent and useful, in
  - Hypertensive emergencies
  - Preoperative hypertensive urgencies
  - Requirement for emergency surgery
  - Refractory hypertension
- o The IV use must be monitored in an ICU setting, preferentially with
  intra-arterial monitoring, and then is followed by oral therapy
- o Useful points
  - Hypertensive plus heart failure (HF) or MI
    - Hydralazine plus nitrites
    - Sodium nitroprusside
    - Nitroglycerine

Hydralazine use has been largely replaced by IV sodium nitroprusside or
nitroglycerine, and by effective and less toxic orally administered anti-
hypertensives.

- Give common or serious adverse effects (AEs) of hydralazine.

  - o ANA-positive lupus-like syndrome
  - o Headache
  - o Nausea / vomiting
  - o Postural hypotension

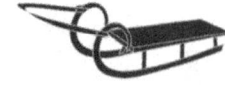

Sodium Nitroprusside

- o Drug of choice for hypertensive emergencies rapid onset / offset of action (immediate / lasts 2-3 min)
    Infusion
        0.5-10 mcg/kg per min
        0.25 mcg/kg per min for renal failure, eclampsia
- o Direct-acting arterial and venous vasodilator

CLINICAL CHALLENGE

A 50 yr old man with compensated cirrhosis is treated for hypertensive emergency with standard increasing doses of sodium nitroprusside. As his serum creatinine concentration rises, on day 3 hr develops delirium, vomiting on metabolic acidosis.

- Give the likely diagnosis, its treatment and prevention.

    - o The development of renal insufficiency ↑ risk of thiocyanate toxicity from accumulation of this metabolite of sodium nitroprusside
    - o Diagnosis can be made by demonstrating serum thiocyanate > 10 mg/dL
    - o The other possibility is that the hepatic dsfunction is leading to cyanide toxicity
    - o Treatment depends upon which chemical is the cause of the clinical presentation
        - Thiocyanate toxicity
            Hemodyalysis
        - Cyanide toxicity
            Nitrates plus thiosulfate
    - o The thiocyanate toxicity could have been prevented by monitoring serum thiocyanate levels
    - o Both toxicities could be reduced in risk by
        - Using low doses of sodium nitroprusside, or
        - Using IV nitroglycerine for the hypertension, because sodium nitroprusside is relatively contraindicated in renal or hepatic failure

---

- Give indications for using IV glycerine rather than IV sodium nitroprusside to treat a hypertensive emergencies.

    - o Hepatic or renal dysfunction
    - o Acute coronary ischemia
    - o After CABG (coronary artery bypass graft)

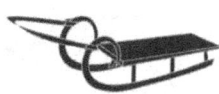

A TRICK QUESTION

In the presence of a hypertensive emergencies associated with acute coronary ischemia, IV nitroglycerine is usually preferred over IV sodium nitroprusside

- Give the reason why this general rule does not apply to an inferior myocardial infarction (MI).

  - An inferior myocardial infarction would involve the right ventricle (RV) and the RV function falls
  - The output from the left ventricle would now be determined not by RV function, but by preload
  - Sodium nitroprusside has its major effect on afterload, while nitroglycerine has its major effect on preload
  - Thus, to optimize LV cardiac output when RV function is impaired, the preload should not be altered so nitroglycerine should be avoided in inferior MI

Labetalol

- α- and β-antagonist used in hypertensive emergencies, especially during
  - Early phase of acute MI
  - During pregnancy
  - During adrenergic crisis
    - CABG
    - Pleochromocytoma
    - Withdrawal of adrenergic agents e.g. clonidine

- May be given as IV bolus or infusion

- Switching from IV to oral labetalol
  - When BP controlled, stop IV
  - When supine DBP begins to rise, begin labetalol 200 mg po then by 200 mg – 400 mg in 6-12 hr, depending on BP

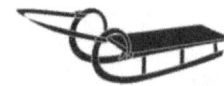

SO YOU WANT TO BE A CARDIOLOGIST!

- Give the name of the beta-blocker that is ideal to use to treat a hypertensive emergency occurring in conjunction with dissection of the aorta.

    o Esmolol is a short-acting β1-adrenergic antagonist (cardioselective) given in the setting of aortic dissection, often in combination with sodium nitroprusside.

- Give the peripherally administered anti-hypertensive drug which is given preferentially in the setting of the perioperative management of solid organ transplantation.

    o Fenoldopam
        - Selective peripheral dopamine
        - Mechanism of action
            - ↑ vasodilation
            - ↑ renal perfusion
            - ↑ naturesis
            - Rapid duration of action (elimination T1/2 < 10 min)

Oral Loading with Clonidine for Urgent Treatment of Hypertension

Dose	Check BP	
0.2 mg po ↓ then	0-1 hr	q 15 min
mg q 1 h for 4 h ↓	1-2 hr	q 30 min
(or DBP ≥ 20 mmHg) ↓ at 6 hr add diuretic ↓ at 8 hr 0.1 mg po bid	5 then	q 60 min

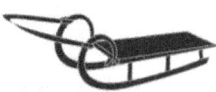

- **Aortic dissection**
  - Acute medical therapy for type B distal dissection [type A proximal acute dissection → urgent surgical correction)
  - IV sodium nitroprusside (SN) plus concurrent IV β1 adrenergic antagonist
    - Give SN to target SBP of 100 to 120 mmHg, or lowest possible BP to maintain perfusion of organs
    - If esmolol not available, use propranolol, a non-selective β-blocker
  - Maintain SBP < 130 mmHg
    - Use antihypertensives with negative inotropic properties:
      - If patient stabilizes after acute therapy, with no aortic rupture or continued dissection
      - BBs, CCBs, centrally acting adrenergic agents (clonidine, methyldopa), reserpine

---

SO YOU WANT TO BE A CARDIOLOGIST!

IV sodium nitroprusside (SN) will rapidly reduce hypertensive associated with a type B (distal) aortic dissection, but SN must be used with an adrenergic antagonist.
- Give the reason why an adrenergic antagonist must be coadministered when sodium nitroprusside is used to rapidly lower hypertension in a patient with type B distal acute dissection.

  - Sodium nitroprusside → ↑ LV contractility (positive inotropic effect) → ↑ shearing forces → ↑ further dissection
  - Beta-blockers such as esmolol or propranolol have negative inotropic effect shearing effect of sodium nitprusside

---

    - Aortic dissection with intolerance to sodium nitroprusside, and / or to BB, use
      - Trimethaphan camsylate, a ganglionic blocking agent with negative inotropic properties (↓ LV contractility)
      - Not 1st line choice because of
        - Rapid loss of effect (tachyphylaxis)
        - Rapid development of sympathetic side effects (sympathalgia), e.g.
          - Blurred vision
          - Urinary retention

- **Diabetes with nephropathy)proteinuria, renal insufficiency)**
  - ACE inhibitors are first-line therapy
    - ↓ proteinuria
    - ↓ end-stage progression of nephropathy to ESRD
    - ↓ rate of MI, CVA, death (in diabetics with CV [cardiovascular] risk but no ↓ LV function
  - ARBs also ↓ progression to ESRD

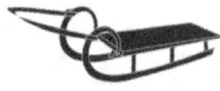

- **Nephropathy but not diabetes**
  - Loop diuretics, especially when serum creatinine > 2.5 mg/dL
    (these patients have ↑ blood volume, and volume-dependent
    hypertension)

- **Left ventricular hypertrophy** (LVH)
  - ACE inhibitors to ↓ LVH and thereby ↓ risk of MI, SCD (sudden
    cardiac death), and all cause mortality

- **Coronary artery disease** (CAD)
  - Unstable angina: BB
    - ↓ progression to MI
  - Acute MI
    - BBs
      - ↓ MR (mortality)
    - BBs
      - ↓ reinfarction
  - CAD +/- LV dysfunction
    - CCBs ↓ MR

A Question

   o You might have wondered why ACE inhibitors are not used in the
      setting of the hypertensive patient with coronary heart disease
   o BBs have been shown to be effective to ↓ progression of unstable
      angina to myocardial infarction, ↓ reinfarction after a MI, and ↓
      mortality rate
   o CCBs reduce mortality rate in persons with coronary artery disease
      with or without LV dysfunction, or mortality after an acute MI
   o The date on the protective benefit of ACE inhibitors is not clear, so
      use a BB or CCB in hypertensive patients with coronary artery
      disease until we learn whether the negative inotropic effect of the
      ACE inhibitors is a problem in this setting.

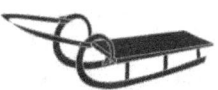

Clinical Tip

- o Sudden cardiac death in patient with hypertension when there is associated
  - LVH (left ventricular hypertrophy) / dilation
  - HF (heart failure)
  - AWS (acute withdrawal syndrome)

- **Heart failure** (HF)
  - o ↑ risk of LV dilation / hypertrophy → SCD (sudden cardiac death)
  - o ACE inhibitors / ARBs
    - ↓ MR in hypertensives with HF
    - ↓ MR hypertensives with acute MI plus HF
    - ↓ recurrent MI
    - ↓ hospitalization

SO YOU WANT TO BE A CARDIOLOGIST!

Nitrates and hydralazine ↓ MR in HF, with or without associated hypertension.
- Give the reason why hydralazine is not given in unstable angina / unstable coronary syndromes.
  - o Hydralazine → reflex tachycardia → ↑ work load and O2 requirements of LV → ↑ risk of demand ischemia

- Give the reason why CCBs are not recommended in the hypertensive patient with HF.
  - o CCBs have a negative inotropic effect and could be harmful in the setting of hypertension plus HF

- **Monoamine oxidase inhibitors** (MAOIs)

  - o MAOIs plus risk drugs / foods → catecholamine excess
  - o MAOI-associated high risk substances
    - Drugs
      - Anti-histamines
      - Levodopa
      - Meperidine
      - Methydopa
      - Sympathetics mimetics
      - Tricyclics

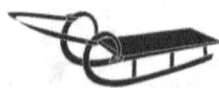

- - Tyramine-risk foods
    - Broad beans
    - Cheese
    - Chicken liver
    - Chocolate
    - Figs (canned)
    - Herring
    - Processed meat
    - Red wine
    - Yeast
  - Antihypertensive drugs safe to use for catecholamine excess state
    - Sodium nitroprusside
    - Labetalol
    - Phentolamine

- **Pregnancy**
  - Types of hypertension which occur in pregnancy
    - Chronic hypertension
    - Preeclampsia
      - Pregnancy > 20 wk
      - Hypertension
      - Proteinuria
      - Edema
      - Coagulopathy
      - Liver function changes
    - Eclampsia
      - As for preeclampsia, plus seizure
    - Transient hypertension
      - Hypertension but no proteinuria or CNS changes
      - Hypertension normalizes within 10 days of delivery
      - BP > 140/90 mmHg before 20th wk
  - Indication for treatment of hypertension in pregnancy (DBP > 100 mmHg)
  - Exclude preeclampsia
  - Non-pharmacological
    - Do
      - ↓ smoking
      - **Stop** alcohol
    - **Do not**
      - ↓ weight
      - Exercise vigorously
  - Pharmacological
    - Methyldopa
    - Labetalol
    - Hydralazine
  - Contraindicated
    - **No** ACE inhibitors (teratogenic)

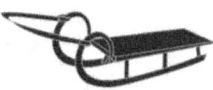

Anti-hypertensive Withdrawal

- o Clinical
  - Withdrawal of any antihypertensive, but especially
    - Clonidine centrally acting adrenergic agent
    - BBs
    - Diuretics
  - Within 24-72 hours after withdrawal of antihypertensive agent
    - CNS
      - Encephalopathy
      - CVA (cerebrovascular accident)
    - CVS
      - MI (myocardial infarction)
      - SCD (sudden cardiac death)

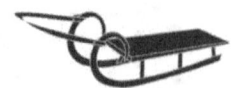

- o Prevention
    - Do not suddenly stop any antihypertensive therapy-taper slowly
    - Taper very slowly of patient has
    - If an antihypertensive is not effective, then add a second class of drug
- o Treatment
    - Mild
        - Antihypertensive drug which was suddenly stopped
    - Moderate / mild
        - Sodium nitroprusside
        - Labetalol

- Given the secondary disorders associated with each of the four major types of lipid abnormality.

Secondary cause	↑ CHOL	↑ TG	↑ CHOL + TG	↑ HDL
o Endocrine				
- Hypothyroidism	+		+	
- Diabetes / metabolic Syndrome		+	+	+
- Lipodystrophies			+	
- Hypertriglyceridemia		+		+
o Kidney				
- Nephrotic syndrome	+		+	
- Chronic renal disease		+		
o Drugs / toxins				
- Alcohol		+		
- Estrogens		+		
- Anabolic steroids				+
- Smoking				+
- Retinoic acid		+		
o GI / liver				
- Moderate / mild				+
- PBC (primary biliary cirrhosis)				
- AN (anorexia neurosa)	+			

Abbreviations: CHOL, cholesterol; TG, triglyceride; HDL, high-density lipoprotein

Clinical Acumen

Fendon xanthomas develop in FH (familial hypercholesterolemia), but not in FCH (familial combined hypercholesterolism).

- Give the type of xanthoma which is pathognomic for serum ↑ CHOL and ↑ TG to 300 mg/dL to 500 mg/dL plus ratio of VLDL / TG > 0.3.

  o The symmetric increase in both cholesterol and triglyceride plus ↑ VLDL / TG suggests dysbetalipoproteinemia
  o The planar xanthomas of the palmar creases is pathognomic for dysbetalipoproteinemia

Patients with primary biliary cirrhosis (PBC) have high levels of serum cholesterol, but they do not have ↑ risk of coronary heart disease (CAD).

- Give the reason why hypercholesterolemia patients with PBC do not have an ↑ risk of CAD.

  o The PBC patient has ↑ HDL-cholesterol, not LDL-cholesterol.

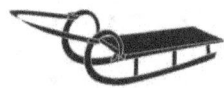

- Give the non-modifiable and modifiable risk factors for coronary artery disease (CAD), and which of these factors modify LDL-cholesterol.

  o Non-modifiable
    - 1° familial history of CAD
      - M < 55 yr
      - F < 65 yr

  o Modifiable
    - Smoking
    - Hypertensive
      - ≥ 140/90 mmHg, or
      - On treatment
    - C-HDL
      - < 40 mg/dL

➢ Risk stratification
  o LDL-cholesterol concentration

National Cholesterol Education Program Adult Therapeutic Panel (ATP) III GuidelinesTable 3-9, page 102

  o Framingham score for prediction of 10-yr risk for coronary heart disease (CHD)

Category of risk	10-yr risk for CHD	Number of non-LDL risk factors
- Very high		
- High		
- Moderate	10% - 20%	≥ 2
- Low		0-1

  o The treatment of hyperlipidemia depends on the serum concentration of LDL-C (low-density lipoprotein cholesterol, and the number of non-LDL-C risk factors for coronary heart disease (CHD).
  o All patients should be started on a TLC (therapeutic lifestyle change) diet when their LDL-C is ≥ 130-160 mg/dL.

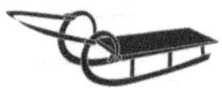

- Give the recommended nutrient composition of the TLC (therapeutic lifestyle change) diet from the Expert Panel on Detection, Evaluation, and Treatment of the High Blood Cholesterol in Adults, from the National Cholesterol Education Program (NCEP) Expert Panel.

Nutrient	Recommended percentage of total calories	Gm/d
o Fat	25% - 35%	
- Saturated	< 7	
- Polyunsaturated	≤ 10	
- Monosaturated	≤ 20	
- Cholesterol	-	< 0.2 /d (< 200 mg/d)
o Carbohydrate	50% - 60%	
o Protein	~ 15%	20 g – 30 g/d

- o Note: this TLC diet is supplemented with weight reduction (daily intake of calories to be sufficient to achieve / maintain "desirable" body weight

- Summary of therapies by risk group
  - o All risk groups, including lower-risk group with LDL-C < 130-160 mg/dL, are placed on TLC diet.
  - o In the patient with the metabolic syndrome, the LDL-C is to be controlled, including the ↑ BMI / WC, ↑ BP, ↑ BS, ↑ TG, ↑ HDL-C
  - o Indications pharmacotherapy to begin

Cardiovascular risk group	LDL-C threshold	Number of risk factors	10-yr for CHD
o Low (> 160)	- ≥ 190 mg/dL - 160-189 mg/dL especially if after 3-mon TLC diet	≤ 1	
o Moderate (> 130)	- ≥ 130 mg/dL, or - 100-129 mg/dL - ≥ 160 mg/dL while on TLC diet	≥ 2	< 10%
o High (> 100)	- ≥ 100 mg/dL, or - < 100 mg/dL		
o Very high (> 70)	- ≥ 70 mg/dL		

- o Note:
  - - The target non-HDL-C (=total C-HDL-C) is 30 mg/dL higher than LDL-C target

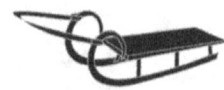

There is a continuum of benefit of statin-associated ↓ LDL-C, with ↓ CV (cardiovascular) risk with greater ↓ LDL-C (Cholesterol Treatment Trialists' (CTT) Collaborators, et al., Lancet 2012, 380: 581-90; Lancet 2010, 376:1670-81)

Abbreviations: BMI, body mass index; BP, blood pressure; BS, blood sugar; CHD, coronary heart disease; (artery disease); HDL-C, high-density lipoprotein; LDL-C, low-density lipoprotein; TG, serum triglyceride concentration; WC, waist circumference

- o The non-coronary heart disease (CHD) risk factors for CHD include
  - Diabetes
  - Cerebrovascular disease
  - Peripheral vascular disease
  - Abdominal aortic aneurysm
- o Consider patient's major risk factors
  - Age
    - M ≥ 45 yr
    - Women ≥ 55 yr
  - 1° family history of early CHD
    - M ≥ 55 yr
    - Women ≥ 65 yr
  - Smoking
  - Hypertension ≥ 140/90, or an antihypertension medications
  - HDL-C < 40 mg/dL

- Give the Adult Treatment Program (**ATP) III Criteria** for the diagnosis of metabolic syndrome.

≥ 3 criteria

o Carbohydrate	- Fasting hyperglycemia ≥ 100 mg/dL
o Lipids	- Fasting triglyceride ≥ 150 mg/dL - Fasting HDL-C
o Obesity (WC)	- M > 40 in - F > 35 in
o Hypertension	- ≥ 130/85 mmHg

Abbreviations: F, female; M, male; WC, waist circumference

- ➢ Monitor therapy to ↓ LDL-C
  - o Goal
    - 6 wk
      - ↓ 30% - 40%
    - 12 wk
      - target LDL-C
  - o If target LDL-C not reached in 3 mon, in conjunction with TLC diet
    - Add second agent

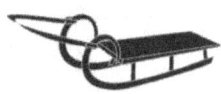

HYPERLIPIDEMIA

Hypertriglyceridemia

- Give the reason why hypertriglyceridemia is important.

  o Independent risk factor for CV disease
  o A component of metabolic syndrome
  o A treatable cause of pancreatitis

Useful background: ATP III classification of hypertriglyceride

ATP III classification	Serum triglycerides, mg/dL
o Normal	< 150
o Borderline	150-199
o High	200-499
o Very high	≥ 500
o Hypertriglyceridemia	
- Severe	1000-1999
- Very severe	≥ 2000

➢ Treatment

  o Treat any associated / causative condition
  - Metabolic syndrome
    ▪ Diabetes / hyperglycemia
    ▪ Hypertension
    ▪ ↑ BMI / waist circumference

  o Non-pharmacological
  - ↓ alcohol, sugars, high-carbohydrate diet
  - TLC (therapeutic lifestyle change) diet
  - ↓ BMI, ↑ exercise
  - Genetic dyslipidemias, including ↑ LDL-C

  o Pharmacological
  - Omega-3 fatty acids plus low-fat (≤ 15% of calories) but
    ▪ Moderate ↑ TG, cotherapy with statin, fibrate, naicid
    ▪ Very severe ↑ TG > 500 mg/dL
    ▪ Either diet with 1-6 g omega fatty acids EPA (eicosapentaenoic acid) plus DHA (docosahexaenoic acid), or ↓ HDL-C

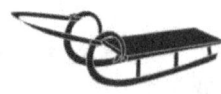

- Drugs
  - Corticosteroids
  - Estrogens: switch from po to transdermal
  - Retinoic acid
- Statins to control ↑ LDL-C in associations with ↑ mild/moderate
  - TG (serum triglycerides)
- For hypertriglyceridemia ≥ 500 mg/dL ("very high")

- **Fibrates** (Fibric acid derivatives)

  - Expected therapeutic benefit of fibrins: expected ↓ concentration of lipids
    - ↓ LDL-C   5-25%
    - ↑ HDL-C   10-35%
    - ↓ TG   30-50%

*In persons with:
            Normal TG → ↓ LDL-C   5-25%
            ↑ TG
                ↑ LDL-C

  - Suggested doses
    - Gemfibrozil 600 mg po bid AC (before meals)
    - Fenofibrate 48-145 mg po per day

  - Common adverse effects
    - Dyspepsia
    - Rash
    - Cholelithiasis
    - Pruritis
    - Rhabdomyolysis

Clinical Caution

  - Gemfibrozil + statin → ↑ risk of rhabdomyolysis
  - Gemfibrozil or fenofibrate → ↑ INR from ↑ effect of warfarin

---

- **Nicotinic acid**

  - Expected therapeutic benefit: expected ↓ concentration of lipids
    - LDL-C   ↓ by ≥ 15%
    - HDL-C   ↑ by ≤ 35%
    - TG   ↓ by 20-50%

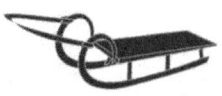

- o Adverse effects
  - Flushing (may be reduced by taking 325 mg ASA 30 min before taking niacin
  - Transaminitis
  - Nausea, bloating
  - Hyperglycemia
  - Gout (hyperuricemia)

Measure blood glucose, uric acid, ALT / AST every 6-8 wk until dose stabilized, then every 4 mon

- o Relative contraindications
  - Liver disease
  - Diabetes (uncontrolled)
  - Gout
  - Active ulcer disease

High Density Lipoprotein Cholesterol (HDL-C)

- o ↓ HDL-C must be correct because
  - ↓ HDL-C is an independent risk factor for CHD (Coronary heart disease)
  - ↓ HDL-C is often associated with
    - ↑ TG (hypertriglyceridemia)
    - Metabolic syndrome
    - Diabetes / insulin resistance
    - Smoking
  - Treatment of ↓ HDL-C is the control of any associated ↑ TG, metabolic syndrome, or ↑ LDL-C

- o Drugs
  - Beta-blockers
  - Anabolic steroids
  - Progestins

- Give the common adverse effects of statins.

  - o CNS
    - Fatigue
    - Malaise
    - Headache

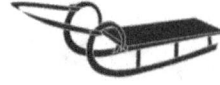

Mastering the Boards: Cardiology   A.B.R. Thomson

- o GI
    - Abdominal pain
    - Bloating
    - ↑ / ↓ stool frequency

- o Muscle
    - Pain / weakness +/- ↑ serum CK (creatinine kinase)
    - ↑ myopathy risk with ↑ intake of grapefruit juice
    - Severe CYP450 associated drug interactions
        - ↑ risk of rhabdomyolysis
        - Examples of fibrates, antibiotics (clarithromycin, erythromycin, ketoconazole,), cyclosporine, protease inhibitors, warfarin, digoxin

- o Liver
    - Transaminitis (↑ ALT, AST 2-3x ULN)
    "....routine periodic monitoring of liver enzymes does not appear to
    - be effective in detecting or preventing serous liver injury"

- o Skin
    - Rash

- o DecompPregnancy / lactation
    - Do **not** use

- o Other drug interactions
    - Simvastatin
        ↑ levels of amiodarone

http://www.fda.gov/Drugs/DrugSafety/UCM293101.htm

- **Bile acid sequestering resins**

    - o By ↓ BA concentration in the intestinal lumen, the "resin: ↓ absorption of cholesterol (CHOL) and thereby ↓ LDL-C 15-30%
    - o If triglyceride concentration is high (> 250 mg/dL), and LDL-C is increased, do not use resin without either a statin or niacin, since by itself the resin would increase further the hypertriglyceridemia
    - o Like the induction of reduced absorption of cholesterol, so also will resins
        - ↓ absorption of the fat soluble vitamins (FSVs), vitamin A, D, E, and K

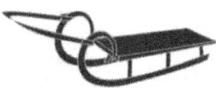

Mastering the Boards: Cardiology   A.B.R. Thomson

- ↓ absorption of certain drugs, such as
  - Amiodarone
  - Glipizide
  - Statins
  - Thyroid hormones
  - Digoxin
  - Thiazides
  - Warfarin
- Colesevelam may ↓ absorption of fewer drugs than do cholestyramine, or colestipol, which must be given 1 h before or 4 hr after other resins

- o Representative po doses
  - Cholestyramine
    - 4 g up to 6 times a day, 1 hr before food
  - Colestipol tab
    - 2 g up to 8 times a day, 1 hr before food
  - Unstable anginaColesevelam
    - 625 mg tabs 3 tid, or tabs od with food
    - Suspension packet per day

Ezetimibe

- o Binds to Nieman-Pick protein in the brush border membrane of the small intestine, thereby ↓ absorption of this transporter-mediated absorption of cholesterol
- o Acts as monotherapy or add-on therapy with a statin (cotherapy)
- o Adverse effects
  When using cotherapy of ezetimbe plus statin, ↑ LE (liver enzymes)
  Do not use in conjunction with moderate / severe liver disease

Summary of expected therapeutic effects of drugs used to treat dyslipidemia

Drug	↓ LDL-C	↓ TG	↑ HDL-C
o Statins	~ 20-60%		
o Niacin	≥ 15%	≤ 35%	
o Ezetimibe	18-25%*		
o Fibrins	5-25%*	30-50%	10-35%

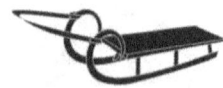

- Give the treatment of low HCl serum cholesterol concentration.

    o Blood lipid concentrations are a surrogate marker for coronary heart disease, and while statins and resins have been shown to ↓ CV events, there is no data to show that increasing low HDL-C levels is associated with improved clinical outcomes except for those arising from associated metabolic syndrome or hypertriglyceridemia, or ↑ LDL-C associated with ↑ TG (serum triglycerides)

- Approach

    o Treat associated conditions
        - Metabolic syndrome
        - Dyslipidemia
    o Life-style changes
        - ↓ BMI
        - ↑ exercise
        - Stop smoking
    o Avoid drugs which may ↓ HDL-C
        - B-blockers*
        - Progestin
        - Androgenic steroids
    o If ≥ 2 non-LDL-C risk factors, calculate Framingham CHD risk score (www.nhlbi.nih.gov)
    o Developing upon Franingham score from non-LDL-C CHD risk factors, patient's risk is grouped

---

SO YOU WANT TO BE A CARDIOLOGIST!

- Give the impact factor for obesity, hyperglycemia, sedentary lifestyle and proinflammatory or prothrombotic factor on the calculation of the value of Framingham CHD risk score.

    o This is a trick question-these factors are not the risk assessment but certainly influence the patient's likely risk.

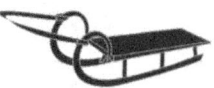

CARDIAC RISK STRATIFICATION

Preoperative assessment of cardiac risk

➢ For urgent conditions, proceed with surgery for life-threatening conditions

➢ For elective surgery, surgical outcome is improved by delaying to improve the following
  o Severe arrhythmia
  o Severe valvular heart disease
  o Decompensated HF
  o Unstable coronary syndrome
    - Severe angina
    - Unstable angina
    - MI < 30 days ago

  o If the patient cannot climb a flight of stairs, or if in doubt, calculate the Revised Cardiac Risk Index (RCRI),

    - RCRI = 0, proceed with any needed surgery

    - RCRI ≥ 3, risk factors ⎤ perform cardiac testing before
                              ⎦ proceeding with surgery

    - Planned vascular surgery

• Calculate the **Revised Cardiac Risk Index** (RCRI) for preoperative cardiac risk assessment.

  o History   -   IHD (ischemic heart disease)
                   -   HF (heart failure)
                   -   CVA (cerebrovascular accident or disorder)
                   -   Diabetes requiring insulin
  o Lab   -   Serum creatinine > 2 mg/dL
  o Surgery   -   Surgery for emergency
                   -   CV surgery
                       ▪ Aorta
                       ▪ Vascular
                       ▪ Peripheral vascular
                   -   Long procedures (fluid shifts, blood loss)

  o Trick
    - The RCRI does not include hypertension, since "hypertension is not an independent predictor of postoperative cardiac complications".

Source: Board Basics 3, 2012, page 51.

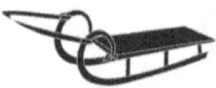

Useful background: American Society of Anesthesiologist Classification of Anesthetic Mortality within 48 hours postoperatively

Class	Physical Status	48-Hour Mortality
I	Healthy persons younger than 80 y	0.07%
II	Mild systemic disease	0.24%
III	Severe but not incapacitating systemic disease	1.4%
IV	Incapacitating systemic disease that is constant threat to life	7.5%
V	Moribund patient not expected to survive 24 hours, regardless of surgery	8.1%
E	Suffix added to any class to indicate emergency procedure	Double risk

Printed with permission: MXSAP IX: Part C, Book 4. *American college of Physician* 1991.

Source: Ghosh AK. *Mayo Clinic Scientific Press* 2008, Table 8-8, page 336.

- Give the cardiac risk stratification for noncardiac surgical procedures.

Cardiac risk	Procedure
o High	- Emergency operations - Elderly patient - Aortic and other major vascular procedures - Peripheral vascular procedures - Prolonged surgical procedures associated with large fluid shifts or blood loss (or both)
o Intermediate	- Carotid endarterectomy - Head and neck operations - Abdominal and intrathoracic procedures - Orthopedic procedures - Prostate operations
o Low	- Cataract extraction - Breast operation - Endoscopic procedures

Adapted from: Ghosh AK. *Mayo Clinic Scientific Press* 2008, Table 8.9, page 337.

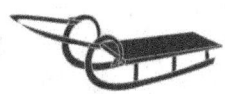

Odds ratios (OR) > 2 for perioperative pulmonary complications.

Risk Factors	Odds ratio
o Patient	
– ASA class $\geq$ II	4.9
– Chronic obstructive pulmonary disease	2.4
– Age (2.3 for 60-69, increasing to 5.6 for $\geq$ 80 years)	
– Total functional dependence	2.5
o Co-morbidities	
– Congestive heart failure	2.9
– Serum albumin <35 g/L	2.5
o Procedure-related	
– Surgical site or type of procedure	6.9
– Open abdominal aortic repair	4.2
– Thoracic	3.1
– Abdominal	2.5
– Neurosurgical	2.2
– Head and Neck	2.1
– Vascular	2.5
– Emergency surgery	2.3
– Prolonged surgery (>3 h)	
o General anesthesia	2.4

Note that the OR < 2 for age 50-59; partial functional dependence, impaired sensorium, smoking; blood transfusion > 4 units.

Abbreviation: ASA, American Society of Anesthesiologists

Adapted from: Ghosh AK. *Mayo Clinic Scientific Press* 2008, Table 18-11, page 341.

"We are inherently critical as scientists, and
inherently kind as physicians."

Grandad

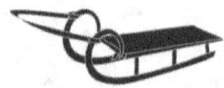

Quality Measures

- Give examples of selected quality measures which could / should be part of the practice of every internist or sub-specialist.

Clinical Condition	Selected Quality Measures
o Acute coronary syndrome (ACS)	– Aspirin at arrival & discharge – B-blocker at arrival & discharge – ACE inhibitor for LVSD
o Heart failure (HF)	– Left ventricular function assessment – ACE inhibitor for LVSD – Smoking cessation advice & counseling
o Community-acquired pneumonia (CAP)	– Oxygenation assessment within 24 h – Pneumococcal screening & vaccination – Antibiotic timing (first dose in < 4 h) – Smoking cessation advice & counseling
o CRC screening	– Risk: age > 50, family history, IBD, smoking, obesity (sporadic, familial polysyndromes) – Adequacy of preparation & sedation – Reporting of cecal landmarks – Withdrawal time – Personal polyp detection rates (M, 25%, F, 15%)

Abbreviation: ACE, angiotensin-converting enzyme; IBD, inflammatory bowel disease (ulcerative colitis, Crohn colitis); LVSD, left ventricular systolic dysfunction; CRC, colorectal cancer

Adapted from: Ghosh AK. *Mayo Clinic Scientific Press* 2008, page 505.

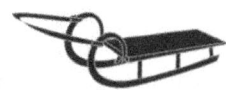

CORONARY ARTERY DISEASE (CAD)

- ➢ Terminology
  - o Coronary artery disease (CAD)
    - Angina pectoris
    - Myocardial infarction (MI)
    - Silent myocardial ischemia
    - Acute coronary syndrome (ACS)
      - ▪ Unstable angina (UA)
    - Heart failure (HF)
      - ▪ NSTEMI (non-ST-segment MI)
      - ▪ STEMI (ST-segment elevation MI)
    - Sudden cardiac death (SCD)

- ➢ Demography
  - o Kills about 15% of persons in developed and in developed and in some developing countries
  - o Risk of having CHD after age 40 yr
    - Men 50%
    - Women 64%
  - o MI incidence
    - New events
      2100 / 10^5 per year
    - Recurrent
      1700 / 10^5 per yr
  - o Women > men for
    - 10 yr incidence of CHD
    - 20 yr MI, SCD
  - o Acute coronary syndrome (ACS)
    - 60% unstable angina (UA)
    - 13% acute STEMI
    - 27% acute NSTEMI
  - o Outcome at 1-yr for UA / NSTEMI
    - Death ~6%
    - Recurrent MI~ 11%
    - Repeat CABG ~ 50%
  - o Mortality
    - Short-term
      STEMI > NSTEMI
    - Long-term
      STEMI = NSTEMI

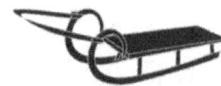

- ➢ Pathophysiology
  - o About ½ of all men and 2/3 of all women who die from CHD had no previous symptoms
  - o Obstruction of coronary artery by atherosclerosis (angiographically significant luminal stenosis)
  - o Majority of acute MI's are from an angioraphically insignificant (< 50% luminal stenosis) plus rupture erosion of a "vulnerable" plaque, which then blocks the lumen of the coronary artery.
  - o Stable angina
    - Disease of microvascular circulation (syndrome x)
      - Not seen on angiography
    - Disease of epicardial arteries
      - Seen on angiography (> 50% obstruction of lumen)

"Epicardial arteries with < 50% obstruction do not usually cause angina"

- Give the exceptions to this general principle.

  - o Epicardial arterial lumen obstruction < 50% plus ↑ demand e.g. sepsis shock
  - o Epicardial lumen obstruction and left main coronary artery disease

- Give the % stenosis, which is usually with pain on exertion, and at rest.

Condition	% stenosis
o Angina	
- With exertion	> 70%
- At rest	> 90%

- ➢ Prevention

- Assess risk

  - o Risk factors
    - Risk evaluation for CHD
      - CHD (coronary heart disease itself)
      - Diabetes
      - PVD (peripheral vascular disease
      - CVA (cerebrovascular accident)
      - AA (aortic aneurysm)

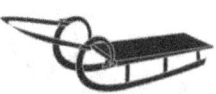

- Risk factors for CVD
  - \> age
  - Hypertension
  - Dyslipidemia
  - Smoking (use of tobacco within 15 yr)
  - 1° family history of CHD
  - Women: past history of preeclampsia / gestational diabetes
  - ↑ BMI / ↑ WC (waist circumference)
  - Comorbidities
    - Diabetes
    - CKD (chronic kidney disease)
    - Autoimmune collagen-vascular
  - ↓ physical activity
  - "poor" duct

- o Risk score
  - GRS (Global Risk Score), for CHD or CVD
  - Note: underestimates absolute ratio in young persons
  - FRS (Framing risk score, for MI or coronary death http://www.framinghamheartstudy.org/risk/gencardio.htm#)
  - Score (systemic coronary risk evaluation) for CVD death
  - RRS (Reynolds risk score) for MI or coronary death

- o Risk categories (based upon GRS)
  - Low
    - \< 10% risk of CHD in next 10 yr undertake plan to maintain cardiac risk
  - Intermediate
    - 10-19% risk of CHD
  - High
    - 20% risk of CHD, or
    - \> 10% risk of CVD events

➢ Risk assessment

- Give tests to reclassify intermediate from high risk for CHD, and for consideration of vigorous preventive measures (eg. ASA, statin, exercise program, DASH diet).

  - o Ultrasound of carotid arteries
    - Intima thickness > 75th percentile

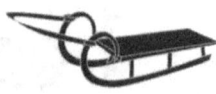

- o ABI (ankle-brachial index) < 9 or > 1.3, suggest presence of peripheral vascular disease, a risk equivalent for CHD)
- o CT scan to determine coronary artery calcium > 400
- o When LDL-C < 130 mg/dL, measure hsCRP (high sensitivity C-reactive protein) > 2 mg/dL

  Men > 50 yr ⎤
  Women > 60 yr ⎦ statin therapy

- o ↑ risk
  - CHD risk > 20%
  - CVD events > 10%

➢ Guidelines

- Give the guidelines from the **American Heart Association for the Prevention of Cardiovascular disease**.

  - o BMI < 25 kg/m^2
  - o Use of tobacco, none
  - o Physical activity intensity
  - o DASH diet (Dietary Approach to Stop Hypertension; please see www.nhlbi.nih.gov/health/public/heart/hbp/dash/new_dash.pdf
  - o Total cholesterol > 200 mg/dL, on no treatment
  - o Blood pressure < 120/80, on no treatment
  - o Fasting blood glucose < 100 mg/dL
  - o Note: these guidelines are promulgated for women

Source: Mosca L, et al. J Am Coll Cardiol 2011; 57: 1404-23.

  - o ASA (aspirin), 75-162 mg/d
    - CVD event risk over 10-yr
      - Men > 10%
      - Women > 20%

➢ Clinical

  - o Angina pain
    - Typical
      - 3 feature
        - Squeezing pressure-like substernal pain
        - Pain brought on by exertion or stress
        - Pain relieved by rest or NTE (nitroglycerin)

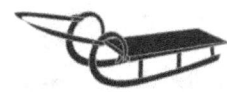

- Atypical
  - 2 feature
- Chronic, stable
  - Predictable onset of pain with a known magnitude of exertion or stress
  - Predictable effect of pain with 5-10 min of rest, or NTE

o Angina equivalents / atypical angina
  - SOB (shortness of breath; dyspnea)
  - Dyspepsia

- Give features of the patient with CAD who is more likely to have atypical angina.

  o Female
  o Males and females with
    - Diabetes
    - CKD (chronic kidney disease)

  o Determine pretest probability (risk category) of CAD based on type of chest pain (Table 4-3 page 16)

Age, year	No symptoms (very low risk, < 5%)		NCCP (low risk, < 10%)		Atypical angina intermediate risk (10-80%)		Typical angina high risk (> 80%)	
	W	M	W	M	W	M	W	M
30-39	< 5	< 5	2	4	12	34	26	76
40-49	< 5	< 10	3	13	22	51	55	87
50-59	< 5	< 10	7	20	31	65	73	93
60-69	< 5	< 5	14	27	51	72	86	94

Abbreviations: F, female; M, males; NCCP, non-cardiac chest pain (chest pain with none of the features of angina)

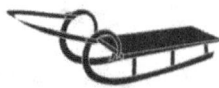

- o Determine clinical severity of angina (CCS class, **Canadian Cardiovascular Society**)

Class	Definition
1	o With strenous / long activity
2	o Moderate - Walk > 2 level blocks - Climb > 1 flight of stair
3	o Mild - Walk < 2 blocks - Climb 1 flight of stair
4	o Any activity, or at rest

Source: Sangareddi V, et al., Coronary Artery Dis 2004; 15: 111-114.

- • Give the usefulness of precardial auscultation for systemic murmurs in the patient with suspected CAD.

  - o AS (aortic stenosis)
  - o HEM (hypertrophic cardiomyopathy)
    - Note: ↑ with Valsalva maneuver
  - o MR (mitral regurgitation)
    - Auscultate for new or worsening murmur

- ➤ Diagnostic testing

  - o Recall that persons at "intermediate risk" may have testing to reclassify their pretest probability of CAD as "high risk":
  - o If patient reclassified to be at high risk or LV dysfunction, proceed to coronary angiography to determine choice of medical or surgical therapy.
  - o Stress testing
    - Exercise
    - Imaging
    - Nuclear perfusion stress testing
    - Echocardiography imaging with exercise or pharmacological stress testing
    - Pharmacological (adenosine, dipyridamole, rogadenoson vasodilators)

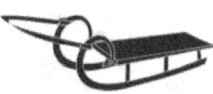

Mastering the Boards: Cardiology   A.B.R. Thomson

- ➢ Indications

  - ○ No known CAD
    - Asymptomatic intermediate risk
      - High-risk job
      - Starting high-risk activity
    - High risk
      - Diabetes
      - Peripheral vascular disease
    - Know CAD
      - Angina despite medical or surgical therapy (CABG)
      - No angina after CABG (controversial)
      - Pre-operatively
      - Post-MI stratification of risk

- ➢ Contraindications

- • Give contraindications of stress testing.

  - ○ Heart   - UA (unstable angina)
    - Unstable angina despite medical therapy
    - MI (active MI within 2 days)
    - Arrhythmias
      - With symptoms
      - Hemodynamic compromise
    - HF (heart failure)
      - With symptoms
    - AS (aortic stenosis)
      - Symptoms, severe
    - Myocarditis
    - Pericarditis

  - ○ Lung   - Pulmonary stenosis

  - ○ Aorta   - Aortic dissection

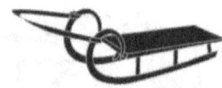

Mastering the Boards: Cardiology   A.B.R. Thomson

Ischemic and Non-ischemic Chest Pain

➢ Testing

- o The typical chest pain of CAD (coronary artery disease) has 3 components
  - Substernal / retrosternal chest pain / discomfort
  - ↑ chest pain / discomfort with exercise or emotional stress
  - ↓ chest pain with rest and/or nitroglycerin
- o For purposes of determining the pretest probability of chest pain for the probability of CAD (coronary heart disease), the chest pain may be classified as typical (Typ), atypical (Atyp) or non-anginal (nonAng).
- o Then use the American College of Cardiology / American Heart Association Task Force on Practice Guidelines to calculate the pretest probability, based on the characteristics of the persons' pain, and their age. Please refer to

www.cardiosource.org/~/media/Images?ACC/Science%20and%20Quality/Practice%20Quality/Practice%20guidelines/s/stable_clean.ashx

Age (yr)	Men			Women		
	Typ	Atyp	NonAng	Typ	Atyp	NonAng
30-39	76	34	4	26	12	2
40-49	87	51	13	55	22	3
50-59	93	65	20	73	31	7
60-69	94	72	27	86	51	14

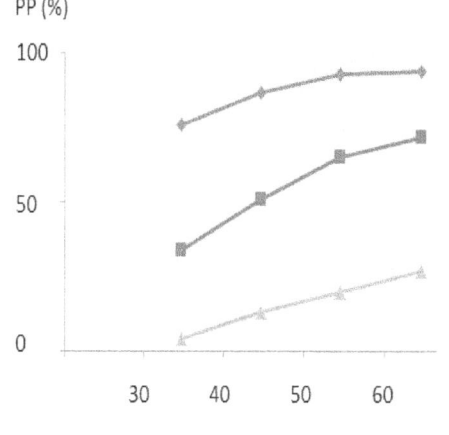

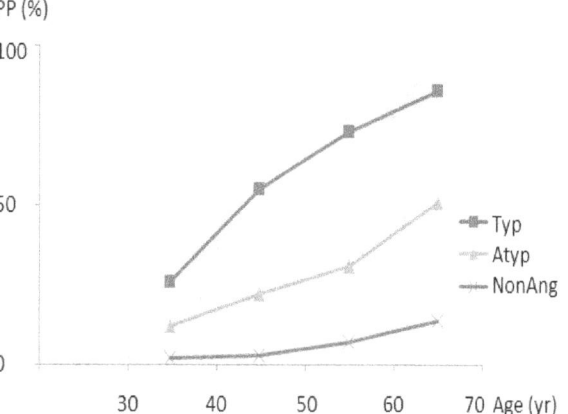

- Give the **characteristic components** of typical angina chest pain

  o Substernal chest pain or discomfort
  o Chest pain is brought on the physical exertion or emotional stress
  o Chest pain is relieved by rest and/or nitroglycerin

<u>Note</u>: the pretest probability of these 3 symptoms rises with age, especially for women.

➢ Treatment

- Give conditions causing **non-ischemic chest pain** which are best treated with

  o CCBs (calcium channel blockers)
    - Coronary vasospasm (prinzmetal angina)
    - Cocaine use
  o BBs (beta blockers)
    - Stress-induced cardiomyopathy
    - Syndrome X
    - HCM (hypertrophic cardiac myopathy)

- Give the clinical diagnostic features of **non-ischemic causes** of acute chest pain for which BBs (beta-blockers) are indicated.

  o Stress-induced cardiomyopathy (takotsubo)
    - Severe emotional or physical stress
    - Angina-like substernal chest pain
    - ↑ serum troponin
    - ST-segment elevation in anterior precardial leads, but coronary angiogram is normal
    - Often seen in post-menopausal women

  o Syndrome X
    - Stress testing → ST-segmnt depression
    - Coronary angiogram is normal
    - After seen in perimenopausal women
    - Harsh systolic murmur which becomes louder with Valsalva maneuver (murmur of AS [aortic stenosis] becomes softer)
    - T-wave is deeply inverted in V2-V4

  o HCM (hypertrophic cardiomyopathy)

Angina pectoris arises from ischemia of the myocardium. However, <u>not</u> all angina arises from coronary artery disease (CAD).

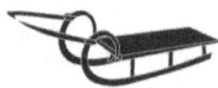

Mastering the Boards: Cardiology   A.B.R. Thomson

➢ Differential

• Give the distinction between classical angina (typical chest pain, atypical chest pain, and non-anginal chest pain).

Type of chest pain	Number of characteristic components
Typical	3
Atypical	2
Non-anginal	0 or 1

➢ Causes

• Give causes of the classical symptom of angina.

  ○ CAD (coronary artery disease)
  ○ AS (aortic stenosis)
  ○ HCM (hypertrophic cardiomyopathy)

Even when the patient has no chest pain(asymptomatic), or has chest pain with only 1 or 2 of the 3 classical angina components (as a marker for CAD), there is a positive pretest probability.

➢ Signs of other causes of chest pain
  ○ Chest wall
    - Muscle strains
    - Myositis
    - Rib fracture or tumour
    - Infection (Coxsackie B)

  ○ Heart
    - Aortic aneurysm, pericarditis

  ○ Lung
    - PE, pleurisy, pneumonia, pneumothorax

  ○ GI
    - GERD, NCCP, PUD, pancreatitis, cholecystitis

  ○ MSK
    - Costochondritis

  ○ Skin
    - Herpes zoster

  ○ Psychological
    - Anxiety

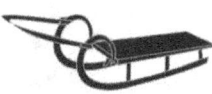

Abbreviations: AE-COPD, Acute exacerabation of chronic pulmonary disease; BP, blood pressure; CHF, congestive heart failure; DS, Down syndrome; GERD, gastroesophageal reflux disease; GI, gastrointestinal; JVP, Jugular venous pressure; L-CHF, left side congestive heart failure; MS, Marfan's syndrome; MSK, musculoskeletal; NCCP, Non cardiac chest pain; PE, pulmonary embolis; PHT, pulmonary hypertension; PR, pulse rate; PUD, peptic ulcer disease; R-CHF, right side congestive heart failure; TS, Turner's syndrome;

Adapted from: Jugovic PJ, et al *Saunders/ Elsevier* 2004, Talley NJ, et al. *Maclennan & Petty Pty Limited* 2003, Table 3.2, page 28

- Give clinical factors which increase the **pretest probability** that atypical or non-anginal chest pain is in fact due to CAD.

  o Previous MI

  o Risk factors for CAD

  o Evidence for artherosclerosis elsewhere
    - PVD (peripheral vascular disease)
    - CVD (cerebral vascular disease)

  o Comorbidities
    - Diabetes
    - Hypertension
    - HF (heart failure)

"Absence of evidence is not

Evidence of absence."

Grandad

 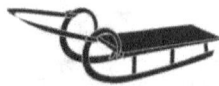

You are given a MCQ scenario where the patient has anginal symptoms or anginal equivalents. Examination shows a new murmur of mitral regurgitation (MR) and S3 and S4 gallops. This suggests acute myocardial ischemia, and you will be provided with additional ECG and biochemical changes to establish from which of the three possible acute coronary syndromes (ACS) the patient is suffering. If there are ST-segment changes, you will be expected to determine the ECG location of the acute MI.

- Give the biochemical markers and ECG changes of the 3 types of acute coronary syndromes acute myocardial ischemia (ACS).

Types of ACS	Troponin, CK-MB biochemical markers	ECG changes Elevation ST segment
o Unstable angina	Normal	– Non-specific changes, or normal

o NSTEMI	↑	– No ST elevation
		– No ST elevation equivalents (new LBBB, or posterior MI)
		– May be
		  ▪ ST depression
		  ▪ Non-specific changes

o STEMI	↑	– ST elevation in ≥ 2 contiguous leads
		– ST equivalents
		  ▪ New LBBB
		  ▪ Posterior MI
		(tall T waves and ST depression in V1-V3)

- Give the ECG changes which help to establish the location of a myocardial infarction.

Location	ST-segment alteration	Involved ECG leads
o Inferior	↑	II, III, aVF
o Anteroseptal	↑	V1-V3
o Lateral and apical	↑	V4-V6 Also, possible ST↑ in I and aVL
o Posterior wall	↓	V1-V3 ST depression Tall R waves
o Right ventricle	↑	V1-V3 tall R waves V4R

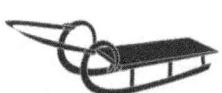

ST segment elevation is an important indication of an acute MI in the correct clinical scenario and/or with abnormal serum biomarkers.

- Give a differential of causes of causes of ST elevation other than STEMI.

  o Normal variation
  o Coronary artery
    - Vasospasm
    - Obstruction
  o LV
    - Aneurysm
  o Muscle wall
    - Stress cardiomyopathy
  o Pericardium
    - Pericarditis

  o Therapeutic aspects of STEMI management would be a very reasonable and expected MCQ. The three areas of focus would be
    - Indications for PCI
    - Contraindications for thrombolytics agents if PCI is **not** available
    - When CABG (cardiac artery bypass graft) surgery is indicated

➢ Of interest
  o Both posterior wall and right ventricles acute MIs have V1-V3 tall R waves, and distinction is made from
  o Both posterior wall and right ventricular acute MIs may be associated with inferior + lateral ST-segment elevation infarctions with unstable angina or NSTEMI, early angiography may be necessary depending upon risk stratification.
    - Because you will be in a position to make this urgent assessment and decision, it is expected that you be able to undertake this risk evaluation.
    - This is done by calculating
      ▪ The TIMI (thrombolysis in myocardial infarction) risk score
      ▪ Determination of the importance of a positive stress when TIMI is low
      ▪ The importance of recurrent angina, elevated serum biomarkers (troponin, CK-MB) and the history of previous revascularization if the TIMI risk is intermediate.

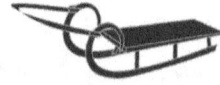

- Give the indications for percutaneous coronary intervention (PCI).
    - STEMI, with PCI performed within 90 min
    - Contraindication for fibrinolytic therapy
    - Previous CABG
    - New onset HF or cardiogenic shock
    - Timing
        - Dual therapy with ASA (aspirin) plus thieno pyridine (e.g. clopidogrel)
        - Non-eluting stent – dual therapy for 1 year, then stop thienopyridine and continue ASA
        - Drug eluting stent – clopidogrel for 12 month or longer

Abbreviations: PCI, percutaneous coronary intervention; CABG, coronary artery bypass surgery; HF, heart failure

- Give the contraindications for thrombolysis

    - Use when PCI is **not** available
    - Heart
        - Cardiopulmonary resuscitation
        - New LBBB
        - NSTEMI > 10 min
        - Asymptomatic, with pain > 24 h ago
    - CNS disorders
        - Previous ICH (intracerebral hemorrhage)
        - Acute ischemic CVA within 3 mon, except within first 3 h
        - 1° / 2° intracranial malignancy
    - ↑ risk of bleeding
        - Closed-head / facial trauma within 3 mon
        - Concurrent warfarin therapy
        - Aortic dissection
        - Active peptic ulcer disease
        - Internal bleeding within 3 week
        - Major surgery within 3 week
        - Hypertension (> 180 / 110 mm Hg) on presentation
    - Pregnancy
    - Note
        - Following thrombolytic therapy a **reperfusion arrhythmia** may develop
        - This reperfusion arrhythmia is often a transient accelerated idioventricular arrhythmia, which does not require additional anti-arrhythmic therapy.

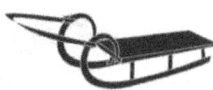

> CABG for STEMI
>   o L. main or L. main equivalent disease
>   o 2- or 3- vessel disease involving LAD artery, plus ↓ LVEF
>   o Cardiogenic shock
>   o Failed
>   – Fibrinolysis
>   – PCI

- Give the **criteria for diagnosing RV/ posterior MI**.

Because RV / posterior MI may be more difficult to diagnose, expect a question on this topic
  o Clinical
  o ECG
    - Tall R waves in V1-V3
    - V4R
    - ST ↑ or ↓

CAD in Diabetics

- Give the benefit of exercise stress testing in the diabetic with suspected CAD (coronary artery disease).
  o Diagnostic and prognostic information
  o Assessment of autonomic function
    - Heart rate recovery often exercise
    - Chronotropic response after exercise

- Give the differences in the therapy for the diabetic vs. the diabetic with CAD (coronary artery disease).
  o Target for LDL
    - In diabetics (<1.81 mmol/L, 70 mg/dL)
    - In non-diabetics (<2.59 mmol/L, 100 mg/dL)
    - SBP < 130/80 mm Hg
  o Avoid using
    - Thiazolidinediones in NYHA functional class III or IV HF (heart failure)
      ▪ ↑ risk of myocardial ischemia)
    - Metformin in recent MI or HF
      ▪ ↑ homocysteine concentration)

Unproven whether GABG or PCI are superior.

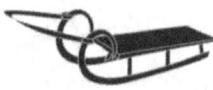

CAD in Women

- Give differences between women and men in the presentation, diagnosis and treatment of CAD.

In women:

- o Presentation
  - More severe
  - More comorbidities
  - Atypical symptoms
    - Fatigue
    - Nausea
    - Dyspnea
  - Possible more microvascular disease

- ➢ Diagnosis
  - o Myocardial perfusion imaging
  - o Scoring assessment Reynolds risk score may be better than Framingham score sex-specific includes hsCRP family history

- ➢ Treatment
  - o Post-menopausal women with CAD
    - Avoid use of HRT (hormone replacement therapy)
  - o Be aware that physician may be less "aggressive" (i.e., less practice guidelines) in the care of women than men with ACSs (acute coronary syndromes)

Reynolds risk score: www.reynoldsriskscore.org

Acute Coronary Syndromes (ACS)

- o NSTEMI (non-ST segment elevation myocardial infarction) has a high longterm morbidity and mortality risk stratification is important to proceed with early angiography and revascularization.
- o "The TIMI (thrombolysis in myocardial infarction) Risk Score is a tool which helps to stratify patients with NSTEMI or unstable angina, using features present at the time of initial assessment in the emergency department.

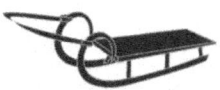

- o "One point is assigned for each feature: some of these are investigation-based, e.g.
    - ↑ cardiac markers, e.g., troponin or creatine kinase-myocardial band)
    - ST segment deviation ≥ 0.5 mm on ECG
    - ≥ 50% coronary artery stenosis
- o Approximately 25% of patients with symptoms suggesting acute cardiac ischemia (ACI) have some other condition
- o For patients with chest pain the response to nitroglycerin does not distinguish those who will prove to have an MI from those who will not.

Adapted from: Graham M, et al. Chapter 31. In: Therapeutic Choices. Grey J, Ed. 6th Edition, *Canadian Pharmacists Association* 2012, page 491.

- On the basis of the TIMI risk score plus additional clinical or laboratory considerations, indicate when early angiography should be performed.

TIMI risk score	Additional considerations	Perform early angiography
0-2	Stress test negative positive	No
3-4	Recurrent angina	Yes
	Elevated troponin, CCK-MB	Yes
	Previous revascularization	Yes
5-7	-	Yes

- o Note
    - Because of the importance of the TIMI risk score or risk stratification for early angiography in unstable angina a NSTEMI, you will be expected to know how to calculate the TIMI risk score from information provided in the MCQ case scenario.

- Give factors used, to calculate the TIMI risk score (give one point for each of the following)d

  - o Age ≥ 65 years
  - o Traditional CAD risk factors ≥ 3
  - o Episodes of angina in past 24 hours ≥ 2
  - o Aspirin use in past 7 days
  - o ↑ biomarkers (troponin, CK-MB)
  - o Coronary obstruction > 50%

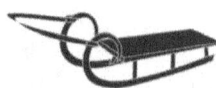

Mastering the Boards: Cardiology   A.B.R. Thomson

- Give the remaining TIMI criteria which may be determined at the bedside.

  o Age ≥ 65 years

  o ≥ 3 cardiac risk factors
    - Hypercholesterolemia
    - Diabetes
    - Hypertension
    - Current smoker
    - Family history of CHD (coronary heart disease)

  o Any ASA use within 7 days

  o ≥ 2 episodes of angina within the last 24 hours

➤ Causes of acute coronary syndrome (ACS)
  o Atherosclerosis (95%)
  Rupture / erosion of on CA → platelet adhesion to subendothelial matrix → platelet

$$\text{partial} \rightarrow \text{NSTEMI}$$
$$\uparrow$$
activation & adhesion → thrombosis → CA obstruction
$$\downarrow$$
$$\text{total} \rightarrow \text{STEMI}$$

  o Reversible
    - Vasospasm of CA (Prinzmetal angina)
    - Wall ballooning syndrome (Takotsubo, stress cardiomyopathy)

Abbreviation: CA, coronary artery

  o Very rare coronary artery causes of MI
    - Embolism (thrombus, infected vegetation)
    - Thrombosis (spontaneous, prothrombotic states)
    - Aneurysm (e.g. Kawasaki disease as a child)
    - Spasm (drugs e.g. cocaine)
    - Arteritis (SLE, PAN, Takayasu)
    - Anomalous coronary artery
    - Dissection, spontaneous

Abbreviations: MI, myocardinal infarction; SLE, systemic lupus erythematosis; PAN, polyarteritis nodosa.

Adapted from: Davey P. *Wiley-Blackwell* 2006, pages 150 and156.

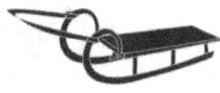

Chest pain 'PQRSTU- A'

Position /location of pain

Quality: crushing (e.g. 'like someone standing on my chest'), dull, burning (suggests epigastric origin), pressing, squeezing, throbbing, knife like (sharp pain suggests chest wall/MSK pain)

Radiation (i.e. does the pain radiate? Where?

Severity: scale of 1-10 (1=mild discomfort, 10= worst pain ever had)

Timing: onset, duration and course

Uniqueness of recent symptoms (i.e. inquire if there was anything different that prompted the patient to seek help e.g. increased duration or severity) precipitating and alleviating factors

Associated symptoms: dyspnea, nausea, cough, palpitations, sweating

Abbreviation: MSK, musculoskeletal

Source: Filate W, et al. *The Medical Society, Faculty of Medicine, University of Toronto* 2005, page 123.

➤ Clinical

• Take a directed history for chest pain.
  o Cardiovascular
  o Coronary artery disease (angina; acute myocardial infarction [STEMI]
    - Acute coronary syndrome [ACS; anstable angina, NSTEMI])
    - Aortic aneurysm/ dissection
    - Pericarditis (including constrictive pericarditis, cardiac tampnade)
  o Pulmonary
    - Pneumothorax, pleurisy, pulmonary embolus, pneumonia
  o Gastroinestinal
    - Esophagitis, peptic ulcer, pancreatitis, cholecystitis
  o Musculoskeletal
    - Costochondrodynia, muscle spasm, nonspecific chest wall pain
  o Other
  o Anxiety, herpes zoster

Abbreviation: MI, myocardial infarction;STEMI, ST elevation MI; NSTEMI, non-ST elevation MI

Adapted from: Jugovic PJ, et al. *Saunders/ Elsevier* 2004, page 118 to120; and Davey P. *Wiley-Blackwell* 2006, page 148.

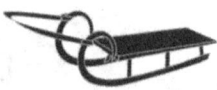

- Take a focused history of clinical features increasing the likelihood of an acute coronary syndrome (ACS).

    o History
        - Profile male over 70 y
        - Pain
            ▪ Accelerating ischemic symptoms over 48 h
            ▪ Ongoing rest pain for > 20 min
            ▪ Recurrent ischemic pain during observation
        - Diabetes

    o Physical examination
        - S3
        - Hypotension
        - Pulmonary edema
        - Peripheral vascular disease
        - Severe arrhythmia
        - Sweating
        - Nausea/vomiting

    o Investigation findings would include
        - Pathologic Q waves; abnormal ST segments; T wave inversion ≥0.02 mV; ST-segment depression > 0.05 mV and increased cardiac biomarkers

Adapted from: Ghosh AK. *Mayo Clinic Scientific Press* 2008, Table 3-25 and Table 3-26, page 101.

- Take a directed focused history to establish the presence of high-risk features in patients with non-ST segment elevation acute coronary syndrome.

    o History
        - Age >75 y
        - Accelerating ischemic symptoms over 48 hrs
        - Ongoing rest pain for >20 min
        - Recurrent ischemic pain during observation

    o Physical
        - Hypotension
        - Pulmonary edema
        - Severe arrhythmia

    o Laboratory
        - Reduced ejection fraction (<40%)
        - ST segment depression >0.5 mV
        - Increased cardiac biomarkers

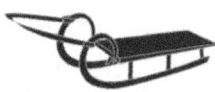

- Give the positive likelihood ratio (PLR) of 7 clinical and 7 ECG features for acute myocardial infarction in patients with undifferentiated chest pain admitted for suspected acute coronary syndrome.

Clinical	PLR
o History	
– Pain in chest or left arm	2.7
– Chest pain radiating to	
▪ Right shoulder	2.9
▪ Left arm	2.3
▪ Left and right arm	7.1
– Chest pain most important symptom	2.0
– Previous history of MI	1.5-3.0
– Pleuritic chest pain	0.2
– Chest pain sharp or stabbing	0.3
– Positional chest pain	0.3
– Chest pain reported by palpation	0.2-0.4
– Nausea or vomiting	1.9
– Diaphoresis	2.0
o Physical exam	
– Third heart sound on auscultation	3.2
– Hypotension (systolic BP <80 mm Hg)	3.1
– Pulmonary crackles on auscultation	2.1
o ECG	
– New ST segment elevation > 1 mm	5.7-53.9
– New Q wave	5.3-24.8
– Any ST segment elevation	11.2
– New conduction deficit	6.3
– New ST segment depression	3.0-5.2
– Any Q wave	3.9
– Any ST segment depression	3.2
– T wave peaking and/or inversion >1 mm	3.1
– New T wave inversion	2.4-2.8
– Any conduction defect	2.7

Abbreviations: ECG, electrocardiography; PLR, positive likelihood ratio; MI, myocardial infarct

Adapted from: Panju AA, et al. *JAMA* 1998; 280:1256-63; Table 35.11, page 413; Simel DL, et al. *JAMA* 2009, Chapter 35, Table 35-5 and Table 35-6, page 467 and Table 35-8, page 472.

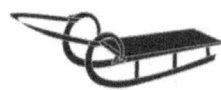

- Take a focused history to determine the risk factors for coronary artery disease.

  - Patient
    - Demography
      - Age
      - Male sex
      - Family history of premature CAD (<55 in men, <65 for primary relatives)

    - Associated disorders
      - Hypertension
      - Diabetes
      - Metabolic syndrome
      - Stress and depression
      - Socioeconomic factors

    - Life style
      - Smoking
      - Sedentary lifestyle
      - Obesity

  - Laboratory
    - Increased LDL: cholesterol level
    - Low HDL cholesterol level
    - Inflammatory markers (e.g. CRP, C-reactive protein)
    - Small, dense LDL
    - Lipoprotein (a)
    - Homocysteine
    - Fibrinogen

Abbreviations: CAD, coronary artery disease; HDL, high-density lipoprotein; LDL, low-density lipoprotein

Adapted from: Ghosh AK. *Mayo Clinic Scientific Press* 2008, page 92.

CCS functional classification of angina

Class	Activity evoking angina	Limits to physical activity
I	Prolonged exertion	None
II	Walking > 2 blocks or > 1 flight of stairs	Slight
III	Walking < 2 blocks or < 1 flight of stairs	Marked
IV	Minimal or at rest	Severe

Abbreviation: CCS, Canadian Cardiovascular Society

Source: Simel DL, et al. *JAMA* 2009, Table 2, page 55.

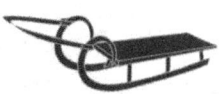

- Perform a focused physical examination to determine if the person with an acute coronary syndrome more likely had disease of the left anterior descending (LAD) versus the right cardiac artery (RCA).

  - LAD
    - Lung
      - Dyspnea
      - Orthopnea
      - Basal crackles
      - Cough
      - Hemoptysis
    - CNS
      - Fatigue
      - Syncope
    - Periphery
      - Hypotension
      - Cool extremities
      - Peripheral cyanosis

  - RCA
    - JVP
      - Elevated JVP
      - Positive hepatojugular reflux
    - Liver
      - Hepatic tenderness
      - Hepatomegaly
      - Pulsatile liver
    - Periphery
      - Peripheral edema

Abbreviations: JVP, jugular venous pressure; LAD, left anterior descending artery; L-CHF, left side congestive heart failure; RCA, right coronary artery; R-CHF, right side congestive heart failure.

Adapted from: Jugovic PJ, et al. *Saunders/ Elsevier* 2004, page 118 to120.

"The superior man is modest in his speech, but exceeds in his action."

Confucius

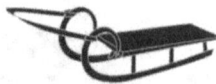

SO YOU WANT TO BE A CARDIOLOGIST!

- In the context of deep vein thrombosis (DVT), give what is Virchow triad.
    - Damage to the vessel wall
        - Trauma
        - Hypoxic blood
        - Drugs
        - Infection
        - Cholesterol
    - ↓ blood flow
    - ↑ blood coagulability

Source: Baliga RR. *Saunders/Elsevier* 2007, pages 100 and 101.

- In the context of the patient with post-myocardial infarction chest pain, give what is Dressler syndrome.
    - Pyrexia, pericarditis, pleurisy

Source: Baliga RR. *Saunders/Elsevier*, 2007, page 101.

- Give the cause and complication of Dressler syndrome.
    - Chest pain, pericardial effusion and fever occureing 3 weeks to 6 months after MI
    - Complications include HF and arrhythmias

Trivia

- The usual cause of ischemic heart disease (IHD) is atheroma in a coronary arteries. Give seven other causes of IHD.

<u>Without narrowing</u>

- Inadequate blood supply
- Left ventricular hypertrophy
- ↓ blood sypply to myocardium
    - Aortic stenosis
    - Mitral stenosis (severe)
    - Pulmonary hypertension (severe)

<u>With narrowing</u>

- Embolism to coronary artery
    - Atrial thrombi
    - Air, fat emboli
    - Embolization of vegetation from infected valve in SBE
- Congenital coronary artery fistula
- Polyarteritis nodosa, giant cell arteritis
- Syphilis (ostial stenosis, ie narrowing or origins of coronary artery)

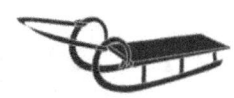

Clinical Tip: Arcus Senilis (AS)

- o A sign of IHD only in men < 50 years who have had a myocardial infarction
- o A tendency for hypercholesterolemia in normal men with AS
- o Otherwise, a debatable sign of IHD

- Give what are the high-risk drugs at the time of hospital discharge.

  - o Heart
    - – Antiarrhythmics
    - – Antihypertensives
    - – Corticosteroids
    - – Diuretics
    - – Warfarin

  - o Diabetes
    - – Oral hypoglycaemic agent & insulin

  - o Pain
    - – Narcotics

  - o Steroids

Adapted from: Ghosh AK. *Mayo Clinic Scientific Press* 2008, Table 13-1, page 505.

➤ Investigation

- Give the uses and cautions in the use of exercise and pharmacologic stress testing for coronary heart disease.

  - o Exercise ECG

    - – Not useful when baseline is abnormal
      - ▪ LVH
      - ▪ LBBB
      - ▪ Pacing
      - ▪ WPWS
      - ▪ ↓ ST > 1 mm

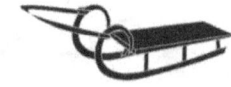

- Criteria
  - ST ↓, ↑
  - ↓ BP
- Sens / Spec
  - 68% / 77%
o Stress echocardiogram

- Useful when
  - Exercise ECG abnormal
  - Area of myocardial risk
  - Measures
    - Valve function
    - Pulmonary pressure

o Criteria
  - Rest EF < 35%
  - Ischemia, > 2 vascular areas
  - EF ↓ with exercise

o Sens / Spec
  - 76% / 78%

"Be an advocate, seek something good for
everyone: seek justice and love"

Anonymous

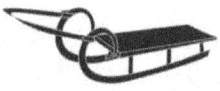

TESTS

Exercise Stress Testing

- o "The test of choice for evaluating most patients of intermediate risk for CAD." (Kizilbash M et al. Washington Manual of Medical Therapeutics, 2014, Chapter 4, page 118. Wolters Kluwer / Lippincott William & Wilkins)

- o Bruce protocol
    - D/C β-blockers, nitrates, nodal blockers
    - ↑ speed / incline q 3 min
    - Endpoints
        - ↓ BP (blood pressure)
        - ↑ ST-segment > 1 mm in several leads
        - Ventricular arrhythmia, sustained

- o Calculate Treamill Score (DTS) to determine annual risk of mortality

DTS score	Annual mortality rate	Risk
5	0.25%	Low
- 10 to 4	1.25%	Intermediate
< -10	> 5%	High

Note: DTS score provides prognosis for persons with chronic angina

- o Performance characteristics for patient with normal resting ECG who reaches 85% of maximal predicted heart rate for age
  Sensitivity and specificity (70%-80%)

Stress Testing with Imaging

Indication for further testing if baseline ECG shows
- Give indications for stress testing with imaging.

    - o Resting changes
    - o LBB (left bundle branch block)
    - o Paced rhythm
    - o LVH (left ventricular hypertrophy)
    - o IVCD (intraventricular or conduction defect)
    - o WPW syndrome (Wolf-Parkinson-White pre-excitation)
    - o Digoxin effects

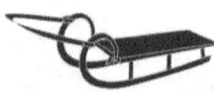

Nuclear Myocardial Perfusion Imaging

- o Thalium-201 or technetium-99m plus stress testing with
- o Advantages: to determine
  - Localization of ischemia
  - Viability of ischemic myocardium
  - Abnormalities of motion of myocardial wall
  - Calculation of ejection fraction (EF)

- o Performance characteristics
  - Sensitivity, 85-90%
  - Specificity, 70%

Echocardiographic Imaging

- o Echocardiographic imaging may be combined with exercise or pharmacologic stress testing to improve performance characteristics ↑ specificity)
  - Sensitivity, 75%
  - Specificity, 85-90%

- o As with any ultrasound investigation, there are ↓ performance characteristics with ↑ BMI (obesity)

Pharmacological Stress Testing

- o Drugs used
  - Vasodilatory drugs
    - ▪ Dipyridamole
    - ▪ Adenosine
    - ▪ Regadenoson
  - Positive inotropic
    - ▪ Dobutamine

- o Used in conjunction with nuclear / MRI perfusion studies

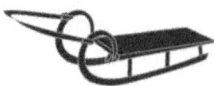

Coronary Angiography

- Give accepted indications for coronary angiography.

- Clinical
  - Angina
    - Unstable despite medical therapy
    - Very high pretest probability of CAD, without previous stress testing, and likely benefit from CABG
  - Myocardial infarction
    - NSTEMI
    - Signs /symptoms
    - ↓ LV ejection fraction
  - Ventricular arrhythmias, serious
  - Sudden cardiac death survivors (SCD)
  - Previous coronary artery bypass grafting (CABG; revascularization surgery)
  - Previous percutaneous coronary intervention (PCI)
  - Suspected / known left main stenosis ≥ 50% stenosis
  - Suspected / known severe 3-vessel CAD

- In conjunction with other testing
  - IVUS (intravascular ultrasound)
    - To access plaque burden at tie of CABG
  - FFR (functional flow reserve)
    - Determine severity of stenosis (flow limiting when 0.8)
  - LV cathetherization
    - LV function
    - LV filling pressure (diastolic function)
    - LV wall measurement
    - Valve gradients
      - Aortic
      - Mitral
    - Abnormalities of aorta

CLINICAL ALERT

- In patient with diabetes or renal insufficiency, consider reducing the 5% risk of contrast-induced nephropathy (CIN):
  - Adequate IV hydration
  - Non-ionic low osmolality contrast solutions
  - Low volume of contrast solution

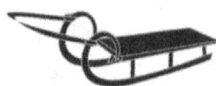

CT Tomography

- o   Useful in persons with
  - Only low-to moderate-risk of CAD, because of its NPV (negative predictive value)
  - Possible congenital anomalies of coronary artery

- o   Limited use in presence of

➢   Treatment of acute coronary syndromes, unstable angina, and NSTEMI
  - o   Algorithm for investigation and management of stable angina
  - o   Substernal chest pain or discomfort
  - o   Treatment choices determined by angiography
    - No lesion
      - Non-ischemic cardiomyopathy
      - Syndrome x
      - Microvascular artery spasm
    - Medical treatment
      - ASA
      - B-blocker
      - Calcium channel blockers
      - Nitrates
      - ACE inhibitors
      - ARBs
    - 1-2 vessels
      - Medical treatment
      - PCI (percutaneous coronary intervention)
        - Refractory to medical Rx
        - High-grade stenosis
        - Severe ischemia
    - Severe 3 vessel disease, or left artery disease
      - CABG
      - PCI

- •   Give forms of **stress testing**, and the usual indications for each

Test	Patient characteristics

o Exercise ECG	- Patient is able to exercise
	- Baseline EGD
	  ▪ Normal, or
	  ▪ Non-specific changes

o Exercise ECG plus myocardial perfusion imaging (or exercise echocardiogram)	- Patient is able to exercise - Previous CABG procedure - ↑ risk of false-positive ECG changes on exercise testing

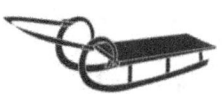

Test	Patient characteristics
○ Myocardial perfusion imaging with vasodilation (or dobutamine chocardiogram)	- Unable to exercise (may consider cardiac angiography) - LBBB - Ventricular pacing

Patients with an ↑ risk of a false-positive ECG changes on exercise testing need to be studied with exercise testing plus myocardial perfusion imaging.

- Give three examples of conditions causing this ↑ risk of **false-positive ECG on exercise testing.**

    ○ Pre-excitation (WPN pattern)
    ○ ST-segment depression > 1 mm on baseline ECG
    ○ Use of digoxin therapy

➤ Dobutamine

For persons who cannot exercise – Take dobutamine (severe baseline hypertension, arrhythmias)

- Echocardiogram

- Nuclear perfusion

    ○ Precautions
        - Withhold β-blockers
        - Do not perform dobutamine tests if baseline
            ▪ Severe hypertension
            ▪ Arrhythmias

➤ Nuclear SPECT perfusion

    ○ Useful when
        - Exercise ECG abnormal
        - Area of myocardial risk
    ○ Prevent false-positive result in LBBB by using vasodilator
    ○ Thallium for rest, technetium for stress
    ○ Criteria
        - TID
        - Thallium uptake into lung
        - Ischemia, > 2 vascular areas
        - EF < 35%

    ○ Sensitivity / Specificity
        - 88% / 77%

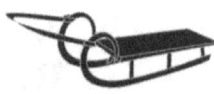

- ➢ Vasodilator Nuclear Perfusion
  - o Prevent false-positive result in LBBB by using vasodilator
  - o Precautions
    - Without caffeine
    - Do not perform if
      - Bronchospasm
      - Use of theophylline
  - o Test vasodilator contraindication
    - Adenosine SSS high degree AV block
    - Adenosine or dipyridamole angina dyspnea flushing

- ➢ PET CT
  - o For "larger" persons
  - o Measures
    - Myocardial
      - Arrhythmias
      - Perfusion
      - Function
      - Viability
      - Blood flow
      - CAC score
  - o Sens / Spec
    - 91% / 82%

Abbreviations: BP, systemic blood pressure; CAC, coronary artery calcium; EF, ejection fraction; LBBB, left bundle branch block; LVH, left ventricular hypertrophy; Sens, sensitivity; Spec, specificity; SPECT, single-photon emission CT; SSS, sick sinus syndrome; TIA, transient ischemic dilation; WPWS, Wolff-Parkinson-White syndrome;

Additional cardiac tests allow identification of coronary artery and vessel narrowing (CA, CCT, CMR), CAC scores, myocardial viability CMR, and therapy (revascularization; CA). These include

- o CA (coronary angiogram)
- o CAC (coronary artery calcium) testing
- o CCT (coronary CT) imaging
- o CMR (cardiovascular magnetic resonance) imaging

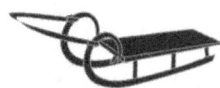

Mastering the Boards: Cardiology   A.B.R. Thomson

- ➤ Treatment

- • Anticoagulation
  - ○ UFA / LMWH (unfractionated or low molecular weight heparin)
  - ○ Cardio-selective beta-blockers (IV unless contraindicated then po indefinitely)
  - ○ Alternatives to UFH / LMWH
    - - Bivalirudin
    - - Fondaparinux

- • Beta-blocker (BB)
  - ○ Contraindications to B-blockers
    - - Pulmonary edema, and/or
    - - Cardiogenic shock
    - - Hypotension SBP < 90 mm Hg
    - - Bradycardia HR < 50 bpm
      - ▪ AV block, second-degree
- • Calcium channel blockers
  - ○ When B-blockers contraindicated → CCBs (calcium channel blockers except nifedipine)
    - - When CCBs not effective → RAN → EEC or SCS

- • IV nitroglycerine
  - ○ **Not** with RV infarction)
  - ○ Angina refractory to nitrates and B-blockers → CCBs
  - ○ Severe post-MI LV dysfunction → eplerenone

- • Diuretics
  - ○ Aldosterone antagonists (spironolactone) have **not** been studied and shown to be effective in ACS

- • ACE inhibitors / ARB
  - ○ Associated
    - - Artherosclerosis
      - ▪ CAD (coronary artery disease)
      - ▪ PVD (peripheral vascular disease)
      - ▪ CVA (cerebrovascular accident)
    - - Diabetes
    - - ≥ 1 more risk factor for CAD
    - - ↓ LF function (EF < 35%)

- • Anti-depressants
  - ○ Screen all post-MI patients for possible depression, since treatment
    - - ↑ sense of well-being
    - - ↓ LOS (↓ hospitalization)
    - - ↓ MR (mortality rate)

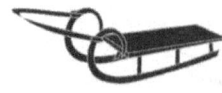

- Statins

- Give two circumstances when treating a person with a normal LDL-cholesterol concentration may benefit from a statin.

  - When a healthy middle-aged person with an ↑hsCRP (high-sensitive C-reactive protein) is treated with a statin within less than 2 yr there is a reduced incidence of a major cardiovascular event

  - When a person with a heart transplant is given calcineurin inhibitor plus statin, there is a ↓ risk of transplant vasculopathy (coronary artery disease of the transplanted heart, manifesting pathologically as diffuse thickening of the intima

---

Clinical Curiosity

  - Statin reduce CV (cardiovascular risk) in persons with CAD (coronary artery disease, and the benefits are proportional to the ↓ LDL.

  - Ezetimibe reduced cholesterol absorption, but even though it ↓ LDL, there is no evidence that ezetimibe
    - ↓ progression of atherosclerosis
    - ↓ future CV events

- Anti-platelet agents

Precious little gem

  If aspirin is contraindicated, ".....use clopidogrel, except if CABG surgery is likely" (ACP Board Basis 3, page 17, 2012)

  - Note: ASA may be used in combination with clopidogrel with
    - Recent MI
    - Stent placement
    - CABG

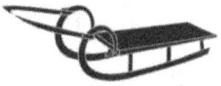

When ASA / CLO are **contraindicated** → PCI / CABG

- Give the contraindications and adverse effects of the drugs / devices used for chronic stable angina.

Drug / Drug Class	Contraindications	Adverse effects
o ASA	Allergy	Bleeding dyspepsia
o CLO		
o BB	Severe bradycardia Severe AV block Severe (decompensated) HF Severe reactive airway disease	Fatigue ↓ sexual function ↓ exercise capacity
o ICCB	Severe systolic dysfunction	Headache dizziness peripheral edema
o LAN	Rx for ED (erective dysfunction)	
o ACEI	Pregnancy, or possible planned / unplanned pregnancy advanced renal disease	Cough
o RAN	↑ QT interval	Use with caution in - Liver disease - Renal disease

- Which of the following is **not** an indication for the use of **clopidogrel** for ACS (you know the answer!)

  - o Unstable angina
  - o NSTEMI
  - o STEMI
  - o Placement of PC stent
  - o CABG surgery planned

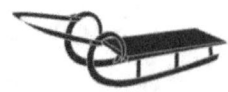

- Intra-aortic balloon pump (IABP)

A patient with acute MI has been stabilized, and first treated in the CCU, then transferred to the general medical ward.

- Give reasons for reconsulting the cardiology service for their consideration for inserting an **intra-aortic balloon pump (IABP)**, or temporary pacing.

    - IABP
        - Angina
            - Refractory
        - VT
            - Intractable
        - Acute murmur*
            - MR
            - VSA
        - Cardiogenic shock

    - Temporary pacing
        - Bradycardia
            - Symptomatic
            - CHB
        - BBB
            - Lorr
        - Asystole
        - Block
            - First-degree AV
            - Indeterminate age bifascicular block

*Note: 2-7 days after acute MI there may occur VS, MR from papillary muscle rupture of the walls of the LV

Abbreviations: MR, mitral regurgitation; VSD, ventricular septal defect VT, ventricular tachycardia

- Coronary artery bypass graft (CABG)

If the patient continues to have angina pectoris and remains refractory to medical therapy, consider CABG.

- Give other **indications for CABG**
    - High-risk criteria an stress testing
    - Large area of ischemic myocardium
        - 3-vessel disease
        - Severe left main disease
    - $\downarrow\downarrow$ EF (LV dysfunction)

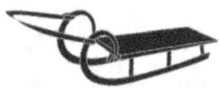

Mastering the Boards: Cardiology   A.B.R. Thomson

Diet

- Give the current recommendations for **lifestyle modification** which are used in the treatment of chronic stable angina.

Used	No longer used
o Smoking - Stop	o Antioxidant vitamins (no)
o Exercise - Increase	o Abnormal lipoproteinemia (no)

o Diet
  - "Healthy heart"
  - LDL cholesterol (> 100 mg/dL)
  - Connection of associated
    ▪ Hypercholesterolemia
    ▪ Glucose intolerance
      (hemoglobin AIC > 7%)
	o ↑ serum homocysteine (using vitamin B12 or folic acid; no)

- o Nine modifiable risk factors are responsible for 90% of the attributable risk for CAD (coronary artery disease and MI (myocardial infarction).

- o In addition are potential predictors, hsCRP (high-sensitivity C-reactive protein)
  - Serum concentration of homocysteine
  - CAC (coronary artery calcium / score (calculated from cardiac CT), and B-mode ultrasound of the carotid artery (for measurement of the intima-media thickness)

- Give the modifiable risk factors for MI, and the approximate odds ratio of each.

Risk Factors, by impact	Approximate Odds Ratio
o Apo B / Apo A1 ratio	3.3
o Smoking, current	2.9
o Stress, psychosocial	2.7
o DM (diabetes mellitus)	2.4
o HBP (systemic hypertension)	1.9
o Obesity, abdominal	1.6
o Alcohol, moderate intake	0.9
o Exercise	0.9
o FF&V (fresh fruit and vegetables) every day	0.7

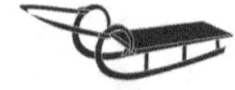

o The cardiac patient "HAS SAD FOE"

H Hypertension
A Alcohol
S Smoking

S Stress
A Apo B / Apo A
D Diabetes

F FF&V
O Obesity
E Exercise

Adapted from: MKSAP 16 2012, Cardiovascular Medicine, Table 6, page 12.

Between days 2 to 7 post-MI, a patient develops sudden
   - Hypotension
   - Loss of pulse
   - ECG: no asystole (cardioelectrical activity continues)

- Give the likely diagnosis:

   o Rupture of the wall of LV
   o If the same person were to develop sudden
      - Hypotension, plus
      - Pulmonary edema
      - Precordial thrill
      - New systolic (holosystolic) murmur (MR [mitral regurgitation] or
         VSD [ventricular septal defect]), from Rupture of papillary muscle

Abbreviations: LV, left ventricle; MR, mitral regurgitation; VSD, ventricular
septal defect

- Give the initial therapy of unstable angina and NSEMI.

➢ Chest pain type

	Unstable angina	NSEMI	STEMI
o ECG	Non-specific	ST ↓	ST ↑
		T ↓	
o Troponin	N	↑	↑
o CK-MB	N	↑	↑
	O--------------------------------→		
	O--→		

 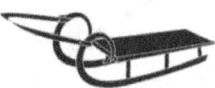

o TIMI score

```
14 d  |-------------------------------------------|
              Risk of death & non-fatal MI


0-2                3-4                5-7
|-----------------------|--------------------------|
Low              Intermediate          High
(8%)                                    (31%)
```

o Initial therapy

Low	Medium-High
Abnormal stress test	GP II b / III a
	Coronary angiogram

Abbreviations:
ASA, aspirin; EF, ejection fraction; GP, glycoprotein; LAN, low-acting nitrate; LMMW, low-molecular weight heparin; PCI, percutaneous coronary intervention; RAN; ranolazine; UFH, unfractionated heparin;

- Give indications for the use of GP IIb / IIIa inhibitor of platelet aggregation (tirofiban, eptifibatide, abciximab)

  o TIMI score 3-7
  o Early coronary angiography with PCI
  o Angina persisting despite initial therapy
  o Dynamic ECG changes
  o DM (diabetes mellitus)
  o HF (heart failure)
  o Not a candidate for early angiography
    - Cancer
    - Elderly

Abbreviations: PCI, percutaneous coronary intervention

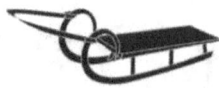

- Give features of STEMI which represent high-risk

  - Age > 75 yr
  - Anterior wall MI
  - ↑↑ ST-elevation
  - HR (heart rate) > 100 bpm
  - SBP (systolic blood pressure) < 100 mm Hg
  - Cardiogenic shock
  - New LBBB (left bundle branch block)

  - For the patient with high-risk STEMI features PCI is preferred to thrombolysis.
  - The available thrombolytic agents include streptokinase, alteplase, reteplase and tenecteplase.
  - If the patient is in a non-PCI facility, then perform thrombolysis, unless there are contraindications.

- Give clinical features which suggest that thrombolytic therapy has been unsuccessful.
  - Chest pain continues
  - ST-segment elevation does not improve (<50% ST – segment fall 60 mm after thrombolysis)
  - Hemodynamic instability (↑ HR, ↓ BP)
  - No reperfusion arrhythmias (accelerate ideoventricular rhythm)

- Give the absolute relative contraindications to thrombolysis for STEMI.

Clinical Condition		Absolute	Relative
○ Head	Ischemic stroke < 3 mon > 3 mon	+	+
	Previous ICH	+	
	AVM (AV malformation)	+	
	Trauma to head / face, within 3 mon dementia	+	

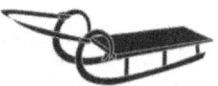

Clinical Condition		Absolute	Relative
○ Aorta	Suspected dissection	+	
○ Hypertension (severe or poorly controlled)			+
○ CPR / major > 10 min			
○ Surgery (< 3 wk)			+
○ Active bleeding		+	
○ Peptic ulcer disease, active			+
○ Puncture site, not compressible			+
○ Bleeding diathesis		+	
○ Anti-coagulants	Current use		+
	Streptokinase allergy		+
	Streptokinase / anistreplase		+

Abbreviation: AVM, AV malformation; ICH, intracerebral hemorrhage

Cardiac Allograft Vasculopathy

In the context of the patient with severe CAD (coronary artery disease), HF (heart failure) and a heart transplantation, give the definition of CAV (cardiac allograft vasculopathy), its clinical presentation, differential and treatment.

➢ Definition

    ○ CAV (cardiac allograft vasculopathy) is the recurrence of coronary artery disease in the cardiac allograft transplantation.

    ○ All of the pro-vasculopathic risk factors present before the first heart transplant are still present.

    ○ Note the unique pathology

       - Diffuse rather than focal thickening of the intima

       - Involvement of large epicardial and small terminal coronary branches

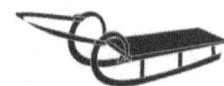

➢ Clinical

- o Atypical cardiac symptoms because of
  - Denervation of transplanted heart
  - Involvement of the large epicardial and small terminal coonary branches

- o Range of symptoms
  - Fatigue
  - ↓ exercise tolerance
  - Shortness of breath
  - New symptoms of HF (heart failure)
  - Heart block

➢ Treatment

- o PCI (percutaneous coronary intervention) and CABG (coronary artery bypass graft) usually not possible

- o Retransplantation

Cardiac (coronary) Angiography (catherization)

- Give the findings from the stress test which would indicate that **cardiac catheterization** is indicated.

  - o Patient inability
    - To exercise or complete the test
    - To ↑ SBP by 10-30 mm Hg
    - To achieve 5 METs (metabolic equivalents) during stress testing

  - o Testing
    - Exercise-induced ST-segment changes (ST elevation, or depression)

  - o Cardiac catherization and coronary angiography are required for persons with a high pre-test probability of CAD, such as
    - these with post-infarction angina
    - These with certain abnormailites on post-MI stress testing
      - Elevation or depression on exercise
      - Unable to reach 5 metabolic equivalents (METs) on exercise – please see previous question).

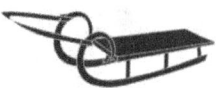

- Give additional **indications for coronary angiography**
  - o Symptoms
    - Angina, class II or IV, despite appropriate therapy
    - Possible coronary spasm
    - History of surviving sudden cardiac death
  - o Exercise test / imaging test
    - Highly positive
    - -Duke treatment score ≤ -11
  - o Echocardiogram
    - ↓ EF (ejection fraction, i.e. LV dysfunction)
  - o Diagnosis **not** clear after exercise testing / imaging

Post ACS-HF

- Give the names of **non-pharmacological** devices or operative procedures used for HF and their indications.

		Treatments	Indications
➤	All stages	o ICD o Heart transplantation	- Cardiomyopathy*, EF ≤ 35% - VO₂ max < 14 mL/kg/min, or < 50% of age-predicted maximum
➤	NYHA II	o Biventricular pacing	- LVEF ≤ 30%, plus QRS > 150 msec - LVEF ≤ 35%, plus QRS > 120 msec

* both ischemic or non-ischemic cardiomyopathy

Abbreviation: ACS, acute coronary syndrome; HF, heart failure; VO_2 max, peak O2 uptake

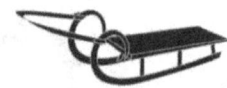

Mastering the Boards: Cardiology   A.B.R. Thomson

- Give the names of the classes of **pharmacological agents used to treat heart failure (HF)** in the post-ACS setting, their indications, and their beneficial outcome(s).

Do <u>not</u> include the treatment of tachycardia, atrial fibrillation, hypertension, or reduced effective circulating blood volume.

	Drug class	Indication	Beneficial outcome
➢ All HF stages	○ ACE inhibitors or ARBs		↓ mortality
	○ B-blocker	- Continue for all stages of HF if stable on previously started BB	↓ mortality
		- Do <u>not</u> stat-in decompensated HF	
		- Do <u>not</u> use if patient has COPD or asthma (may use metoprolol)	
	○ Candesartan	- Diastolic HF	↓ hospitalization
	○ CCBs – Not used for HF		
➢ NYHA III – IV	○ Patient inability	- For persons intolerant to ACEI / ARBs	↓ mortality*
	○ Hydralazine plus nitrates		
	○ Spironolactone (or eplereone)		↓ mortality
	○ Patient inability	- Do <u>not</u> use in presence of renal disease	↓ symptoms
	○ Digitalis		↓ hospitlizations
	○ CCBs are not used for HF		

* only in Africa-origin patients

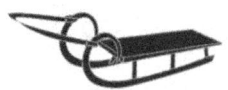

A patient with chronic stable angina follows advise for the modification of lifestyle, and well as a B-blocker which effectively maintained to resting heart rate at 55-60 bpm.

- Give the types of CCBs (calcium channel blockers) which may be added, their main cardiological benefit, and with which class of CCBs dose-adjustment is necessary if **Ranolozine** is added.

CCB class	Relative effects		
	Contractility	Conduction	Vasodilation
Dihydropyridines	-	-	+
Non-dihydropyridines*	+	+	-

Verapamil and diltiazem are examples of non-dihydropyridine agents which interfere with the metabolism of ranolazine, increasing the blood concentration of ranolazine by up to 50%, unless the dose of ranolazine is reduced appropriately.

ACE inhibitors or ARBs are used for ACSs under selected circumstances.

STEMI – associated Complications in Peri-Infarction Period After Successful Reperfusion

➤ Arrhythmias

- o Sinus bradycardia — Inferior wall
- o Sinus tachycardia — Anterior wall
  - < 24 h self-limited
  - > 24 h poor prognosis
- o AF (atrial fibrillation, transient) — Pericarditis
- o Complete heart block
  - Inferior wall
    - Transient
    Pacing, temporary
  - Anterior wall
    - Large infarct
      - Pacing, permanent
      - Poor prognosis

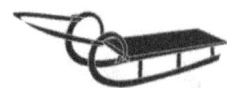

- ➤ HF (heart failure)
  - o Large infarcts
  - o LV dysfunction
  - o Rx
    - ↓ preload
    - ↓ afterload
      - Diuretics
      - ACE inhibitors
      - PA catheter and hemodynamic monitoring

- ➤ Cardiogenic shock
  - o Atherosclerosis (95%)
  - o Extensive contractile dysfunction
  - o RV infarction
  - o Extensive LV infarction
  - o LV free wall rupture
  - o LV thrombus
  - o VSD (ventricular septal defect)
  - o MR (mitral regurgitation)

Left Ventricular (LV) Thrombus

  - o Anterior STEMI
  - o ~15%
  - o Often apex of LV

SO YOU WANT TO BE A CARDIOLOGIST!

- Give the findings in a PA (pulmonary artery) catheter study in 5 of the following structural complications post-STEMI.

o LV infarction	- ↑ RA pressure
	- ↑ RV pressure
	- Tracing
	- ↓ pressure
o Severe LV infarction	- CI < 2 L/min per m^2
	- Wedge ↑ pressure > 18 mm Hg tracing
o LV free wall rupture	- CI < 2 L/min per m^2
	- Diastolic pressure RV = LV
o VSD	- Wedge tracing
	- ↑ V waves
	- O_2 saturation increases from RA to RV

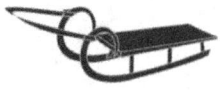

Rupture of LV Free Wall

> Clinical
> o Day 3-7 post-STEMI
> o Typical older women
> o Typically
>   - First MI, and
>   - Anterior wall
> o Pericardial effusion / tamponade
>   - ↑ JVP
>   - ↓ BP
>   - Distant heart sounds
> o High mortality

> Treatment
> o Emergency pericardiocentesis
> o Surgical repair
> o High mortality

When should you suspect **RV infarction**

- o RCA (right coronary artery) proximal to origin of acute marginal vessels

- o Remember
  - RV dysfunction leads to LV dysfunction

- o Triad
  - ↓ BP (hypotension)
  - Lungs clear
  - ↑ JVP (jugular venous pressure)

- o ECG
  - V3R, V4R   ↑ ST > 1 mm

- o Treatment
  - Revascularization (PCI, or thrombolysis)
  - ↑ fluids
  - Dopamine or dobutamine

- Give the management of the patient who develops ↑ Cr_s (serum creatinine) concentration while on an ACE inhibitor or on the anti-atrial fibrillation antiarrhythmic drugs "amiodarone".

  - o Stop the drug if there is a decline in the glomerular filtration rate

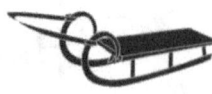

POST MYOCARDIAL INFARCTION COMPLICATIONS

To be considered here
- o Acute Pericarditis
- o Aneurysm
- o Arrhythmias
- o Cardiogenic Shock
- o Cocaine-use STEMI
- o Dressler syndrome
- o Free wall Rupture
- o ICD (Implantable Cardioverta-defibrillator)
- o In-stent Restenosis (ISR) and Stent thrombosis (ST)
- o Ischemic Mitral Regurgitation (MR)
- o Papillary Muscle Rupture
- o Recurrent Chest Pain
- o Right Ventricular (RV) Myocardial Infarction
- o Transcutaneous and Transvenous Pacing
- o Ventricular Pseudoaneurysm
- o Ventricular Septal Rupture

Acute Pericarditis

➤ Demography
- o Seen in ~15% of STEMI patients, usually 1-4 days after MI

➤ Clinical
- o Chest pain
  - Pleuritic
  - Worse when lying down, better when sitting up
- o Friction rub, with or without effusion

➤ ECG
- o Diffuse
  - ↑ ST-segment
  - ↓ PR fragment

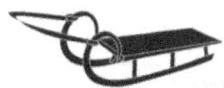

Mastering the Boards: Cardiology   A.B.R. Thomson

> Treatment
  o ASA, NSAIDs, colchicine plus ASA, corticosteroids

- Give the major cardiac related reasons why corticosteroids must be **used with caution** in acute post-NSTEMI pericarditis.
    o ↓ healing of infarct
    o ↑ risk of free wall rupture

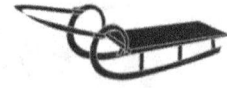

Aneurysm

➢ Pathophysiology
  ○ Infarction → thinning of myocardial wall → aneurysm

➢ Complications
  ○ Mural thrombus
  ○ Rupture

➢ Diagnosis
  ○ ECG
    - ↑ ST segment

  ○ Diagnostic imaging
    - Echocardiogram
    - MRI
    - Ventriculography

➢ Treatment
  ○ Anticoagulation
    -      Especially with LV thrombus or chronic atrial fibrillation
      ▪ UFA / LMWH
      ▪ Warfarin for 3-6 mon
  ○ Surgical correction
    -      Associated heart failure (HF)
    -      Failed medical therapy associated ventricular arrhythmias

Arrhythmias Post-MI

➢ Classification

  ○ Conduction block   - AV block
                             - IV (intraventricular) conduction delay
      ▪ Monofascicular block
      ▪ Bi- / trifascicular block → complete heart block

  ○ Sinus arrhythmia   - Sinus bradycardia
                             - Sinus tachycardia

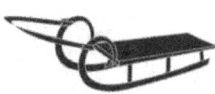

- o Atrial arrhythmia
  - - Atrial fibrillation / flutter
  - - Accelerated junction rhythm

- o Ventricular arrhythmia
  - - Ventricular premature depolarization (VPDs)
  - - Accelerated ideoventricular rhythm (AIVR)
  - - Ventricular tachycardia (VT)
  - - Ventricular fibrillation (VF)

➤ Most common sites of MI causing arrhythmias

- o Anterior MI
  - - Mobitz II second-degree block
  - - Third-degree block

- o Inferior MI
  - - Mobitz I second-degree block
  - - Accelerated junctional rhythm (especially with digitalis toxicity)

CLINICAL ALERT

- • Give the clinical significance of persistent unexplained post-MI sinus tachycardia.

  - o Sinus tachycardia which persists in the post-MI period and is not explained by anxiety, pain, fever, heart failure, may be due to poor ventricular function, and is associated with ↑ mortality rate

---

➤ Treatment
- o Treat associated conditions
- o Pharmacotherapy for specific arrhythmia
- o Procedures
  - - Transcutaneous pacing (TCP)
  - - Transvenous pacing (TVP)
  - - Implantable cardioverter-defibrillator (ICD)

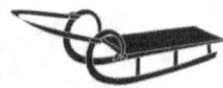

Cardiogenic Shock

➢ Definition
   o "…. Hypotension in the setting of inadequate ventricular function to meet the metastatic needs of the peripheral tissue".

Kizilbash M, et al., The Washington Manual of Medical Therapeutics, 34th Edition, 2014. Wolters Kluwer

   o Signs of organ hypoperfusion
   o CNS changes
   o Diaphoresis
   o Shortness of breath (dyspnea)
   o Renal failure, progressive

➢ Demography
   o Uncommon post-MI, but mortality rate > 50%

➢ Associations
   o Older
   o Diabetic
   o Prior MI
   o Current anterior MI

➢ Diagnosis
   o Early diagnostic angiography
   o Echocardiogram
      - LV function
      - Wall motion
      - Pericardial tamponade
      - Mechanical complication
         ▪ Aneurysm
         ▪ Pseudoaneurysm (ventricular)
         ▪ Free wall rupture
         ▪ Ventricular septal rupture

   o Measurements
      - > 20 mmHg
      - ↓ SBP (hypotension)

Kizilbash M, et al., The Washington Manual of Medical Therapeutics, 34th Edition, 2014. Wolters Kluwer; Figure 4-5, page 146.

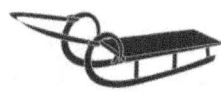

➤ Treatment
- o Inotrope
  - SBP > 90 mmHg
    - ▪ Dobutamine
  - SBP < 70 mmHg
    - ▪ Dopamine plus norepinephrine / phenylephrine

  - SBP < 80 mmHg but dopamine
    - ▪ Not effective, or
    - ▪ ↑↑ tachycardia but no
    - ▪ Renal insufficiency
    - ▪ Milrinone

Adapted from: Kizilbash M, et al., The Washington Manual of Medical Therapeutics, 34th Edition, 2014. Wolters Kluwer; Table 4-22, page 168.

- Give mechanical support devices other than IABC or surgery that may be considered in cardiogenic shock.

  - o LVDD LV assist device
  - o Extracorporeal membrane oxygenation
  - o Cardiac transplantation

Cocaine-use STEMI

➤ Demography
  - o 3 h to several days after use of cocaine, chest pain may develop from vasospams

➤ Pathophysiology
  - o ↑ stimulation of both α- and β-adrenergic receptors
    - Vasospasm
    - Demand ischemia
    - Thrombus formation

➤ Treatment
  - o Same as per non-cocaine STEMI (O2, ASA, UFA / LMWH, nitrates, benzodiazepines) but no beta blockers of any kind, non-selective or selective
  - o In addition to nitrates to ↓ vasospasm, the α =adrenergic antagonist phentolamine, or calcium channel blockers may be used.
  - o Failure to loose symptoms with above medical therapy
    - Primary PCI
    - Fibrinolysis if PCI cannot / should not be performed.

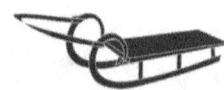

Dressler Syndrome

The pericardial pain of Dressler syndrome occurs 1-8 wk post-MI, and is treated similar to post-MI pericarditis, including **non-use** of

- o Wk 1 – NSAIDs
- o Wk 1-4 – Corticosteroids
- o At anytime – Heparin

- Give the components of the autoimmune disorder.

    - o Heart   - Pericardial pain
                     - Pericardial effusion (sometimes)

    - o General   - Fever
                     - Malaise

    - o Lab'   - ↑ WBC (white blood count)
                     - ↑ ESR (erythrocyte sedimentation rate)

Free wall Rupture

➤ Pathophysiology
    o Acute hemodynamic shock in first post-STEMI week, especially after anterior or inferior wall MI

➤ Clinical
    o Risk factors
        - Drugs
            ▪ NSAIDs   ⎤ early use
            ▪ Corticosteroids ⎬
            ▪ Fibrinolytics late use ⎦
        - Women with hypertension and first, large transmural MI

➤ Treatment
    o Even with emergent surgical repair, mortality rate > 90%

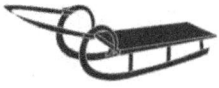

In-stent Restenosis (ISR) **and Stent thrombosis** (ST)

➢ Demography
   o ISR occurs months after coronary angiography (CA) plus placement of a stent
   o ST
      - Acute
         ▪ Within 24 hr
      - Subacute
         ▪ 1-30 days
      - Late
         ▪ 1-2 month

➢ Pathophysiology
   o ISR
      - Hyperplasia of intima over 6-9 mon after CA + stent → progressive
   o ST
      - ↓ endothelial repair
      - Non-adherence to anticoagulation, antiplatelets P2Y12 inhibitors
   o Incidence at 1 yr
      - No BMS (restrnosis of target lesion after balloon angiography) ~ 40%
      - BMS ~ 25%
      - DES ~ 5%

➢ Risk factors
   o Table 4-20, page 162; Kizilbash M, et al., The Washington Manual of Medical Therapeutics, 34th Edition, 2014. Wolters Kluwer

➢ Treatment
   o ISR
      - DES
      - Not recommended
         ▪ Atherectomy
         ▪ Brachytherapy
   o ST
      - PCI plus aspiration od thrombus, plus stent replacement
      - If not due to cessation of antiplatelet, then
         ▪ Assess for possible resistance to clopidogrel 10 mg /d, or ticagrelor), 90 mg bid
         ▪ Use clopidogrel 150 mg plus cilostazol

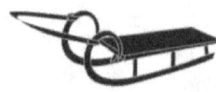

Ischemic Mitral Regurgitation (MR), and Papillary Muscle Rupture

➢ Pathophysiology
  o Acute posterior MI
  o Progressive worsening of MR → dilation of LV → annular dilation of mitral valve

Note: Even a small STEMI or NSTEMI may cause papillary muscle rupture
➢ Clinical
  o Sudden unexplained deterioration

GEMS

- When to suspect ischemic MR after STEMI when there is no murmur of MR (as in ~ 50% of cases):

  o Suspect ischemic MR in the patient with STEMI if there is
    - Heart failure (HF), or
    - Acute pulmonary edema
    - Hyperdynamic LV function ......or without an obvious cause such as LV dysfunction

- Why does ischemic MR rarely affect the anterior papillary muscle?

  o The anterior papillary muscle has a dual blood supply
  o Associated with ↑ mortality rate

➢ Diagnosis
  o Echocardiogram (TEE is superior TTE)

➢ Treatment
  o Stable patient
    - ↓ afterload
    - ↑ vascularization
  o Unstable, or failed medical therapy
    - Urgent surgery

Abbreviations: TEE, transthoracic echocardiogram; TTE, transthoracic echocardiogram

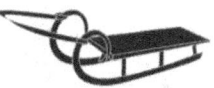

Recurrent Chest Pain

➢ Etiology

    o Cardiac-   - Ischemia
                              ▪ Recurrence of ischemia
                              ▪ Extension of infarction
                    - Arrhythmias
                    - Mitral regurgitation
                    - Acute stent thrombosis
                    - Rupture
                    - Shock (cardiogenic)
                    - Pericarditis

    o Lung   - PE (pulmonary embolism)

➢ Treatment
    o Standard therapy for STEMI
    o Treat any associated condition (e.g. PE, arrhythmia, ischemic MR)
    o Repeat coronary angiography
    o IABP (intra-aortic balloon pump)

Right Ventricular (RV) Myocardial Infarction

➢ Demography
    o RV MI
        - Seen in 50% of those with acute inferior MI
        - 50% have hemodynamic compromise

➢ Clinical
    o ↑ JVP
    o JVP ↑ with inspiration (Kussman) sign
    o R-S3 / S4
    o Hypotension /cardiogenic shock

CLINICAL CHALLENGE

• Give the circumferences under which right ventricular (RV) dysfunction is associated with pulmonary rates (pulmonary edema).

    o While the lung fields are often clear with RV-MI, this is not the case if there is associated heart failure (HF) or mitral regurgitation (MR)
    o May be associated heart block and AV dyssynchrony

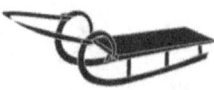

- ➤ Pathophysiology
    - o RA pressure > 10 mmHg
    - o LV filling pressure N / ↓
    - o Cardiac index ↓ (< 2.5 L/kg per min)

CLINICAL TIP

- o The finding of a normal right atrial (RA) pressure in RV-MI does not necessarily mean that the RV function is not impaired.
- o The RA pressure may increase after the patient has been given IV fluids

---

- ➤ Treatment
    - o Invasive hemodynamic monitoring to guide IV fluid volumes, especially if hypotension persists
    - o Inotropic support
        - Dobutamine, or
        - IABP (intra-aortic balloon pump)
    - o Sequential pacing for associated heart block and AV dyssynchrony

Transcutaneous and Transvenous Pacing

- Give indications for transcutaneous pacing (TCP) and for transvenous pacing (TVP).

    - o AV node
        - Symptomatic bradycardia
        - Second degree AV block, Mobitz type II (sudden AV conduction block with no progression delay of conduction)
        - Complete heartblock (CHB)
        - Recurrent sinus pausesNew trifascicular block
        - LBBB plus pulmonary artery cathetherization (LBBB → CHB)

    - o Asystole

    - o Ventricular
        - Frequent recurrent VT
        - Implantable cardioconverter-defibrillators (ICDs)

- Give the indications for placement of an ICD.

    - o ↓ LV function ≥ 40 days post-STEMI
        - E section fraction (EF) < 30%, or
        - EF < 35% in NYHA class 2 or 3
    - o Recurrent ventricular tachycardia (VT) or ventricular fibrillation (VF)

Note: even when there is ↓ EF in the first 40 days after STEMI, there is no proven benefit from ICD; the benefit of ICD for ↓ EF or VT / VF is > 40 days

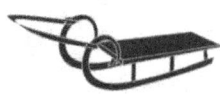

Ventricular Pseudoaneurysm

- o Incomplete rupture of wall of ventricle → blood contained in pericardium
- o Diagnosis TTE with contrast, or TEE
- o Surgical repair to ↓ risk of subsequent rupture of wall of myocardium

Ventricular Septal Rupture

➤ Demography
- o 3-5 days post anterior MI

➤ Pathophysiology
- o Rupture across or along wall septum

➤ Clinical
- o Unexplained heart failure
- o New systolic murmur (holosystolic)

➤ Treatment
- o Stability ↓ afterload, inotropic, IABC, surgical closure after 1 wk
- o Non surgical patient percutaneous device closure of septal rupture

Timing of post-STEMI complications

- o Day
1-2	– Accelerated ideoventricular rhythm (AIVR)
1-4	– Acute pericarditis
3-5	– Ventricular septal rupture
1-7	– Free wall rupture
1-30	– Subacute atent thrombosis

- o Week
1-8	– Dressler syndrome

- o Month
1-12	– Late stunt thrombosis

Frequency of common post-STEMI complications

- o 50% after acute inferior MI – RV-MI
- o 25% Recurrent chest pain after fibrinolytic therapy
- o 20% Atrial fibrillation / flutter
- o 15% Acute pericarditis
- o 12% Recurrent chest pain after PCI
- o 5% Ventricular fibrillation

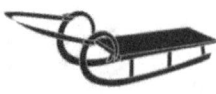

VALVULAR HEART DISEASE

HEART MURMURS

Useful background: "Rules" of Cardiac Murmurs !

- o When giving your summary of a cardiac murmur, state that the type murmur (lesion), the likely etiology, and the functional status (severity of lesion, associated dysrhythmia, CHF).

- o "Gold"
  - Judge murmurs by the company they keep
  - A soft or absent S_2 is pathological

- o "Silver": Pathologic murmurs
  - All diastolic murmurs
  - All holosystolic or late systolic murmurs
  - All continuous murmurs (span the entire cardiac cycle)

- o "Bronze": mechanism of production of murmurs
  - Abnormal size, shape, edge of the area through which flow is occurring
  - Low blood viscosity
  - Hyperdynamic heart syndrome

- o "Tin"
  - Murmur that extends into S_2 is usually pathologic; a murmur in early or mid systole is usually benign and due to ejection through semilunar aortic and pulmonary valves

Source: Mangione S. *Hanley & Belfus* 2000, page s 240 and 241.

- o Effect of drugs on murmurs
  - Drugs increasing arteriolar resistance will decrease systolic ejection murmurs and increase regurgitant murmurs at all valves. Vasodilators have the opposite effect.

Source: Burton JL. *Churchill Livingstone* 1971, page 7.

- o Effects of respiration on murmurs
  - Inspiration increases stroke volume of R ventricle, therefore increases intensity of TS, TI and PS
  - Inspiration increases vascular volume of lungs and decreases stroke volume of L ventricle, therefore decreases intensity of MS, MI, AS and AI
  - Inspiration decreases L → R shunts

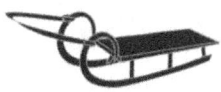

Visual Presentation of Various Cardiac Murmurs

- Normal heart tones

- Early systolic murmur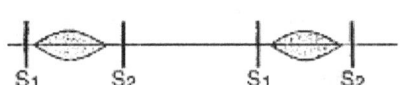

- Midsystolic murmur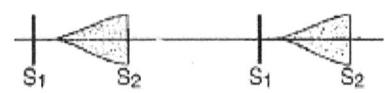

- Late systolic murmur

- Late systolic murmur and click ©
  of mitral valve prolpapse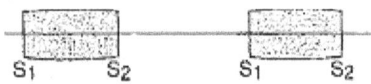

- Holosystolic murmur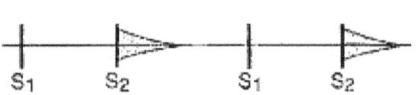

- Early diastolic murmur of aortic
  regurgitation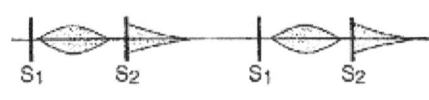

- Early diastolic murmur of aortic
  regurgitation and aortic flow
  murmur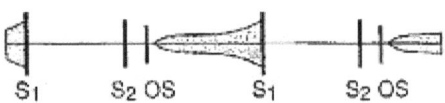

- Opening snap (OS) and diastolic
  rumble of mitral stenosis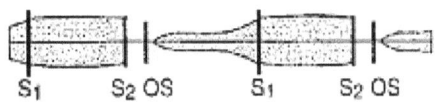

- Opening snap, diastolic rumble of
  mitral stenosis, and mitral
  regurgitation

- Continuous murmur of
  arteriovenous fistula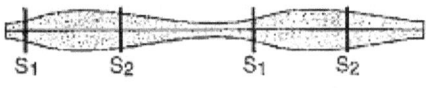

- Continuous murmur of venous
  hum or mamary soufflé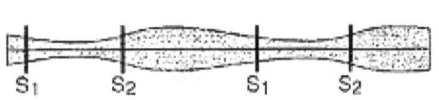

Printed with permission: McGee SR. *Saunders/Elsevier* 2007, Figure 39-1, page 457.

- Give the murmur grades.

Grade (out of "6")	Intensity	Thrill
1	Very faint, often not audible in all positions or by beginners	-
2	Quiet, usually audible by all listeners	-
3	Moderately loud	-
4	Loud	+
5	Very loud, audible with stethoscope partly off chest	+
6	Loudest, audible with stethoscope removed from contact with chest	+

Source: Filate W, et al. *The Medical Society, Faculty of Medicine, University of Toronto* 2005, Table 9, page 61.

➢ Useful tips: Murmurs
  o The length and intensity of a murmur do not necessarily reflect severity
  o Diastolic murmurs usually represent valvular disease
  o Systolic murmurs are caused by:
    - Structural valve disease
    - Dilation of heart valve (e.g., LV dilation – AR, MR), or dilation of large vessel (dilation of aorta from artherosclerosis; dilation of pulmonary artery from PHT)
    - Pressure difference
    - Rapid flow
    - Ruptured papillary muscle, or the (VSD)
    - Floating tissue – bacterial endocarditis

  o Intensity
    - High pitched
      ▪ Large pressure difference across small orifice (e.g. AR)
    - Low pitched
      ▪ Small pressure difference across large orifice (e.g. MS)

Abbreviations: AR, aortic regurgitation; LV, left ventricle; MR, mitral regurgitation; MS, mitral stenosis; PHT, pulmonary hypertension; VSD, ventricular septal defect

Source: McGee SR. *Saunders/Elsevier* 2007, Box 39-2, pages 466 and 467.

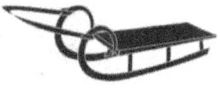

- Give the heart sounds of non-valvular origin (continuous murmurs).

Murmur	Location	Radiation	Quality	Pitch	Associated signs
o Pericardial friction rub	Variable, 3rd ICS	Little	Scratchy	High	3 phases: mid-systolic, mid diastolic, pre systolic
o Patent ductus arteriosus (PDA)	2nd LICS	Left clavicle	Harsh, machinery like	Medium	Loudest in late systole fades in diastole, often silent interval in late diastole
o Venous hum	Above medial third of right clavicle	1st-2nd ICS	Humming, roaring	Low	Soft murmur without a silent interval, loudest in diastole

Abbreviations: ICS, intercostal space; LICS, left intercostal space

Source: Filate W, et al. *The Medical Society, Faculty of Medicine, University of Toronto* 2005, Table 11, page 62.

- Give the heart murmurs of valvular origin.

Murmur	Location	Radiation	Quality	Pitch	Associated signs

- **Midsystolic murmurs**

|﹐|‖‖﹐|

S1   S2

Murmur	Location	Radiation	Quality	Pitch	Associated signs
o Aortic stenosis (AS)	2nd RICS	Neck	Harsh	Medium	Ejection sound, ↓ S_2, S_4, narrow pulse pressure, slow rising and delayed pulse
o Pulmonic stenosis (PS)	2nd-3rd LICS	Neck, back	Harsh	Medium	Ejection sound, S_4

Murmur	Location	Radiation	Quality	Pitch	Associated signs
o MV prolapse (MVP)	Apex	Axilla			Mid-systolic click
o Hypertrophic cardiomyopathy (HCM)	3rd-4th LICS	LLSB → apex, base	Harsh	Medium	S_3, S_4 sustained apical impulse- two palpable components, carotid pulse rises quickly

- **Pansystolic murmurs**

|||||||
|S1   S 2|

Murmur	Location	Radiation	Quality	Pitch	Associated signs
o Mitral regurgitation (MR)	Apex	L axilla	Blowing	High	↓S1; S3, S4 present, laterally displaced diffuse PMI
o Tricuspid regurgitation	LLSB	RLSB	Blowing	High	S3, ↑JVP
o VSD	3rd-5th LICS	Wide	Harsh	High	Vary with severity

- **Diastolic murmurs**

OS

|||ıⅠ|
|S1   S2|

Murmur	Location	Radiation	Quality	Pitch	Associated signs
o Aortic regurgitation (AR)	2nd-4th LICS	Apex, RSB	Blowing	High	Ejection sound, S3, S4, laterally displaced PMI, wide pulse pressure, bounding pulse, midsystolic flow murmur or Austin Flint murmur
o Mitral stenosis (MS)	Apex	Little/ None	Rumbling	Low	↑S1, OS after S2, RV impulse, often assoc. with AV disease

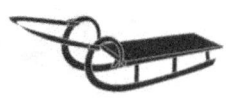

Abbreviations: R/LISC, Right/left intercostals space; R/LLSB, right/left lateral sternal border; JVP, jugular venous pressure; PMI, point of maximal impulse; OS, opening snap; RV, Right ventricle; AV, Aortic valve

Printed with permission: Filate W, et al. *The Medical Society, Faculty of Medicine, University of Toronto* 2005, Table 10, pages 61 and 62.

- Take a directed history for the cause of a patient's cardiac murmur.

o Ideopathic	- Flow, dilation, distortion, anemia, hyperthyroidism - Dissecting aortic aneurysm - Hypertrophic obstructive cardiomyopathy (HOCM)
o Inherited	- Cyanotic, acyanotic heart disease - Marfan's, Turner's, Down syndrome
o Infection	- Syphilis - Subacute bacterial endocarditis (SBE)
o Immune / Inflammation	- Lupus (Libman Sachs murmur) - Ankylosing spondylitis - Rheumatic heart disease
o Infiltration	- Carcinoid tumor - Tumor - Atrial myxoma
o Trauma	
o Metabolic	- Coronary artery disease (CAD) - Papillary muscle rupture, ventricular septal defect (VSD)

Abbreviations: CAD, coronary artery disease; HOCM, hypertrophic obstructive cardiomyopathy; SBE, subacute bacterial endocarditis; VSD, ventricular septal defect

Adapted from: Burton JL. *Churchill Livingstone* 1971, page 9.

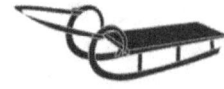

- Perform a focused physical examination of the precordium for the site of optimal ausculatation of normal and abnormal heart sounds and murmurs.

  o Pulmonary area
  - 1-3 LICS, at manubrium, medial LIC area
  - Posterior thorax, T4,5, 2-3 cm to either side of spine

  o Aortic area (Erb's point, 3 LICS)
  - 3 LICS, sterna edge, across manubrium to 1-3 RICS

  o Descending thoracic area
  - Posterior thorax, T2 – T16, 2-3 cm to either side of spine

3-5 LICS
RVE (PHT,L-CHF)

o Tricuspid area (RV)
  - 3-5 LICS, 2 cm. R&L
  - RVE → extend laterally
o RA
  - 4-5 RICS, 2 cm. to right of sternum
  - TR

o Mitral area (LV)
  - 3-5 LICS, 2 cm medial & lateral to LAAL
  - LVE → extends medially
  - RVE → extends to L. axilla

o Aortic area
  - AS, AR
  - A2, Aortic ejection click
  - Systemic hypertension
  - Dilated aortic aneurysm

o Pulmonary area
  - PS, PR, flow, PDA
  - P2, pulmonary ejection click
  - PHT

o Mitral area
  - MS, MR, AS, AR, IHSS, functional diastolic rumble
  - A2, S3, S4

o Tricuspid area
  - TS, TR, PR, VSD
  - RV S3,S4
  - TV opening sanp

o Descending thoracic area
  - Coarctation of aorta
  - Aortic aneurysms

Abbreviations: AO, aorta; AR, Aortic regurgitation; AS, aortic stenosis; ICS, intercostal space; IHSS, idiopathic hypertrophic subaortic stenosis; L-CHF, left sided congestive heart failure; LA, left atrium ; LICS, left intercostal space; LV, left ventricle; LVE, left ventricular enlargement; MR, mitral regurgitation; MS, mitral stenosis; PA, pulmonary artery; PDA, patent ductus arteriosis; PHT, pulmonary hypertension; PS, pulmonary stenosis; RA, right atrium; RICS, right intercostal space; RV, right ventricular; RVE, right ventricular enlargement; TR, Tricuspid regurgitation; TS, tricuspid stenosis; TV, tricuspid valves; VSD, ventricular septal defect

Adapted from: Mangione S. *Hanley & Belfus* 2000, pages 239 and 240; Filate W, et al. *The Medical Society, Faculty of Medicine, University of Toronto* 2005, Table 7, page 58.

- Give the performance characteristics for physical examination for murmurs from valvular heart disease.

Finding	PLR
o Abnormal heart examination	
- Detecting any valvular heart disease	18.3
o Characteristic systolic murmur	
- Detecting AS	3.3
- Detecting mild MR or worse	5.4
- Detecting moderate to severe MR	3.3
- Detecting MVP	12.1
- Detecting mild TR or worse	14.6
- Moderate to severe TR	10.1
- Detecting VSD	24.9
o Characteristic diastolic murmur	
- Detecting mild AR or worse	9.9
- Moderate to severe AR	4.3
- Detecting PR	17.4

Abbreviations: AR, aortic regurgitation; AS, aortic stenosis; PLR, positive likelihood ratio; MR, mitral regurgitation; MVP, mitral valve prolapse; NS, not significant; PR, pulmonary regurgitation; TR, tricuspid regurgitation; VSD, ventricular septal defect

Adapted from: McGee SR. *Saunders/Elsevier* 2007, Box 39-1, page 460.

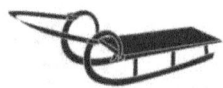

- Give the maneuvers to improve auscultation of heart sounds and murmurs.

Position		Effect
o Clenching fists	↑systemic arterial resistance	↑ some left sided murmurs MR, AR, VSD; ↓ AS
o Leaning forward and holding breath		↑ AS, AR, pericardial rubs
o Lying in left lateral decubitus positions; (use bell of stethoscope)		S3, S4, MS
o Raising leg	↑venous return	↑ right sided murmur, TR, PS
o Standing	↓ venous return / vascular tone	↑ MVP, HCM; ↓ AS
o Squatting	↑ venous return / vascular tone	↓ MVP, HCM; ↑ AS

Abbreviations: AS, aortic stenosis; AR, aortic regurgitation; HCM, hypertrophic cardiomyopathy; LLD, left lateral decubitus; MR, mitral regurgitation; MS, mitral stenosis; MVP, mitral valve prolapse; PS, pulmonary stenosis; TR, tricuspid regurgitation; VSD, ventricular septal defect

Adapted from: Filate W, et al. *The Medical Society, Faculty of Medicine, University of Toronto* 2005, page 63.

Non-pathological Murmurs

➢ Pathophysiology
  o Due to rapid flow across the mitral or tricuspid valve or to distension of the left ventricular wall

➢ Clinical

- Take a direct history and perform a focused physical examination to determine if a systolic murmur is benign (i.e. non-pathological).

  o History
    - Family history
      ▪ Family members with heart disease

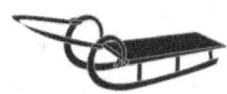

- Past medical history
  - Ante-and perinatal history
  - Infancy and childhood
- Personal history of
  - Central cyanosis
  - Feeding difficulties
  - Poor weight gain

○ Cardiovascular exam (characteristics of murmur)
- No other abnormality detected
- No thrill
- Usually short, of low frequency and early in systole
- Localised to apex or pulmonary area
- Intensity varies with change in posture
- Short, soft (grade III/ IV, or less) diastolic murmur
- Loudest at the apex or left sternal border
- No fixed splitting of S2
- Follows immediately after a physiologic S3
- No S4
- Heard in normal young people
- No supportive evidence of organic heart disease
- Soft mid-diastolic murmur
- Located at base of heart
- No radiation of murmur
- 1 or 2/6 (no louder)
- No associated diastolic murmur
- Associated with Still's murmur (precordial vibratory murmur)
- Valsalva maneuver - both pulmonary ejection and Still's murmur disappear

Source: Burton JL. *Churchill Livingstone* 1971, page 10.

- Give the performance characteristics for a Significant Systolic Murmur vs. Functional Systolic Murmur.

Clinical sign	PLR	NLR
○ Holosystolic murmur	8.7	0.19
○ Loud murmur	6.5	0.08
○ Plateau-shaped murmur	4.1	0.48
○ Loudest at the apex	2.5	0.84

Abbreviation: NLR, negative likelihood ratio; PLR, positive likelihood ratio

Source: Simel DL, et al. *JAMA* 2009, Table 33-10, page 444.

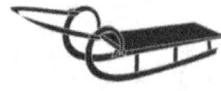

Functional Murmur
- o Absence of
  - \- On palpitation
    - ▪ Systolic thrill, over the suprasternal area
    - ▪ Abnormal apical impulse
  - \- On auscultation
    - ▪ Holosystolic or diastolic murmur (a purely diastolic murmur should be considered organic until proved otherwise)
    - ▪ Presence of ejection clicks/sounds
    - ▪ Fixed splitting of S_2

➢ **Precordial vibratory murmur** (Still murmur): Most commonly heard between the ages of 2 and 6 years

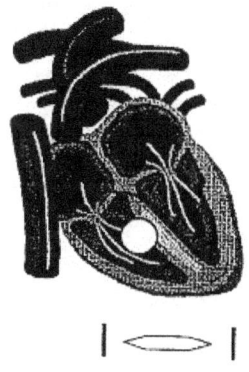

- o Short, soft (I-II/VI) mid systolic murmur
  - \- Low frequency, coarse, twangy
  - \- Starts after S_1, left lower sternal border
  - \- Changes with position
  - \- Rarely radiate to the neck (rarely)
- o Softens or disappears on standing, reappears on squatting
- o Differentiate from VSD

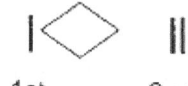

1st   2nd

➢ **Pulmonary ejection systolic murmur**

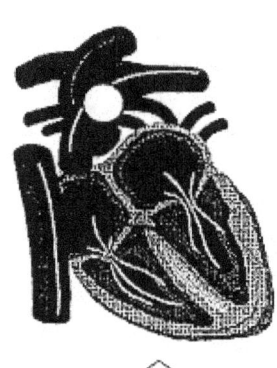

- o Location
  - \- Pulmonary area (2-3 L -ICS; also can be heard over the aortic area, [left sternal border], apex, or neck [left side])
  - \- Loudest at the second or third left interspace
- o Early systolic ejection murmur
  - \- Early to mid systolic
- o Short, soft, high frequency, blowing crescendo-decrescendo murmur
- o Increased in supine position
- o Normal P2, no diastolic murmur, no clicks, heaves or thrills
  - \- Most commonly heard in thin adolescents
- o Differentiate from ASD and PS
  - \- S2 normally split and of normal intensity

1st   2nd

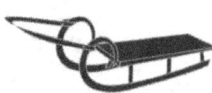

➢ Carotid arterial bruit

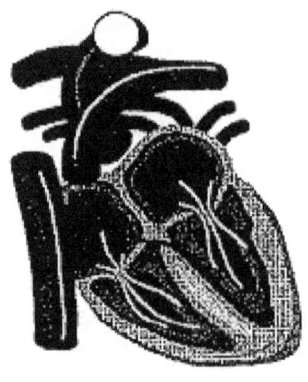

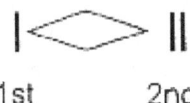

1st   2nd

- o Loudest over carotid artery, at base of the heart, or right supraclavicular area (opposite to aortic stenosis, which is loudest over the second right ICS)
- o Harsh, crescendo-decrescendo, ejection systolic murmur
- o No precordial or suprasternal notch thrill
- o ↓ with
  - Hyperextension of the shoulders toward the back
  - Compression of the subclavian artery
- o Unaffected by Valsalva manoeuvre

➢ Venous hum

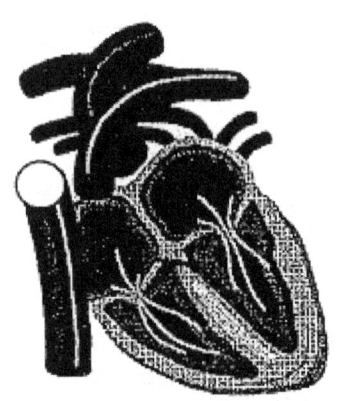

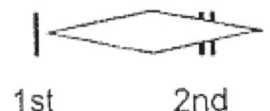

1st   2nd   1st

- o Maximal in early diastole
- o Continuous murmur
- o Location
  - Infraclavicular, loudest at the right supraclavicular area or upper right sternal border
- o Loudest in upright position
- o ↑ with Sudden release of the jugular veins
- o Disappears when lying down
  - ↓ in supine position
  - Compression of the jugular veins
- o Differentiate from PDA
  - Thrill palpable over the jugular veins

➢ **Mammary soufflé**
  o Usually present in late pregnancy or early lactation
    - Varies from day to day; disappears after lactation period
  o Continuous murmur related to the cardiac cycle
    - In some patients may be primarily systolic
  o Loudest at the third or fourth interspace (either side or bilateral)
  o Unaffected by Valsalva murmur

➢ **Straight back/pecutus excavatum** (due to close proximity of
      pulmonary artery)
  o Mid-systolic ejection murmur
  o Short, crescendo-decrescendo
    - Grade I-III/VI
  o Loudest at the left upper sternal border
  o Louder in held exhalation
  o S2 usually widely split
    - P2 (less commonly A2) can be loud
  o ASD or PS by diagnostic, but chest x-ray

Abbreviations: ASD, atrial septal defect; ICS, intercostal space; PDA, patent
ductus arteriosus; PS, pulmonary stenosis; VSD, ventricular septal defect

Adapted from: Mangione S. *Hanley & Belfus* 2000, pages 246 to 250;
Permission granted: McGee SR. *Saunders/Elsevier* 2007, Box 34.1, page 402.

- Give the mechanism for the development of functional tricuspid
  regurgitation with cardiomyopathy and with pulmonary hypertension.

Condition	Mechanism
o Cardiomyopathy	- RV dilation
o Pulmonary hypertension	- ↑ RV pressure

- Give the basis for the systolic and diastolic cardiac murmur associated
  with ASD (atrial septal defect).

  o Systolic   ↑ PA (pulmonary artery) flow

  o Diastolic   ↑ flow through tricuspid valve

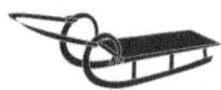

Mastering the Boards: Cardiology   A.B.R. Thomson

Maneuvers and Heart Murmurs

- Perform dynamic maneuvers which increase or decrease the intensity/ duration of three systolic cardiac murmurs.

Maneuvre	Lesion			
	Hypertrophic cardiomyopathy	Mitral valve prolapse	Aortic stenosis	Mitral regurgitation
o Valsalva strain phase (decreases preload)	↑	↑	↓	↓
o Squatting or leg raise (increases preload)	↓	↓	↑	↑
o Hand grip (increases afterload)	↓	↓	↓	↑

Adapted from: Talley NJ, et al. *Maclennan & Petty Pty Limited* 2003, Table 3.10, page 61, and Ghosh AK. *Mayo clinic Scientific Press* 2008, Table 3-1, page 42.

Maneuver	Technique	When to note change in murmur
• Normal respiration	- The patient breathes normally in & out	▪ During inspiration & expiration
• Maneuvers affecting venous return		
o Valsalva maneuver (↓ venous return)	- The patient exhales against closed glottis for 20 seconds	▪ At end of the strain phase (i.e., at 20 seconds)
o Squatting-to-standing (↓ venous return)	- The patient squats for at least 30 seconds & then rapidly stands up	▪ Immediately after standing

Maneuver	Technique	When to note change in murmur
o Standing-to-squatting (↑ venous return)	- The patient squats rapidly from the standing position, while breathing normally to avoid a Valsalva maneuver	▪ Immediately after squatting
o Passive leg elevation (↑ venous return)	- The patient's legs are passively elevated to 45 degrees while the patient is supine	▪ 15-20 seconds after leg elevation

- Maneuvers affecting systemtic vascular resistance

o Isometric handgrip exercise (↑ afterload)	- The patient uses one hand to squeeze the examiner's index and middle fingers together tightly	▪ After 1 minute of maximal contraction
o Transient arterial occlusion (↑ afterload)	- The examiner places blood pressure cuffs around both upper arms of patient and inflates them to pressures above the patient's systolic blood pressure	▪ 20 seconds after cuff inflation

Permission granted: McGee SR. *Saunders/Elsevier* 2007, Table 39-2 page 467.

- Give the likelihood ratios for the overall examination for detecting valvular disease.

	LR for Valvular Disease	
	PLR	NLR
o Cardiologists	38	0.31
o Emergency department physicians	14	0.21
o Overall	15	0.25

Abbreviations: CI, confidence interval; PLR, positive likelihood ratio; NLR, negative likelihood ratio.

Adapted from: Simel DL, et al. *JAMA* 2009, Table 33-13, page 446.

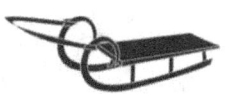

- Give the performance characteristics for Systolic Murmurs and Maneuvers.

Finding	PLR

o Louder with transient arterial occlusion
  - Detecting mitral regurgitation or
  ventricular septal defect
	48.7

o Softer with amyl nitrite inhalation
  - Detecting mitral regurgitation or
  ventricular septal defect
	10.5

Source: McGee SR. *Saunders/Elsevier*, 2007, Box 39-2, page 467.

- Give the likelihood ratios of individual findings for identifying systolic murmurs that are clinically significant*.

Clinical Sign	PLR	NLR
o Systolic thrill	12	0.73
o Holosystolic murmur	8.7	0.19
o Loud murmur	6.5	0.08
o Plateau-shaped murmur	4.1	0.48
o Loudest at the apex	2.5	0.84

Abbreviations: CI, confidence interval; LR, likelihood ratio; PLR, positive likelihood ratio, NLR, negative likelihood ratio.

*Moderate to severe aortic stenosis or mitral regurgitation, congenital shunt, or intraventricular pressure gradient.

Note that radiation of the murmur to carotids has a PLR < 2, and is not included here.

Adapted from: Simel DL, et al. *JAMA* 2009, Table 33-14, page 96.

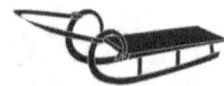

- Perform a focused physical examination of the precordium, and from the timing of the murmur, give the differential of the lesion.

Timing of murmur	Differential of the lesion

- Systolic
  - Pansystolic
    - MR
    - TR
    - VSD
    - Aortopulmonary shunts

  - Mid
    - AS
    - Pulmonary stenosis (PS)
    - Hypertrophic cardiomyopathy
    - ASD

  - Late
    - Mitral valve prolapse
    - Papillary muscle dysfunction (due usually to ischemia or hypertrophic cardiomyopathy)

- Diastolic
  - Early
    - AR
    - Pulmonary regurgitation (PR)

  - Mid
    - MS
    - TS
    - Atrial myxoma
    - Austin Flint murmur of AR
    - Carey Coombs† murmur of acute rheumatic fever

  - Late (Presystolic)
    - MS
    - TS
    - Atrial myxoma

- Continuous
  - PDA
  - AS+AR
  - MS+AR
  - MS+PR
  - Venous hum
  - Aortopulmonary septal defect
  - Rupture of sinus of Valsalva into RV or RA
  - 'Mammary soufle' (in late pregnancy or early postpartum period)
  - Bronchial artery anastamosis in pulmonary atresia
  - Pericardial friction rub

Venous hum: above clavicle and down over upper sternum: ↑ by turning head, ↓ by jugular compression; distinguish from PDA (patient ductus arterious)

Abbreviations: AR, aortic regurgitation; AS, aortic stenosis; ASD, atrial septal defect; MR, mitral regurgitation; MS, mitral stenosis; PDA, patent ductus arteriosus; PR, pulmonary regurgitation; RA, right atrium; RV, right ventricle; TR, tricuspid regurgitation; TS, tricuspid stenosis; VSD, ventricular septal defect

Adapted from: Talley NJ, et al. *Maclennan & Petty Pty Limited* 2003, page 58. The combined murmurs of aortic stenosis and aortic regurgitation, or mitral stenosis and mitral regurgitation, may sound as if they fill the entire cardiac cycle, but are not continuous murmurs by definition.

- ➤ Causes of Continuous Murmurs
    - o Venous hum
    - o Mitral regurgitation murmur with aortic regurgitant murmur
    - o VSD with aortic regurgitation
    - o Pulmonary arteriovenous fistula
    - o Rupture of the sinus of Valsalva
    - o Coronary arteriovenous fistula
    - o Arteriovenous anastomosis of intercostal vessels following a reactured rib

Source: Baliga RR. *Saunders/Elsevier*, 2007, page 81.

- • Give the differences in the diastolic murmurs of Austin Flint, and Graham Steell.

    - o Austin Flint
        - - Mitral diastolic murmur (MS-like) occurring with severe aortic regurgitation
        - - The regurgitating blood from the AR Roughens the aortic cusp of the mitral valve, causing MS- like murmur
        - - Syphilis never affects the mitral valve, so an Austin Flint murmur can be diagnosised, whereas AR from other causes (atherosclerosis; SBE; aneurysm- dissecting, or Marfan's; Aortic valve – bicuspid, ruptured cusps, surgery) may be producing true MS.

    - o Graham Steell
        - - Severe pulmonary hypertension causes load muumur of pulmonary regurgitation

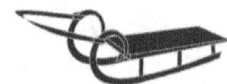

- Perform a focused physical examination of the precordium, which will help to distinguish between

    o Pleural rub (vs pulmonary rales)
    - ↑ by pressure to chest wall with stethoscope
    - Present in inspiration and expiration
    - Not cleared by coughing

    o Pericardial rub (vs cardiac murmur)
    - ↑ by pressure on chest wall
    - ↑ by expiration
    - ↑ by lying on L or R side
    - Sound changes from day –to- day

    o Pericardial effusion (vs cardiac tamponade [restricted diastolic filling])
    - ↑ dullness of precardium
    - ↓ apex impulse
    - ↓ heart sounds
    - Pressure on adjacent structures
    - Ewart's sign (compression of lung near left scapula results in dullness, bronchial breathing, increased tactile vocal fremitus)

    o Tamponade
    - ↑ JVP
    - ↓ SBP
    - Pulsus paradoxicus (shock, laboured breathing, ventiliation)
    - Absence of cardiomegaly

Abbreviations: JVP, jugular venous pressure; SBP, systolic blood pressure

Permission granted: McGee SR. *Saunders/Elsevier* 2007, Box 34-1, page 402.

- Give whether an early ejection click (EC) occur with muscular narrowing above or below the aortic or pulmonary valves.

    o No, only with stenosis at the valve
    o So, no EC with HOCM

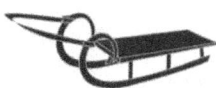

- Useful background: Select features of systolic murmurs

    o In the holosystolic murmur, the murmur begins just after the first heart sound (S_1) and continues throughout the systole.
    o In the late systolic murmur, the murmur begins at the middle of the systole or later and ends at the second heart sound (S_2).
    o In an early peaking murmur, peak intensity is before the middle of the systole. In a mid or late peaking murmur, peak intensity is at the middle of the systole or later.

Source: Simel DL, et al. *JAMA* 2009, Figure 33-1.

TRICKS TO HELP DIFFERENTIATE CARDIAC MURMURS

- Give what makes the murmur louder.

    o Inspiration
       - R. side murmur
    o Valsalva
       - HCM
       - MVP
       - Murmur becomes longer and moves closer to S1
    o Change position
       - Squat → stand – HCM
       - Stand → squat – AS
       - Turning on left side – MV murmurs
       - Leaning forward – AV, PV murmurs

- Give pregnancy-associated **changes in auscultation of the precordium**.

    o ↑ S1 from ↑ P2
    o Fixed splitting of S2
    o S3

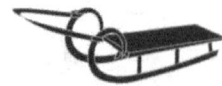

Valvular Heart Disease

➢ Pathophysiology

- o It is not the stenosis or regurgitation which is so important, as is the nature of the resulting remodeling and hypertrophy

- o Stenosis → ↑ afterload of ventricle → concentric hypertrophy (remodeling) of ventricle → diastolic dysfunction → only then does systolic dysfunction develop (↑ LV filing pressure)

- o Regurgitation → ↑ overload of ventricle → eccentric remodeling of ventricle → ↑ ventricular volume with NO ↑ filling pressure early, but later → ↓ systolic function

➢ Clinical

- o Associations
  - Aortic valve lesions
    - Angina ↓ flow in coronary artery
    - Hypertrophy → subendocardial ischemia
    - Syncope (↓ CO reserve)
  - Mitral valve lesions
    - Atrial fibrillation

- o Assessment of severity:
  - Stenosis (Doppler-derived velocities)
    - Pressure gradients
    - Area of valve
  - Regurgitation jet
    - ROA (regurgitation orifice area)
    - Vmax (maximum jet velocity)
    - VCW (width of the narrowest segment of the regurgitant jet)
    - Signal strength
    - Regurgitant
      - Area of orifice
      - Volume

- o Assessment tools
  - Vmax (maximum aortic jet velocity)
  - MVA (mitral valve area)
  - VCW (venacontracta width; width of the narrowest segment of the regurgitatnt jet)
  - EF (ejection fraction)

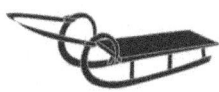

For reference purpose only

• Give the assessment of the severity of the following valvular heart disorders.

	Vmax (m/s)	MVA (cm²)	MPG (mm Hg)	PASP (mm Hg)	ROA (cm²)	RV (mL/beat)	MG (mm Hg)	AVA (cm²)
Aortic stenosis (Vmax, MG, AVA)								
Mild	< 3						< 2.5	> 1.5
Moderate	3-4						25-30	1.0-1.5
Severe	> 4						>40	<1
Mitral stenosis (MVA, MPG, PASP)								
Mild		>1.5	<5	<30				
Moderate		1.0-1.5	5-10	30-50				
Severe		<1.0	>10	>50				
Aortic regurgitation (VC, ROP, RV)								
Mild				<0.3	<0.10	≤ 30		
Moderate				0.3-0.6	0.10-0.29	30-59		
Severe				>0.6	≥ 0.30	≥ 60		
Mitral regurgitation (VC, ROA, RJ, RF)								
Mild				< 0.3	<0.20	<30	<30	
Moderate				0.3-0.69	0.20-0.39	30-59	30-49	
Severe				> 0.70	≥ 0.40	≥ 60	>50	

Abbreviation: AVA, aortic contracta area; MG, mean gradient; MVA, mitral valve area; MPG, mean pressure gradient; PASP, pulmonary artery systolic pressure; RF, regurgitant fraction; ROA, regurgitant orifice area; RV, regurgitation volume; VC, vena contracta width; Vmax, maximum aortic jet velocity

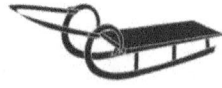

Mastering the Boards: Cardiology   A.B.R. Thomson

> Classification
- Early
    - Begins with the second heart sound (S_2).
    - Decrease in intensity (decrescendo) and disappear before the first heart sound (S1)
    - Can continue through diastole.
- Mid diastole
    - Begins clearly after S_2 (in mitral stenosis, classically after an opening snap [OS]).
- Late
    - Begins in the interval immediately before S_1.
    - In mitral stenosis, the mid diastolic murmur may merge with the late diastolic (presystolic) murmur.

Abbreviations: OS, opening snap

Source: Simel DL, et al. *JAMA* 2009, Figure 32-2, page 421.

> Causes
- Mitral or tricuspid stenosis
    - The degree of stenosis indicated by duration of murmur, not intensity
    - Mitral stenosis- use bell, lightly applied at apex with patient on L side after exercise. Presystolic accentuation is often a sign of pure stenosis, but is absent in atrial fibrillation
    - Tricuspid stenosis- murmur louder on inspiration
    - Mitral or tricuspid distortion eg Carey-Coombs murmur of active rheumatic carditis

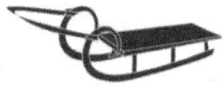

- o Mitral Stenosis
    - Calcification of mitral annulus and leaflets
    - Rheumatic heart disease
    - Rheumatoid arthritis
    - Systemic lupus erythematosus
    - Malignant carcinoid
    - Congenital stenosis

- o Conditions that Simulate Mitral Stenosis
    - Left atrial myxoma
    - Ball valve thrombus in the left atrium
    - Cor triathriatum (a rare congenital heart condition where a thin membrane across the left atrium obstructs pulmonary venous flow).

Adapted from: Mangione S. *Hanley & Belfus* 2000, pages 266 to 269.

- Give the typical location of maximal intensity and radiation for various types of abnormal systolic murmurs.

Location of maximal intensity	Radiation	Typical for
o Second R.ICS	- Right carotid artery - Right clavicle	AS
o Fifth or sixth L.ICS	- Left anterior axillary line - Left axilla	MV-P
o Mid left thorax		
o Lower L.SB	- Lower R.SB - Epigastrium - Fifth ICS, mid left thorax	TR
o Fifth L.ICS	- Lower L.SB	HCM

Abbreviations: HCM, hypertrophic cardiomyopathy; ICS, intercostal space; MV-P, mitral valve prolapse; SB, sternal border; TR, tricuspid regurgitation

Source: Simel DL, et al. *JAMA* 2009, Table 33-2, page 435.

- Give the causes of systolic ejection murmur at the base of the heart.

- o Aortic stenosis (AS)
    - Valvular
    - Supravalvular
- o Aortic sclerosis
- o Pulmonary stenosis
- o HOCM

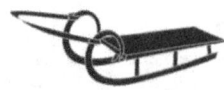

Aortic Stenosis (AS)

➢ Types
   o There are several causes of obstruction of the outflow from the left ventricle (LVOT, left ventricular outflow tract obstruction). While sclerosis of the aortic valve will cause turbulent flow and a systolic murmur like aortic stenosis (AS), there is no pressure gradient.
   o Outflow obstruction may be just above or just below the AV, and may be fixed or dynamic such as HCM (hypertrophic cardiomyopathy) with obstruction
   o There are 3 major types of aortic stenosis

Characteristics	Calcification/ degeneration	Congenital aortic valve	Rheumatic aortic stenosis
o Demography			
- Prevalence	USA 2% of persons > 65 4% of those > 85	1% to 2% of the population	Commonest cause world wide
- Mean age of presentation	Mid-70's	Mid 60's	30's to 50's
o Calcification and bone formation of valve	Yes	Yes	-
o High rate of aortic valve replacement (AVR)	-	Yes	-
o High rate of endocarditis	-	Yes	-

➢ Useful bacground
   o Confirmed by narrow pulse pressure and thrill (patient leaning forward in expiration)
   o Increased flow rate
   o Valve distortion without stenosis
   o Post valvar dilatation eg hypertension
   o Coarctation murmur is later in systole and may extend to 2nd sound
   o Calcific degeneration of a tri-leaflet aortic valve is a degenerative process of atherosclerotic-like changes, which begins as aortic sclerosis.

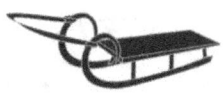

- Give types of defects of the aortic valve which result in the murmur of AS.

  o Congenital bicuspid AV
    - May be associated with dilation o the arch of the aorta*

  o AV sclerosis (thickening of tricuspid valve, but with no obstruction of the outflow)

  o AV calcification of tricuspid valve

  o Pseudostenosis

Note*

  - Post-stenotic dilation of aortic arch may give a boot-shaped appearance of the heart

  - AS must be distinguished from HOCM (please see earlier)

  - Dobutamine increases cardiac output

  - If the calculated area of the AV increases with dobutamine, diagnose pseudostenosis

---

SO YOU WANT TO BE A CARDIOLOGIST!

- In the context of a murmur suggesting AS (aortic stenosis), give the components of the Heyde syndrome.

  o Turbulent blood flow across stenosic AV which disrupts von Willebrand proteins, leading to acquired von Willebrand disease and GI bleeding.

➢ Causes
  o Congenital, degenerative, rheumatic (bicuspid semiluminar valve)
  o Valvular, supravalvular, subvalvular
  o Arterial pulse
    - Valvular: small amplitude (parsus) with slow upstroke (tardus) may be associated thrill best heard over carotid artery
    - Supravalvular: amplitude of pulse higher R>L –sided vessels
    - Subvalvualr: brick pulse, with palpable double systolic impulse (pulsus bisferiens)

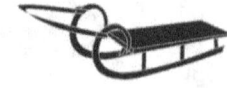

- ➤ Valvular Aortic Stenosis Impulse (Pulsus Bisferiens)
  - o PMI – normal in AS, unless LV hypertrophy and L-CHF or AS plus aortic regurgitation
  - o Precardial thrill – palpable, does not reflect severity of AS
  - o Murmur budest in "sach area" 2nd right intercoatal space (aortic area) down to 5/6th intercoatal space at the left mid clavicular line
  - o Crescendo – decrescendo murmur; louder and longer murmur with later peak is more severe soft or absent A2 and audible or palpable S4, suggests more. If murmur becomes softer, suspect obesity or COPD, or CHF.

- ➤ Subvalvular Aortic Stenosis (HOCM)

- ➤ Supravalvular Aortic Stenosis
  - o Males, with associated congenital abnormalties
    - Typical Facies
    - Patulus lip
    - Deep, husky voice
    - Hypercalcemia
  - o Pulse and BP stronger on right than left side (R > L)
  - o No aortic ejection click
  - o May be an associated murmur of aortic regurgitation

Adapted from: Mangione S. *Hanley & Belfus* 2000, pages 254 to 259.

- ➤ Complications of aortic stenosis
  - o Sudden death occurs in 10-20% of adults and 1% of children. It has been rarely documented to occur without prior symptoms.
  - o Ventricular arrhythmias (more common than supraventricular arrhythmias)
  - o Heart block (may occur because of calcification of conducting tissues).
  - o Systemic embolization (disintegration of the aortic valve or concomitant aortic atheroma).
  - o Infective endocarditis
  - o Hemolytic anemia

Adapted from: Baliga RR. *Saunders/Elsevier* 2007, page 21.

  - o The initial sclerosis progresses over time

	Annual change
- Mean aortic transvalvular gradient	↑ 7 mm Hg
- Effective enface area	↓ 0.1 cm^2

  - o Associated mitral annular calcification → MR (mitral regurgitation)

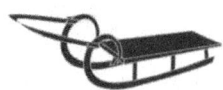

- Perform a focused physical examination for AS.

  - Pulse
    - Normal, when gradient across the aortic valve is < 50 mm Hg
    - ↓ pulse pressure (in severe AS)
    - ↓ pulse volume (pulsus parvus)

      - Slow upstroke (pulsus tardis)
      - Anacrotic notch during upstroke
      - Bisferious pulse (AS plus AR)

  - Heart sounds
    - Normal S_2 – mild AS
    - ↓ S_2
      - Valvular stenosis
      - More severe AS
      - Reversed splitting of S_2 (longer LV systole)
    - S_3
      - LV systolic dysfunction
      - ↑ LV filling pressure

  - Apex
    - Displaced with LVD

  - Aortic area
    - Thrill (may also be palpated over carotids)
    - More prominent when sitting and in expiration

  - Murmur
    - Systolic
      - Crescendo – decrescendo (ejection)
      - Base of heart
      - Murmur over right clavicle
      - Radiation to carotids and to right clavicle
      - Loudness does not reflect severity o AS (ie magnitude of gradient, or cross-sectional area)
    - Diastolic
      - Often associated with aortic regurgitation(AR)

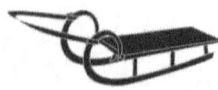

Precordium- Basal systolic thrill; apex displaced anteriorly and laterally.

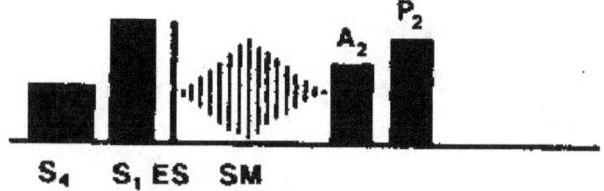

S_4 S_1 ES   SM

Carotids- slow upstroke to a delayed peak. Auscultation- A2 diminished or paradoxically ejection systolic murmur radiating to carotids. Cold extremities. Reversed S2-P2-A2 in severe AS (paradoxican splitting)

- Give the performance characteristics of the physical examination for detecting aortic stenosis.

Finding	PLR	NLR
o Slow carotid upstroke	9.2	0.56
o Murmur radiating to right carotid	8.1	0.29
o Reduced or absent S_2	7.5	0.50
o Murmur over right clavicle	3.0	0.10
o Any systolic murmur	2.6	0
o Reduced carotid volume	2.0	0.64

Abbreviation: NLR, negative likelihood ratio; PLR, positive likelihood ratio.

Source: Simel DL, et al. *JAMA* 2009, Table 33-11, page 445.

- Perform a directed physical examination to distinguish between the systolic murmur of aortic sclerosis (no pressure gradient; due to stiff or dilated aortic root) and aortic stenosis (AS).

		Aortic Stenosis	Aortic Sclerosis
o	Symptoms		
	- Dizzy, syncopy, chest pain, dyspnea	+	-
o	Pulse		
	- Slow, small volume	+	-
o	Apex beat PMI	+	-
o	Precordial thrill	+	-
o	Heart sounds (S_2, A_2)	↓	↑
o	Murmur		
	- Short peaks in first half of systole		+

Adapted from: Mangione S. *Hanley & Belfus* 2000, page 252,254; Baliga RR. *Saunders/Elsevier* 2007, page 19.

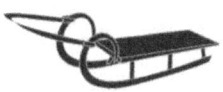

Aortic stenosis (AS) (at the aortic area)

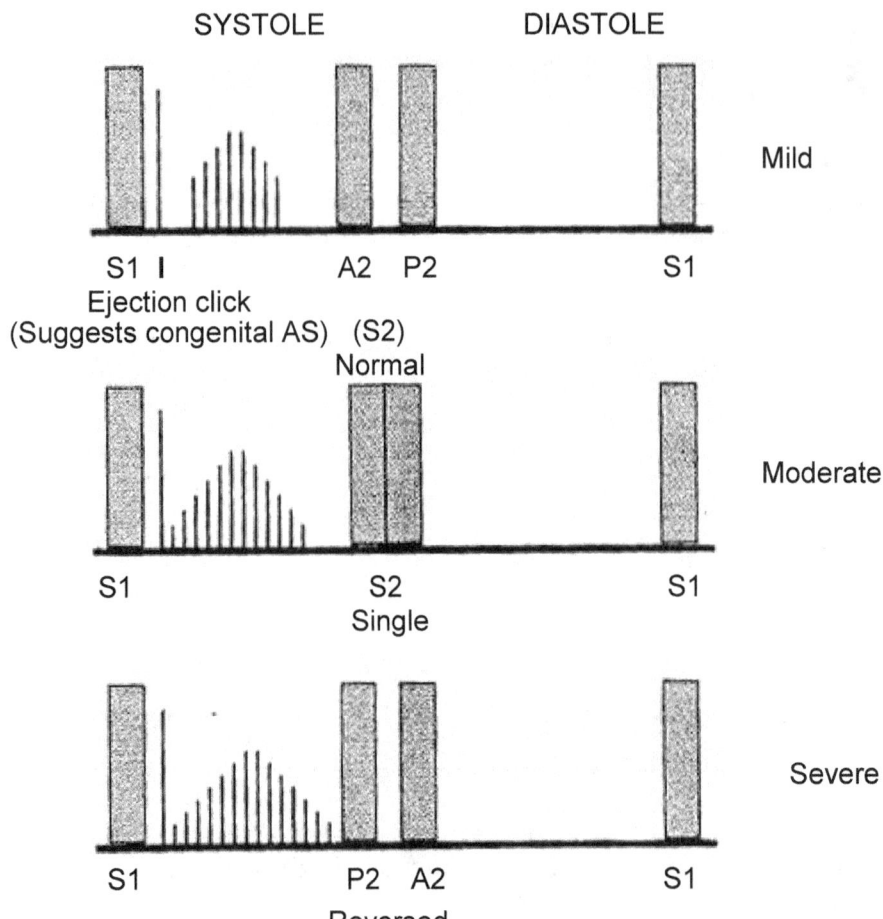

- o Soft S_2
- o Reversed A_2 / P_2
  (narrow or reverse split S_2)
- o S_4

- o Narrow pulse pressure
- o Systolic thrill
- o Heaving apex beat
- o L- CHF

Adapted from: Talley NJ, et al. *Maclennan & Petty Pty Limited* 2003, Figure 3.31, page 77.

- Perform a focused physical examination to distinguish hypertrophic obstructive cardiomyopathy (HOCM) from aortic stenosis (AS).

	HOCM	AS
o Pulse	- Jerky - Rapid upstroke - Double impulse in systole	▪ Anacrotic (plateau) ▪ Single impulse
o Heart sounds		▪ ↓ A_2 ▪ Ejection click
o Thrill	- No	▪ Yes

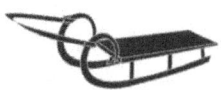

	HOCM	AS
○ Murmur		
- Timing of onset systolic murmur	Begins in mid-systole	Immediately after S1
- Midsystole	+	-
- Intensity of murmur:		
– Valsalva maneuver	↑	↓
– Squatting	↓	↑
○ Associated MR*	75%	Rare

*MR murmur HOCM ends before A2, and may be from MVP (mitral valve prolapsed)

MR, initiated regurgitation; S1, first heart sound; A2 the A2 components of S2, the second sound

Abbreviations: AS, aortic stenosis; HOCM, hypertrophic cardiomyopathy; L-SE, left sterna edge; MR, mitral regurgitation; PMI, point of maximum impulse

Adapted from Mangione S. *Hanley & Belfus* 2000, pages 256 to 258.

- Perform a focused physical examination to access the severity of AS.

  - ○ Heart sounds
    - ↓ S_2
    - S_2 narrow/ split
    - S_4
  - ○ Apex
    - Thrill during LV systole
    - Heave
  - ○ Pulse
    - ↓ pulse pressure
  - ○ Signs of HF

Source: Baliga RR. *Saunders/Elsevier* 2007, page 18.

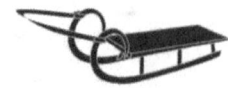

- Give the performance characteristics of physical examination of severe aortic stenosis (AS).

  - The finding of S_4 gallop, a murmur best heard over the 2nd intercostal space, or a murmur radiating into the neck have no value to predict the presence of severe AS.

Finding	PLR
o Arterial pulse	
- Delayed carotid artery upstroke	3.7
- Reduced carotid artery volume	2.3
- Brachioradial delay	2.5
o Apical impulse	
- Sustained apical impulse	4.1
- Apical carotid delay	2.6
o Heart sounds	
- Absent A2	4.5
- Absent or diminished A2	3.6
o Murmur	
- Late peaking (midsystole or beyond)	4.4
- Prolonged duration	3.9

Abbreviation: ICS, intercostal space; PLR, positive likelihood ratio

Note: The finding of S4, murmur loudest over aortic area (2nd ICS), and transmission of the murmur to the neck are not mentioned here because their PLR are < 2.

Adapted from: McGee SR. *Saunders/Elsevier* 2007, Box 40-1, pages 477 and 478.

Trick Question

- Give what S_2 indicates about the cause and severity of AS.

  - S_2 normal – mild AS
  - S_2 splitting reversed – prolonged LV systole (electrical or mechanical prolongation)
  - ↓ S_2 – valvular stenosis*
  - Single S_2 (no A_2, only P_2) – valve leaflets – fused, fibrosed

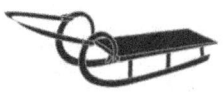

SO YOU WANT TO BE A CARDIOLOGIST!

The presence of aortic stenosis (AS) is decreased with any murmur radiating to the right carotid artery.
- Give 4 symptoms or signs which increase the likelihood that a systolic murmur is AS.

    o History   - Effort syncope
                      - Slow rate of increase of carotid pulse

    o Physical   - Reduced carotid volume
                      - Slow rate of increase of carotid pulse
                      - Murmur loudest at second right intercostals space
                      - Apical-carotid delay, or brachioradial delay
                      - Decreased or absent S_2
                      - Peak murmur intensity late or mid systolic
                      - Valve calcification on chest radiograph

Adapted from: Simel DL, et al. *JAMA* 2009, pages 437 and 438.

➢ Pathophysiology
    o AV obstruction
    o LVH

Abbreviations: IVP, intraventricular pressure; LV-EF, left ventricular ejection fraction; LV, left ventricular; LVEDP, left ventricular end diastolic pressure; LVH, left ventricular hypertrophy

- Give an explanation to the way in which LaPlace's law helps to understand why LVH (left ventricular, ↑thickness of wall of LV) occurs in aortic stenosis (AS).

    o LaPlace Law
    o Obstruction to outflow from LV caused by AS → ↑ IVP → ↑ LV wall stress
    o To attempt to normalize the tendency to ↑ LV wall stress, the ↑ wall thickness rises, and lowers the LV wall stress, as per LaPlace's Law.

➢ Clinical
    o Classic as triad of symptoms
        – Syncope
        – Angina
        – HF (heart failure)

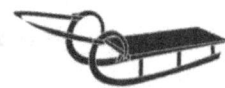

- Perform a focused physical examination for aortic stenosis (AS).

    o Pulse
        - Weak upstroke and late peak (aka pulsus parvus tardus), best palpated in carotid artery

    o Auscultation
        - Heart sounds
            ▪ ↓↓ S2 (↓↓ or absent A2)
            ▪ Ejection click
            ▪ S4
        - Precordium
            ▪ Systolic murmur
                - Harsh
                - Crescendo – decrescendo
            ▪ Right upper sternal border
            ▪ Radiates into neck (carotids) and into left axilla

- Give characteristic found on physical examination which suggest that the degree of LV outflow obstruction from the aortic stenosis is severe.

    o Pulsus parvus et tardus
    o A2 ↓↓ / absent
    o Late time to peak of harsh
    o Crescendo – decrescendo murmur

SO YOU WANT TO BE A CARDIOLOGIST!

- Give characteristics which distinguish the Gallavardin ↓ murmur of mitral regurgitation (MR), which mimics the murmur of aortic stenosis (AS), from the classical murmur of AS.

Characteristics	Gallavardin murmur of MR	Classical AR
o Site where best heard	Heard	Right upper sternal border
o Radiation into left axilla	No	Yes
o ↑ intensity with slowing HR	No	Yes

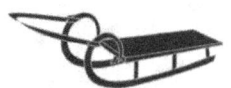

Mastering the Boards: Cardiology   A.B.R. Thomson

➢ Diagnostic testing

- o ECG
  - – LAE (left arterial enlargement)
  - – LVH (left ventricular hypertrophy)

- o Chest x-ray
  - – LVH
  - – Cardiomegaly
  - – Calcification
    - ▪ Aortic valve
    - ▪ Aorta
    - ▪ Coronary arteries

- o Transthoracic echocardiography (TTE)
  - – Morphology of AV 2 or 3 leaflets (bicuspid vs. trileaflet)
  - – Function / hemodynamics
    - ▪ AV area
    - ▪ Mean transvalvular gradient
    - ▪ Mean peak jet velocity

- o ECG exercise testing
  - – Exercise symptoms, capacity, blood pressure increase (normally > 20 mmHg)

SO YOU WANT TO BE A CARDIOLOGIST!

In the context of the patient with aortic stenosis (AS) an area of the aortic valve (AV) < 1.0 cm^2 suggest severe AS.

- Give ways to distinguish true severe AS from pseudo-severe AS.

Parameter	Truly severe	Pseudo-severe AS
o Area of V, cm^2	< 10	< 10
o Mean transvalvular gradient, mmHg	> 40	< 30 to 40
o Ejection fractions (EF)	↓	Normal
o BNP	↑↑	↑

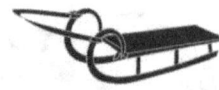

CLINICAL CHALLENGE

- For each of the function / hemodynamic measures obtained from TTE, give the values WAICH suggest that the aortic stenosis (AS) is severe.

  o AV area < 1.0 cm^2
  o Mean transvalvular gradient > 40 mmHg
  o Mean jet velocity > 4.0 m/sec

---

  o Transesophageal echocardiography (TEE)
    – Used if necessary to clarify findings of TTE

  o Dobutamine stress echo
    – Distinguish true from pseudo- severe AS
    – Determination presence of "contractile reserve"

  o Cathetherization
    – Exclude CAD (coronary artery disease) in high-risk patient with AS scheduled to have aortic valve replacement (AVR)
    – Access severity of AS (when non-invasive tests are unclear)

  o CT angiography
    – Exclude CAD low-risk patient (in place of cardiac catherization) in AS patient scheduled to have AVR surgery

  o BNP (brain naturetic peptide)
    – Predictive use

Patient	Prediction
▪ Asymptomatic	- Symptom-free survival
▪ Pre-operative	- Post-operative survival - Functional class - LV function
▪ Low-flow, low-gradient AS	- Survival

➢ Treatment
  o Treat associated conditions e.g. IABP (intra-aortic balloon pump) in severe AS awaiting surgery
  o Bridge to AVR
    – IABP (intra-aortic balloon pump) in severe AS awaiting surgery
    – Balloon aortic valvular valvuloplasty (BAV)
    – Nitroprusside
  o Transcatheter (transfemoral ortransapical, through left thoracotomy) aortic valve replacement (AVR)

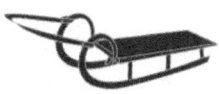

The timing for valve replacement, or other invasive procedures for valve repair (such as percutaneous balloon valvotomy for mitral stenosis or valve repair for mitral or tricuspid regurgitation) depends upon symptoms, LVEF (left ventricular ejection fraction), LV dilation, and PASP (pulmonary artery systolic pressure).

- Give the **indications for valve intervention** in the following valvular disorders.

Valve disorder	Symptoms	LVEF (%)	LV dilation (mm)	PASP (mm Hg)	Additional considerations
o Aortic stenosis	+	<50			↓ BP with exercise
o Aortic regurgitation	+	<50	End-systolic, >55 End diastolic, >75		
o Mitral stenosis	+			At rest, ≥50 With exercise, ≥60	
o Mitral regurgitation	+	<60	End-systemic > 40	At rest, ≥50 With exercise, ≥60	New onset atrial fibrillation

- Give the negative prognostic factors for prosthetic heart valves.

  - o Heart failure
  - o Non-streptococcal endocarditis, especially *Staph. aureas*, fungal endocarditis
  - o Infection of a prosthetic valve
  - o Elderly patients
  - o Valve ring or myocardial abscess

Note: "AS is a surgical disease; currently there are no medical treatments proven to decrease mortality or to delay surgery" (The Washington Manual of Therapeutic 34th Edition, 2014. Edited by Godara H, et al. Chapter 6, Shah J and Lindman BR, page 194-219)

Clinical Caution: Medical Care of AS prior to AVR requires correct and careful treatment

  - o Hypertension
    - Undertreatment → ↑ load on LV
  - o Diuretics
    - Overtreatment → ↓ preload → hypotension
  - o IABP
    - Only for severe AS

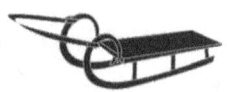

> SO YOU WANT TO BE A CARDIOLOGIST!
>
> - Give the ACC / AHA guidelines – class I indications for AVR in severe AS.
>
>   - Symptoms
>   - CABG 9coronary artery bypass graft)
>   - Surgery on
>   Other heart valves
>   - EF < 50% (systolic dysfunction)
>
> Abbreviation: EF, ejection fraction

➢ Prognosis
  - Progressive ↓ area of aortic valve

  - Asymptomatic
    - SCD < 1% per year

  - Symptoms when AV < 1 cm^2

  - Factors predicting SCD / death
    - ↑ peak aortic jet velocity
    - Calcification of AV
    - Associated coronary artery disease

Abbreviations: SCD, sudden cardiac death

Syncope in AS

➢ Mechanism
  - The left ventricle is suddenly unable to contract (transient electro-mechanical dissociation) against the stenosed valve.
  - Cardiac arrhythmias (bradycardia, ventricular tachycardia or fibrilation)
  - Marked peripheral vasodilatation without a concomitant increase in cardiac output, particularly after exercise.
  - Transient electro-mechanical dissociation
  - Peripheral vasodilation

  - Arrhythmia
    - Bradycardia
    - Tachycardia
    - Ventricular fibrillation

Source: Baliga RR. *Saunders/Elsevier* 2007, page 20.

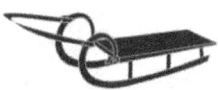

Mixed Aortic Lesions (AS plus AR)

➢ Causes
  o < 60 years
    - Rheumatic
    - Congenital

  o 60 to 75 years
    - Calcified bicuspid aortic valve, especially in men

  o > 75 years
    - Degenerative calcification
    - In the aortic and mitral valve apparatus

  o Others
    - Infective endocarditis
    - Collagen degenerative disorder (e.g. Marfan syndrome)

➢ Importance of S_2
  o Normal S_2
    - Strong evidence against the presence of critical aortic stenosis

  o Soft S_2
    - Valvular stenosis (except in calcific stenosis of the elderly, where the margins of the leaflets usually maintain their mobility)
    - Single second heart sound
    - When there is fibrosis and fusion of the valve leaflets

  o Reversed splitting of the S_2
    - Mechanical or electrical prolongation of ventricular systole

  o Indication of more severe AS
    - Loud S_2
    - Delay of peak of crescendo-decrescendo ejection systolic murmur with increasing severity of aortic stenosis.
    - Crescendo-decrescendo murmur begins after the first heart sound (or after the ejection click when present)
    - Peaks in mid or late systole
    - Ends before the second heart sound; this peak is delayed

Adapted from: Baliga RR. *Saunders/Elsevier* 2007, page 19 and 22.

➢ Investigation of suspected AS
  o Exercise test   - When there are no symptoms
                          - If hypotensive response (indicating LV dysfunction) → urgent AV replacement
                          - If symptoms, do **not** do exercise testing

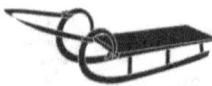

- Echocardiography
  - Valve are
  - Transvalvular gradient
  - This test may underestimate transvalvular gradient, especially with ↑ LV dysfunction

- Coronary angiography
  - All suspected AS patients > 35 year who are being considered for valve replacement

➤ Treatment
  - Valve replacement
    - Symptoms
    - LVEF < 50%
    - ↓ systolic BP with exercise
  - For ↑ operative risk
    - Repeated balloon valvulopasty
  - Replace ascending aorta if > 5 cm
    - Transcatheter aorta valve implantation

- Give the unique circumstances when **percutaneous balloon valvuloplasty** is indicated for AS.

  - Young patient
  - Congenital bicuspid valves
  - No calcification of bicuspid valve
  - Survival without aortic valve replacement is 2-3 yr once development of
    - Angina
    - Syncope
    - Heart
    - Failure

- Give the criteria for selection of AS patients for AV replacement.

  - Symptoms
  - Exercise stress testing showing hypotension / LV dysfunction
  - Patients requiring CABG surgery

I THINK I BETTA BE A GENERALIST!

- In the presence of aortic stenosis (AS) or hypertrophic cardiomyopathy, what is the Brockenbrough- Braunwald- Morrow (B-B-M) sign?
  - ↓ pulse pressure after an extrasystolic beat.

- Give the types of muscular dystrophy in which most frequently involve myocardial.
  - Pseudohypertrophic muscular dystrophy
  - Dystrophia myotonia

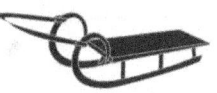

Pulmonary Stenosis (PS)

➢ Causes
  o Congenital (commonest cause)
  o Carcinoid tumour of the small bowel
  o Functional, especially in young people
  o

Source: Baliga RR. *Saunders/Elsevier*, 2007, page 81

➢ Types
  o Narrowing which may be
    - Valvular
    - Subvalvular
    - Supravalvular

➢ Clinical

• Perform a focused physical examination for pulmonary stenosis (PS).

  o May be very soft especially if associated with VSD

  o Increased flow rate ASD, VSD, TAPVD (total anomalous pulmonary venous drainage), hyperdynamic circulation

  o Post valvar dilatation, eg pulmonary hypertension
  o General inspection   -   Plump face

  o JVP   -   'a' wave

  o Peripheral pulse   -   Normal

  o Palpation   -   LSE heave

  o Heart sounds   -   ↓ S_2 (from ↓ A_2)
                           -    S_2 split
                           -    Ejection click

  o Murmur   -   Ejection systolic
                           -    Upper LSE, left lung posteriorly
                           -    For infundibular PS, murmur heard best at 3rd – 4th L-ICS (aka the Erb point)

  o Skin   -   Cyanosis, clubbing (Fallot tetralogy)

  o Signs of HF, SBE

  o Signs of eponymous syndromes

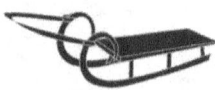

- ○ Ejection click (from post-stenotic dilation)

- ○ Loud splitting of P_2

- ○ Soft P_2

Abbreviation: ASD, atrial septal defect; HF, heart failure; L-ICS, left intercostals space; SBE, subacute bacterial endocarditis; TAPVD, total anomalous pulmonary venous drainage; VSD, ventricular septal defect

Adapted from: Davies IJT. *Lloyd-Luke LTD* 1972, pages 32 to 39.

- ○ Severity of PS

Pathophysiology	Mild	Moderate	Severe
- Pulmonary valve area, cm^2/m^2	>1.0	0.5 – 1.0	< 0.5
- Transvalvular gradient, mm Hg	< 50	50 – 80	>80
- Peak RV systolic pressure, mm Hg	< 75	75 - 100	>100

Adapted from: Baliga RR. *Saunders/Elsevier* 2007, page 81.

- • Perform a focused physical examination to determine the severity of pulmonary valve stenosis.

Clinical	Mild	Severe
○ ↑ JVP	N	A wave
○ RV impulse	-	+
○ Ejection click decreasing with inspiration	+	
○ Ejection click	+	Disappears
○ Systolic murmur	+	+++
○ P2	Delayed	Disappears
○ RV S4	-	+

- • Give the clinical findings which suggest subvalvular PS.

    - ○ No ejection click
    - ○ Often associated with a VSD

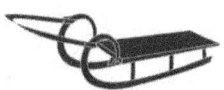

- Give how valvular pulmonary stenosis (PS) can be distinguished from on a chest X-ray.

  o Only valvular PS has post-stenotic dilation.

- Give why blood cultures usually negative for growth in the patient with PS.

  o Embolization is to the lungs, not to the peripherial blood

- Perform a directed physical examination to distinguish between the systolic murmur of pulmonary stenosis (PS) and aortic stenosis (AS).

	AS	PS
o Site of maximal intensity	Apex, or 2nd R-ICS	L. sternal border
o Intensity		
o Inspiration	—	↑
o Expiration		
- Effect on murmur	↑	—
- Effect on ejection click	—	↓
o Standing	↓	↑
	Late ↑	Early ↑
o After release of Valsalva maneuver		
o S2	Paradoxical splitting of S2	Widened physiologica S2
o S4 inspiration	Expiration	Inspiration

Systotic Regurgitation causes: mitral regurgitation (MR), tricuspid regurgitation (TR), ventricular septal defect (VSD), patent ductus arteriosus (PDA)

Abbreviations: AS, aortic stenosis; ICS, intercostal space; R, right; L, left; ICS intercostals space PS, pulmonary stenosis

Adapted from: Mangione S. *Hanley & Belfus* 2000, pages 258 and 259.

  o Pulmonary valve balloon valvuloplasty

	Mean gradient
– Asymptomatic	>40 mm Hg
– Symptomatic	>30 mm Hg

  o Pulmonary valve regurgitation may occur after valvuloplasty

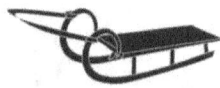

➢ Treatment

- Give causes of the combined aortic and mitral valve disease.

  o Rheumatic valvular disease

  o Infective endocarditis

  o Collagen degenerative disorder, e. g. Marfan syndrome

  o Calcific changes in the aortic and mitral valve apparatus

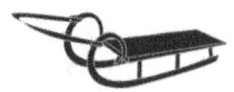

- Give the performance characteristics of the physical examination performed by experts for detecting Hypertrophic cardiomyopathy (HOCM also known as IHSS, idiopathic subaortic stenosis).

	PLR	NLR
o Decreased intensity with passive leg elevation	8.0	0.22
o Decreased or unchanged intensity with standing to squatting	4.5	0.13

Abbreviations: PLR, positive likelihood ratio; NLR, negative likelihood ratio

Source: Simel DL, et al. *JAMA* 2009, page 439.

SO YOU WANT TO BE A CARDIOLOGIST!

- Give the complications of HOCM.

  - o Sudden cardiac death
  - o Atrial fibrillation
  - o Infective endocarditis
  - o Systemic embolization

- Give the most pathophysiological abnormality in HOCM.

  - o Diastolic dysfunction

Prosthethic Heart Valves

Useful background

- o Mechanical valves last longer than biosynthetic valve, but require life-long anti-coagulation

- o Biosynthetic valves do not require long-term anti-coagulation

- o Prosthetic MV are less durable and are more likely to be associated with thromboembolic disease, as compared with AV

- o The bioprosthetic (pig, cow) tissue prosthetic valves do not require anti-coagulation as do the mechanical valves, which also has the disadvantage of sudden severe failure of the valve, and risk of endocarditis

- o Please refer to subspecialty sources (e.g. UpToDate) for relative advantages and disadvantages of the various types of prosthetic valves, and the required aspirin and warfarin therapy

Abbreviations: AV, aortic valve, MV, mitral valve

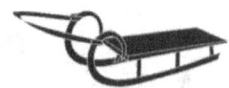

- o In patients with a prosthetic cardiac valve aspirin (ASA) is given, and the goal of anti-coagulation is to maintain the INR at 2.0 to 3.0.
- o However, in those at high risk of thromboembolism, the target INR is increased to 2.5 to 3.5.

- Give the characteristics of the patient with a prosthetic valve who is considered to be at high risk, and in whom the INR should be adjusted to between 2.5 and 3.5.
  - o The patient with a mechanical (not bioprosthetic) AV or MV, plus one additional factor is considered to be at a high risk of thromembolic disease. These additional factors include.
    - The patient
      - ▪ Previous-thromboembolism
      - ▪ A hypercoagulable disorder
    - The heart
      - ▪ AF
      - ▪ LV dysfunction
      - ▪ Multiple prosthetic valves

Abbreviations: AF, atrial fibrillation; LV, left ventricle

After valve replace, a thrombus with thromboembolism may develop, bleeding may occur as a result of the anticoagulation required for a mechanical valve, the valve may become infected (endocarditis), or deteriorate.

- ➢ Clinical
  - o Prosthetic valve heart sounds

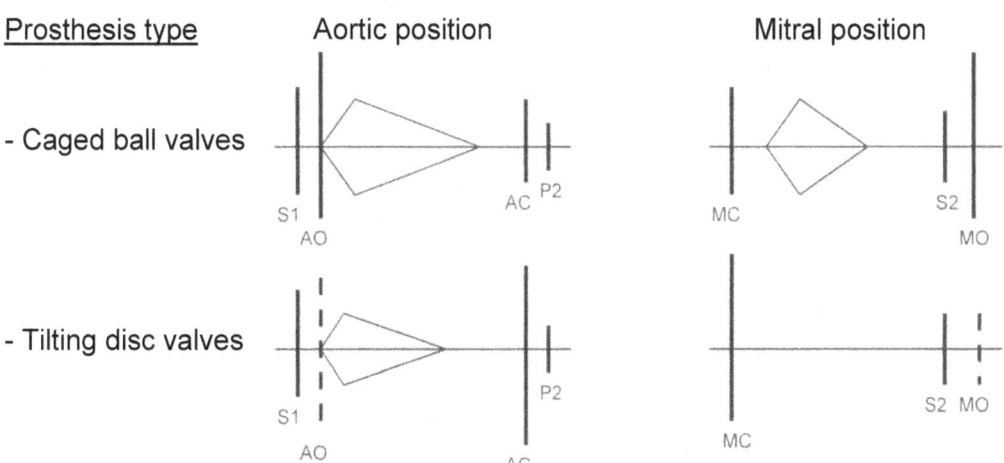

Abbreviations: AC, closure sound of aortic prosthesis; AO, opening sound of aortic prosthesis; MC, closure sound of mitral prosthesis; MO, opening sound of mitral prosthesis; P$_2$, pulmonary component of second heart sound; S$_1$, first heart sound; S$_2$, second heart sound

Adapted from: McGee SR. *Saunders/Elsevier* 2007, Figure 38-2, page 449.

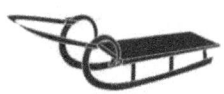

- Give the clinical features which suggest that there is malfunction of a prosthetic heart valve.
  o New cardiac symptoms
  o New cardiac murmur
  o Thromboembolism
  o Hemolytic anemia with schistocytes

- Perform a focused physical assessment for prosthetic heart valves.

  o Mitral Valve
    - Recognized by their site, metallic first heart sound, normal second heart sound and metallic opening snap
    - Systolic murmurs are often
    - Diastolic flow murmurs may be heard normally over the disc valves
  o Aortic Valve
    - Be recognized by their site, normal first heart sound and metallic second heart sound
  o Both mitral and aortic
    - Both the first and second heart sounds will be metallic
    - The presence of a systolic murmur does not indicate valve dysfunction
    - The presence of an early diastolic murmur indicates a malfunctioning aortic valve
  o Complications
    - Thromboembolism
    - Valve dysfunction, including valve leakage, valve dehiscence and valve obstruction due to thrombosis and clogging
    - Bleeding (such as upper gastrointestinal hemorrhage) due to anticoagulants
    - Hemolysis at the valve, causing anemia
    - Endocarditis (prosthetic valve endocarditis)
      ▪ <2 months of surgery: develops as a result of intraoperative contamination of the prosthetic valve or as a consequence of a postoperative nosocomial infection
      ▪ >2 months of surgery: after transient bacteremia (minor skin or upper respiratory tract infections or following dental or urinary manipulations). The non-cardiac manifestations resemble those of native valve infective endocarditis

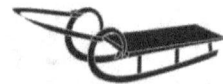

- Structural dysfunction
  - Fracture
  - Poppet escape
  - Cuspal tear
  - Calcification
- Non-structural dysfunction
  - Paravalvular leak
  - Suture/tissue entrapment
  - Noise

- Give the conditions that can simulate clinical manifestations of infective endocarditis.

  - Atiral myxoma
  - Non-bacterial endocarditis
  - Systemic lupus erythematosus (SLE)
  - Sickle cell disease

Adapted from: Baliga RR. *Saunders/Elsevier* 2007, page 61-63; Talley NJ, et al. *Maclennan & Petty Pty Limited* 2003, Table 3.14, page 81.

"Harsh words are heavy and often fall with a big thud,
but a kind word will bounce on and on..."

Anonymous

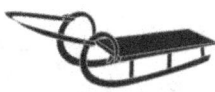

MITRAL REGURGITATION (MR)

➢ Types

- o Mitral valve
  - Annulus
  - Leaflets

- o Subvalvular apparatus
  - Chordac tendinae
  - Papillary muscle

- o Organic
  - Leaflets
  - Chordae tendinaee

- o Functional
  - Ventricular dysfunction
  - Annulus dilations
    - ▪ Ischemia
    - ▪ Dilated
- o Left atrium and ventricle

➢ Pathophysiology
- o Inferior or inferior-posterior STEMI
- o Annular dilation
- o Rupture of papillary muscle
- o Rupture of chordae tendineae
- o And, obviously, a murmur of MR that was present pre-STEMI

➢ Causes (in adults)
- Acute
  - o Coronary artery disease
  - o Rupture of the papillary muscle (often with MI)
  - o Endocarditis
    - Perforation of the MV leaflet
    - Ruptured clordate tendinae
  - o Trauma
  - o Myxomatous degeneration of the MV

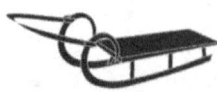

- Chronic
    - Mitral valve leaflets
        - Annular calcification
        - Endocarditis
            - Infection
            - Chordal and papillary muscle damage often from coronary artery disease
            - Rheumatic heart disease
            - Prolapse
            - Annular clacification
            - Connective tissue disease
            - Congenital cleft
            - Drug related
    - Heart
        - Cordial and papillary muscles
            - MV prolapse (MVP)
            - Rupture of chordae
            - Myocardial infarction
            - Papillary muscle rupture
        - Myocardium
            - Regional ischemia or infarctions
            - Dilated cadiomyopathy (coronary artery disease)
            - Hypertrophic cardiomyopathy
        - Left ventricular dilatation
    - ASD (ostium primum, cleft of mitral valve)
    - Partial AV canal
    - Post – surgical correction of transposition of great vessels
    - Connective tissue disorders
- Causes (in infants)
    - Endocarditis fibroelastosis
    - Congenital abnormality of anomalous left coronary artery arising from the pulmonary artery
    - Myocarditis
    - Marfan syndrome

Adapted from: Baliga RR. *Saunders/Elsevier* 2007, page 9 and Ghosh AK. *Mayo Clinic Scientific Press* 2008, Table 3-6, page 47.

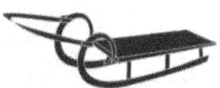

➢ Clinical

    ○ Symptoms   - Orthopnea
                    - PND (paroxysmal nocturnal dyspnea)
                    - Peripheral edema

Mitral regurgitation (at the apex)

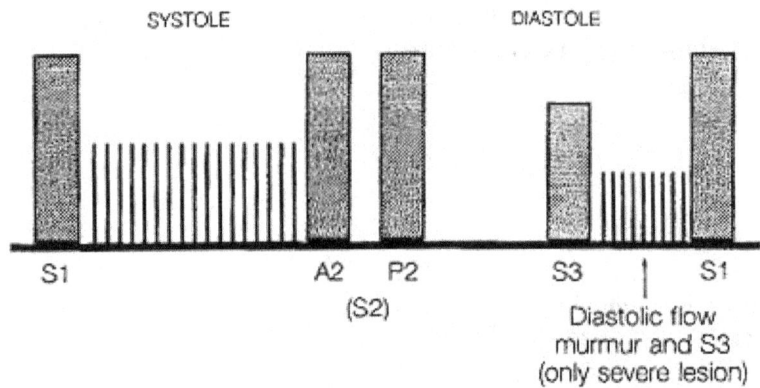

Adapted from: Talley NJ, et al. *Maclennan & Petty Pty Limited* 2003, Figure 3.29, page 75.

- Perform a focused physical examination for MR.

    ○ Peripheral pulse – rapid upstroke of short duration (↑ BV regurgitating into LA causes ↓ LV ejection time)

    ○ Apex beat
        - Position: down and out
        - Character: forceful
        - Precordium- Apical systolic thrill, apex displaced to left.

    ○ Heart sounds
        - ↓ S_1
        - ↑ S_2 (if PHT present)
        - S_3 present
        - S_1 ↓ or absent (murmur may replace S_1).
        - S_3 due to increased left ventricular end diastolic volume. Auscultating an S_3 does not reflect the severity of MR, nor does a systolic regurgitant wave in the neck weins reflect the severity of TR.
        - Auscultation- Apical systolic regurgitant murmur following a ↓ S1 radiating to axilla
        - S3 due to ↑ left ventricular end diastolic volume
        - S1 ↓ or absent (murmur may replace S1)
        - Diastolic flow murmur in severe MR

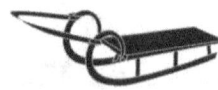

- o Murmur
  - Apical systolic regurgitant murmur following a ↓ S_1 radiating to apex
  - Pansystolic, loud
  - Left sternal edge (LSE)
  - Transmitted to axilla
  - Use diaphragm for best detection
  - Expiration for ↑ loudness
  - Diastolic flow murmur in severe MR
  - In tall persons (eg. Marfan's syndrome, maximal intensity of MR murmur is close to left sternal border)
- o Distinguish from other causes of pansystolic murmurs
  - Continuous with the 2nd sound
  - Mitral regurgitation- propagated into axilla
  - Tricuspid regurgitation –increases with inspiration
  - VSD- 3rd or 4th LICS. Thrill in 90 per cent
  - PDA- usually in 2nd LICS. Murmur may be absent, pansystolic or continuous
- o Radiation
  - Left axilla or left interscapular area
  - With ruptured chordate tendinae
    - Anterior: mid-thoracic spine, or top of head (!)
    - Posterior: into the carotids
  - Left axilla or left interscapular area
  - With ruptured chordate tendinae

Abbreviations: LICS, left intercostal space; PDA, patent ductus arteriosus;

Adapted from: Davies IJT. *Lloyd-Luke LTD* 1972, pages 32 to 39.

- ➢ Treatment
  - o Stabilize
  - o Intra-aortic balloon pump
  - o Nitroprusside and diuretics
  - o Emergent surgical intervention

- o In the STEMI post-infarction period, it is important to distinguish between the complications of MR (mitral regurgitation) and VSD (ventricular septal defect).
- o Both MR and VSD have a pansystolic murmur along left sternal edge.

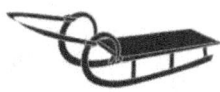

- o Both have V waves on wedge pressure tracing. Both are treated with stabilization and intra-aortic balloon pump.

		MR	VSD
o	Site of MI	- Often anterior wall	Inferior, or inferior-posterior wall
o	Thrill	-	+
o	Radiation		Apex Axilla
o	Electrocardiography	- Flail mitral leaflet - Pupillary muscle lead may be attached to mitral valve leaflet - Severe MR	High velocity L→R shunt systolic turbulence in RV
o	Treatment-stabilize	+	+
	- Intra-aortic balloon pump	Nitroprusside Diuretics	Vassopressin
	- Surgery	Repair mitral valve	Repair VSD

- Perform a focused physical examination to distinguish between the systolic murmur of mitral regurgitation due to dysfunctional papillary muscle dysfunction (PMD) versus ruptured chordate tendinae (RCT).

	PMD	RCT
o Flash pulmonary edema		
o Loud S3	-	+
o Loud S4 (3/6 or more)	-	+
o Decreased early systolic murmur	-	+
o Murmur radiates into carotids	-	+

Rupture of chordate tendinae (usually with infective endocarditis)

Source: Mangione S. *Hanley & Belfus* 2000, page 261.

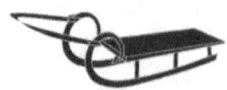

- Perform a physical focused physical examination to distinguish between the murmur of MR caused by rupture of the chordate tendinae (RCT) versus papillary muscle dysfunction (PMD).

Physical sign	RCT	PMD
o Flash pulmonary edema	- Yes	▪ No
o Timing of MR murmur	- Starts immediately after S1 - Decreases in mid systole	▪ Starts at mid systole ▪ Crescendo pattern ending at S2
o Radiation	- Into carotids	▪ Left axilla
o S4	- Yes	▪ No

Adapted from: Mangione S. *Hanley & Belfus* 2000, page 261.

SO YOU WANT TO BE A CARDIOLOGIST!

- How do you make the diagnosis of MR, in the absence of a murmur? (In the patient with a thick chest, well aerated lung tissue and a large RV, even severe MR may not have an audible murmur of MR).
    - o Large L-atrium and L-ventricle
    - o S_2 widely split

- Perform a physical focused physical examination to determine the severity of mitral regurgitation (MR).

    - o Displased of apex (PMI) from large LV
    - o Louder and longer apical systolic murmur
    - o Loud S_3
    - o Early loud diastolic flow murmur after S_3
    - o S_2 widened, unless pulmonary hypertension is present and the S_2 split is narrow
    - o In mitral regurgitation (MR), the louder the murmur, the more severe the regurgitation.

Abbreviation: LV, left ventricle; PMI point of maximal impulse of apex of LV.

Source: McGee SR. *Saunders/Elsevier* 2007, Box 42-1 pages 494 and 495; Simel DL, et al. *JAMA* 2009, Table 33-12, page 445.

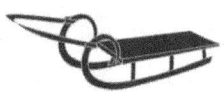

- Give the performance characteristics of physical examination for determining the severity of characteristics systolic murmur of moderate to severe mitral (MR) and tricuspid regurgitation (TR).

  o Auscultating the murmur of mitral regurgitation (MR) has a positive likelihood ratio (PLR) of 4.4 that the MR is moderate – to – severe

  o For tricuspid regurgitation (TR), palpating a pulsative liver has a PLR of 3.9 that the regurgitation is moderate – to – severe.

Finding	PLR
o Mitral Regurgitation (MR)	
- Detecting MR	4.4
o Tricuspid regurgitation (TR)	
- Pulsatile liver	3.9

  o Auscultating an S_3 does not reflect the severity of MR, nor does a systolic regurgitant wave in the neck weins reflect the severity of TR.

Abbreviations: PLR, positive likelihood ratio; MR, mitral regurgitation; TR, tricuspid regurgitation

Adapted from: McGee SR. *Saunders/Elsevier* 2007, Box 42-1, page 497.

- Perform a focused physical examination to determine the severity of aortic regurgitation.

  o Pulse
  - Wide pulse pressure

  o Heart sounds
  - Soft S_2
  - Presence of S_3

  o Murmur
  - Duration of the decrescendo diastolic murmur
  - Austin Flint murmur (an apical, low-pitched, diastolic murmur caused by vibration of the anterior mitral cusp in the regurgitant jet, and is heard at the apex.)

  o Associated signs – L-HF

Adapted from: Baliga RR. *Saunders/Elsevier*, 2007, page 15.

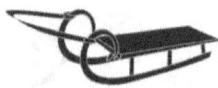

- Perform a physical focaused physical examination to distinguish between the murmur of tricuspid regurgitation (TR) and mitral regurgitation (MR).

Sign	Tricuspid regurgitation	Mitral regurgitation
○ Pulse	Normal	Jerky, or normal
○ JVP		
- V' wave	↑	Normal
- Deep Y descents (Lancisi's sign)		
○ Palpation		
- Left parasternal heave	+	+
○ Auscultation		
- Parasystolic murmur	+	+
- Intensity on inspiration	↑	↑↑
- Valsava	In 3 sec	In 1 sec
- Radiation	To liver	To axilla
- AJR	+	-

Abbreviations: JVP. Jugular venous pressure; AJR, abdomino jugular reflux test

Adapted from: Baliga RR. *Saunders/Elsevier*, page 9; Mangione S. *Hanley & Belfus* 2000, pages 264 and 265.

➤ Treatment

- Give the treatment of MR.

  - Acute MR
    - Vasodilator (nitroprusside) to ↓ MAP to ≤ 60 mm Hg (↓ afterload)
    - Diuretic
    - Nitroglycerine for continued syndromes (e.g. orthopnea)
    - If hypotension persists
      - Dobutamine (inotropic agents, to ↑stroke volume [SV])
      - Amrinone
      - Milrinone
    - If no response to vasodilators and ionotropes
      - IABP (intra-aortic balloon pump)
    - Surgery
      - MV repair or replacement for symptoms despite medical therapy
      - LVEF < 55%, with/without symptoms
      - LVEF dilation > 45 mm, with / without symptoms

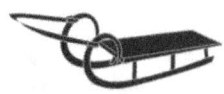

- o Chronic   - Diuretics
  MR   - ACEI / ARB2
                - BB
                - Digoxin
                - Warfarin anticoagulation
                - Surgery

Abbreviation: BB, beta-blocker; AF, atrial fibrillation; MR, mitral regurgitation; LV, left ventricle; ACEI, ACE inhibitor; ARB, angiotensin receptor blocker

- Give the indications for mitral valve repair / replacement.
  - o Symptoms
  - o LVEF < 60%
  - o LV end-systolic diameter > 40 mm
  - o Pulmonary artery systolic pressure
    - ↑ at rest ≥ 50 mm Hg
    - With exercise ≥ 60 mm Hg
  - o MR from LV dilation / dysfunction from ischemia may be helpful more by stenting or CABG revascularization, than from mitral valve repair / replacement
  - o Leaflets ≥ 5 mm
  - o Flail leaflets (no coaptation)

Acute MR

➤ Causes / associations
  - o Rupture chordae tendineae
  - o Rupture papillary muscle
  - o Infective endocarditis

➤ Pathophysiology
  - o ↑LAP
    - PH / pulmonary edema

  - o ↑ LVEDP
    - → ↑ LV preload
    - ↑ HR
    - Total SV
    - ↑ EF (maintain normal forward SV / CO
    - → ↑ LV dilation
    - LVH
    - ↑↑↑ MR
    - ↓ EF

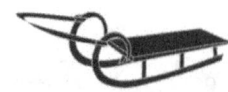

Mastering the Boards: Cardiology   A.B.R. Thomson

- ○ ↑↑ flow LV → LA
    - – → ↓ forward SV →
    - – ↓ SBP (hypotension, shock)
    - – ↓ forward SV / CO
    - – ↓ EF

Abbreviations: CO, cardiac output; EF, ejection fraction; LAP, left atrial pressure; LV, left ventricle; LVEDP, LV end-diastolic pressure; PH, pulmonary hypertension; SBP, systolic blood pressure; SV, stroke volume;

Chronic Degenerative MR

- ➢ Demography
    - ○ Prevalence ~ 1.0 – 2.5% of population
    - ○ F:M, 2:1
    - ○ Familial or non-familial
    - ○ Common indication for mitral valve (MV) surgery (together with mitral valve prolapse syndrome (MVPS)

- ➢ Causes / associations
    - ○ Primary (fibrinoelastic deficiency, aka Barlon disease)
    - ○ Secondary to inherited connective tissue disease
        - – Marfan syndrome
        - – Ehlers-Danlos syndrome
        - – Osteogenesis

- ➢ Pathology
    - ○ Myxomatous proliferation, and cartilage formation
    - ○ Leaflet (one or both leaflets), chordac tendineae +/- annulus

Rheumatic MR

- ○ Leaflets and chordae tendineae
- ○ MR (mitral regurgitation or MR plus MS (mitral stenosis)

- ➢ Clinical
    - ○ Heart sounds
        - – Early A2
        - – Split S2 (because of early A2)

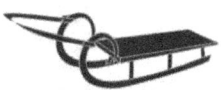

- o Murmur of MR
  - – Apical holosystolic; radiation to
    - ▪ Axilla
      - - Usual
    - ▪ Anterior chest wall
      - - Prolapse posterior leaflet of MV
    - ▪ Posterior chest wall
      - - Prolapse anterior leaflet of MV
- o Other signs of HF (heart failure)

- ➢ Diagnostic testing
  - o Chest x-ray
    - – Enlarged
      - ▪ Left atrium
      - ▪ Pulmonary arteries
    - – Pulmonary edema
    - – Cardiomegaly
  - o ECG
    - – LAE (left atrial enlargement)
    - – LVE (left ventricular enlargement)
    - – LVH (left ventricular hypertrophy)
    - – AF (atrial fibrillation)
    - – Q wave
      - ▪ Pathological in ischemic MR from previous myocardial infarction
  - o Transthoracic echocardiography (TTE)
    - – Assess etiology
    - – Size, LA, LH
    - – Severity
      - ▪ LV dysfunction (EF < 60%)
  - o Tranesophageal echocardiography (TEC)
    - – Assess ↑ detail than
      - ▪ Endocarditis
      - ▪ Guide to MV repair
  - o 3-dimension (D) echocardiography
    - – Assess ↑ detail
      - ▪ Guide to MV repair (especially for periprosthetic valve MR)
  - o Echocardiogram with exercise (EF [ejection fraction])
    - – Assess
      - ▪ LV function
      - ▪ Severity with exercise
      - ▪ Pulmonary artery pressure with exercise

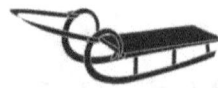

- o Catheterization
  - – Right heart catheterize (LHC)
    - ▪ LA filling pressure
    - ▪ Pulmonary hypertension
    - ▪ Pulmonary capillary wedge pressure (PCWP) giant "V" waves suggest severe MR
  - – Left heart catheterization (LHC)
    - ▪ Assessment of coronary arteries
    - ▪ Guide therapy, if associated CAD [coronary artery disease]
- o CT angiography (CTA)
  - – Guide therapy associated coronary artery disease
- o MRI
  - – Assess
    - ▪ LV function (EF)
    - ▪ Severity of MR
      - – Viability of myocardiac MR associated with ischemic disease
- o Nuclear scan
  - – Assess LV function (EF) if echo studies non-diagnostic viability of myocardium if MR associated with ischemic disease

- ➢ Treatment

- • Acute
  - o ↓ afterload
    - – Nitroprusside IV
    - – IABP (intra-aortic balloon pump)
  - o Mitral valve repair or replacement surgery for severe MR

- • Give the reason while treatment of acute MR-associated HF (heart failure) should not include the use of B-blockers.

  - o B-blockers decrease the heart rate (HR)
  - o The compensatory mechanisms to maintain normal forward SV /CO is by way of ↑ HR and ↑ contractility

- • Chronic
  - o Degenerative
    - – Asymptomatic normal LV function
      - ▪ No therapy, regardless of severity

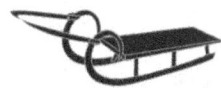

- o Functional
  - - Usual treatment for ↓ LV function
  - - Benefit

	↓ severity of MR	↓ mortality
o B-blockers	+	+
o ACE inhibitor	+	+
o Cardiac resynchronization therapy	+	-

- o Placement of clip on percutaneous anterior and posterior MV leaflets

Surgery

- o MV repair recommended over replacement for severe MR
- o Acute
  - – Symptoms
- o Chronic
  - – Asymptomatic
    - • EF (ejection fraction) 30% - 60%, +/-
    - • ESD (end-systolic dimension) ≥ 40 mm
  - – NYHA II-IV symptoms
    - • EF < 30%, ± ESD > 55 mm
  - – Ischemic / post-infarction, and dilated cardiomyotomy (DCM) is a ventricular problem, so role of annuloplasty is nuclear

- • Give factors, which are associated with ↑ perioperative mortality from surgery for MR (mitral regurgitation).
  - o ↑ age
  - o Associated
    - – CAD
    - – AF
  - o Symptoms NYHA function class
  - o Ejection fraction < 60%

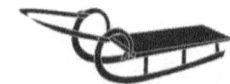

AORTIC REGURGITATION (AR)

➢ Pathophysiology

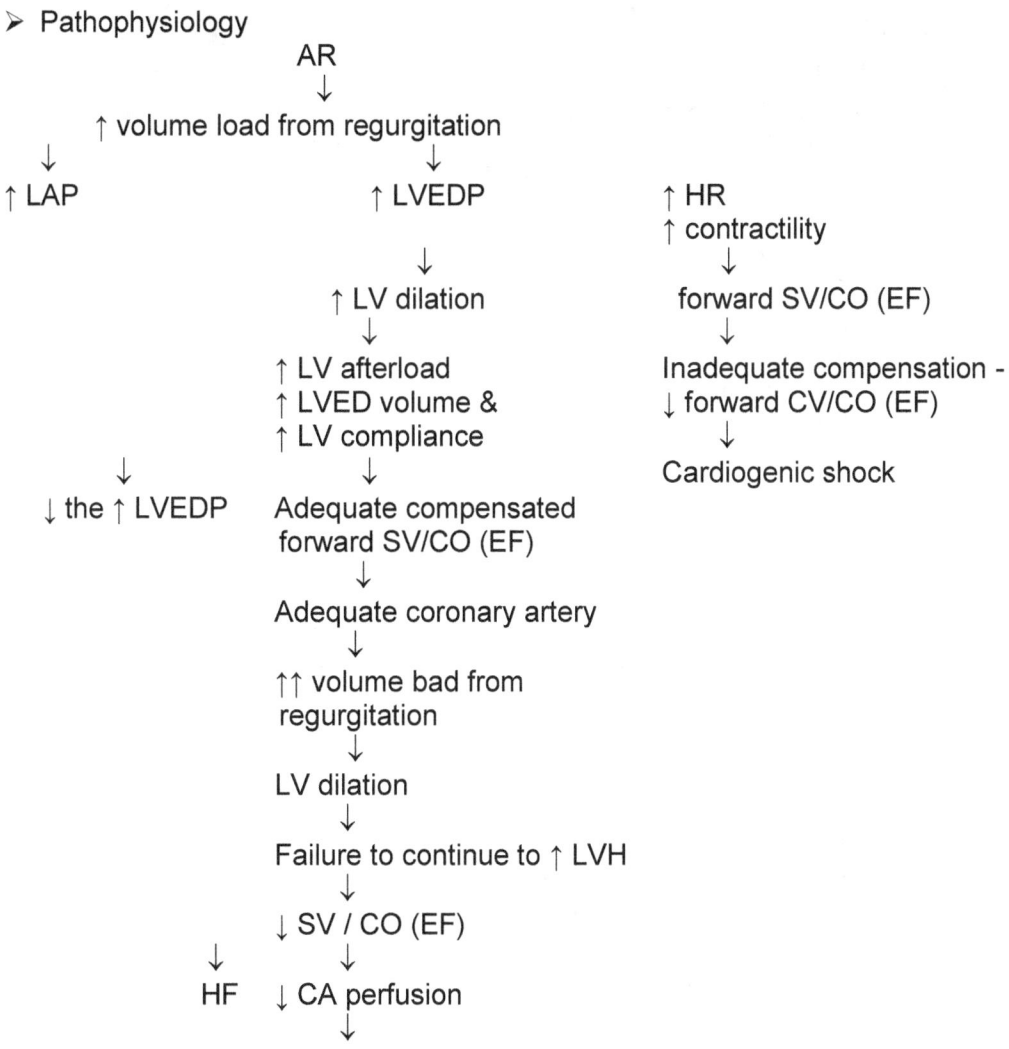

Abbreviations: CA, coronary artery; CO, cardiac output; EF, ejection fraction; HR, heart rate; LAP, left atrial pressure; LV, left ventricle; LVED, left ventricular and diastole; LVEDP, left ventricular and diastolic pressure; LVH, left ventricular hypertrophy; SV, stroke ventricle

- ➤ Causes / associations
  - ○ Acute
    - – Trauma
    - – Dissection of ascending
    - – Infection
      - ▪ Endocarditis
  - ○ Chronic
    - – Aortic valve
      - ▪ Rheumatic fever
      - ▪ Degeneration
        - - Calcification
        - - Myxomatous
      - ▪ Bicuspid valve
      - ▪ Infective endocarditis
      - ▪ Inherited
        - - Marfan syndrome
    - – Subaortic valve stenosis
    - – VSD (ventricular septal defect) plus prolapse of aortic cusp
    - – Aorta
      - ▪ Dissection, ascending aorta
      - ▪ Ideopathic dilation
      - ▪ Syphilitic aortitis
      - ▪ Giant cell aortitis
    - – Hypertension
    - – Collagen vascular disease
      - ▪ Rheumatoid arthritis (RA)
      - ▪ Ankylosing spondylitis (AS)
      - ▪ Reactive arthritis
      - ▪ Whipple disease

  - ○ Inherited/ congenital
    - - Bicuspid aortic valve
    - - Marfan syndrome

  - ○ Idiopathic
    - - Dilation of aortic root and annulus
    - - Cystic medial necrosis
    - - Ruptured sinus of valsalva

  - ○ Infection
    - - Rheumatic fever
    - - Bacterial endocarditis
    - - Syphilis

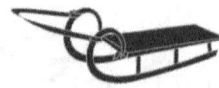

- o Inflammatory
  - MSK
    - Ankylosing spondylitis
    - Reiter syndrome
  - Rheumatoid arthritis

- o Cardiac
  - Atherosclerosis
  - Hypertension
  - Aortic dissection
  - Rupture of sinus of valsalva
  - Non-functioning prosthetic valve

- o Trauma

- o Failure of prosthetic valve

- o Conditions associated with aortic valve leaflet abnormalities
  - Marfan syndrome
  - Rheumatoid arthritis
  - Ankylosing spondylitis

- o Diseases that affect the aortic root
  - Hypertension
  - Syphilis
  - Inherited connective tissue disorders
  - Aortic aneurysm (dissection of descending aorta
- o Misdiagnosed AR
  - Easily confused with similar murmur of pulmonary regurgitation or tricuspid regurgitation (Graham Steell murmur): early diastole, 2nd L-ICS due to pulmonary hypertension.
  - Sudden onset AR is different from chronic AR by having a soft/absent S1, and a diastolic murmur which is never holodiastolic (only early-to-mid diastole)

Abbreviaton: AR, aortic regurgitation

Adapted from: Baliga RR. *Saunders/Elsevier* 2007, page 14 to 16; Simel DL, et al. *JAMA* 2009, page 430.

- o Acute Aortic Regurgitation
  - Infective endocarditis
  - Aortic dissection
  - Trauma
  - Failure of prosthetic valve
  - Rupture of sinus of Valsalva

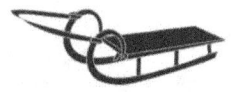

SO YOU WANT TO BE A CARDIOLOGIST!

- Give the 7 causes of systolic murmur which may accompany the typical diastolic murmur of AR.
  - Severe AR, or concurrent AS (i.e. AR+AS)

- Give the causes of a **diastolic murmur** auscultated on the right- and left-side of the sternum.

  - R-side   - Secondary to dilation of aortic root

  - L-side   - AV valve disease (normally murmur is just after A2 if A2 can be heard, and is associated with ↓ PP (pulse pressure), as well as ↓ S1, ↓ A2 and S3.

➢ Clinical

- Acute
  - History
    - Cardiogenic shock
    - Severe dyspnea
  - Physical
    - ↑ pulse / heart rate
    - ↑ (wide) pulse pressure short, soft, 3rd ICS
    - Murmur diastolic
      - Systolic flow murmur
    - Signs of
      - Infective endocarditis
      - Marfan syndrome
      - Aortic dissection

- Chronic
  - History
    - Compensated asymptomatic
    - Decompensated
      - HF (heart failure)
      - Angina

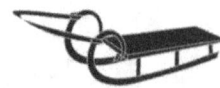

- o Physical
  - Palpitation
  - Auscultation
    - Diastolic
      - Decrescendo
      - LSB
      - Leaning forward
      - End of expiration
    - Systolic flow murmur
    - Austin Flint murmur

- Perform a focused physical examination to access the severity of AR.

  - o Heart sounds
    - $\downarrow S_2$
    - S_3
    - S_1, S_2 usually normal
    - $\uparrow S_2$ pulmonary hypertension
    - $\downarrow S_2$ severe AR
    - S_3 (bicuspid aortic valve, or severe AR)

  - o Pulse
    - $\uparrow$ Pulse pressure

  - o Apex
    - Extensive outward displacement from LVH/ LVD (cor bovinum)

Aortic regurgitation (at the left sternal edge)

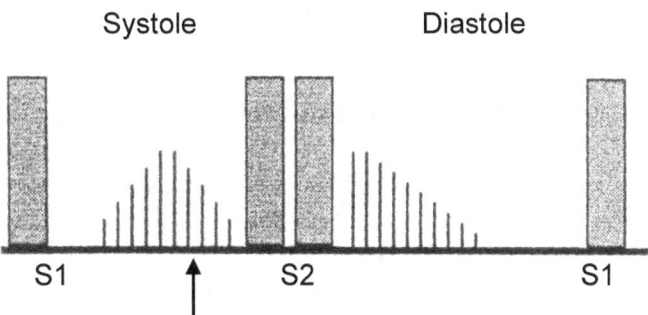

Flow murmur

Source: Talley NJ, et al. *Maclennan & Petty Pty Limited* 2003, Figure 3.32, page 79; Baliga RR. *Saunders/Elsevier* 2007, page 16; Burton JL. *Churchill Livingstone* 1971, page 9 and Mangione S. *Hanley & Belfus* 2000. page 251.

- o Carotids   - Double systolic wave

- o Head & neck   - Head-nodding (in timed with systole; de Musset's sign)
  - Eyes – Argyll Robertson pupils (syphilis)
  - Uvula – movement (timed with systole; Muller's sign)
  - Palate – high arch (Marfan's syndrome)
  - Carotids – Corrigan's sign (visible pulsating carotids)

- o Murmur   - Diastole, early
  - High-pitched
  - LSE
  - Leaning forward, at best heard end of expiration
  - Diastole, mid
    - Apex of heart
    - May fill all diastole
    - Low-pitched
  - Austin Flint murmur
    - Mimicking MS, but with no OS
    - Seen in severe AR
    - The regurgitant jet of blood in AR causes the anterior cusp of the mitral valve to vibrate
  - Systole
    - Base of heart
    - Ejection-like crescendo – decrescendo murmur
  - Presence of Austin Flint murmur

- o Pulse   - Large volume, rapid fall
  - Wide pulse pressure

- o MSK   - Hands – rheumatoid arthritis
  - Capillary – pulsation in nail beds (Quincke's sign)
  - Arm span > height (Marfan's syndrome)
  - Back – ankylosing spondylitis

- o Signs of L-HF   - Length of murmur is proportional to the severity of the lesion

Abbreviations: L-HF, L-sided heart failure; LSE, left sterna edge; LVD, left ventricular dilation; LVH, left ventricular hyperteophy; OS, opening snap

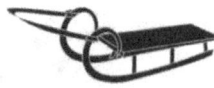

- Take a directed history and perform a focused physical examination for aortic regurgitation.

    o General
      - Dyspnea
      - Fatigue
      - Exercise intolerance
      - Night sweats

    o Heart
      - Shock
      - Arrhythmia
      - Chest pain
        - Dissection
        - Infarct
      - Palpitations

    o Lung
      - Pulmonary edema

    o History to establish
      - Cause and
      - Complications

Abbreviation: LSB, left sterna border; LV, left ventricle; LVH, left ventricular hypertrophy; RSB, right sternal border

Adapted from: Ghosh AK. *Mayo Clinic Scientific Press* 2008, Table 3-3, page 44.

XXXXXXXXXXXXXXXXXXXXXXXXXXXXXXXXXXXXXXXXXXXXXXXX

SO YOU WANT TO BE A CARDIOLOGIST!

- In the context of Aortic regurgitation, give what is the "Hill" sign.

    o Higher systolic pressure in the leg than in the arm, and
    o An indicator of severity of aortic regurgitation

XXXXXXXXXXXXXXXXXXXXXXXXXXXXXXXXXXXXXXXXXXXXXXXX

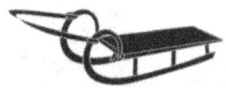

SO YOU WANT TO APPLY FOR A CARDIOLOGY RESIDENCY!

Stump Your Staff – See if they know more than four of the eponymous signs of aortic regurgitation

o De Musset sign: head nodding in time with the heartbeat
o Corrigan sign: prominent carotid pulsations
o Quincke sign: capillary pulsation in the nail beds- it is of no value, as this sign occurs normally
o Mueller sign: pulsation of the uvula in time with the heartbeat
o Duroziez sign: systolic and diastolic murmurs over the femoral artery on gradual compression of the vessel
o Traube sign: a double sound heard over the femoral artery on compressing the vessel distally; this is not the 'pistol shot' sound that may be heard over the femoral
o Hill sign: increased blood pressure in the legs compared with the arms

Source: Talley NJ, et al. *Maclennan & Petty Pty Limited* 2003, page 78.

Useful back: Aortic or pulmonary regurgitation (PR)

> o Aortic regurgitation – often missed. Listen with diaphragm all down L sternal edge for soft 'whispered R' murmur with patient leaning forward in expiration
> o Pulmonary regurgitation (PR)- usually due to pulmonary hypertension (PHT)
> o Austin-Flint due to Aortic Incompetence mimics mitral stenosis (MS)
> o Graham Steell due to mitral stenosis, mimics pulmonary regurgitation (PR)

➢ Continuous ('Machinery murmur')
    o Patent ductus arteriosus (PDA)
    o Aortico-pulmonary septal defect
    o Pulmonary AV fistula
    o Bronchial artery anastomosis in pulmonary atresia
    o Venous hum
    o Combined AS and AR, or MR and AR

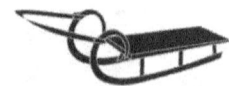

Mastering the Boards: Cardiology   A.B.R. Thomson

- Perform a focused physical examination for Marfan Syndrome.

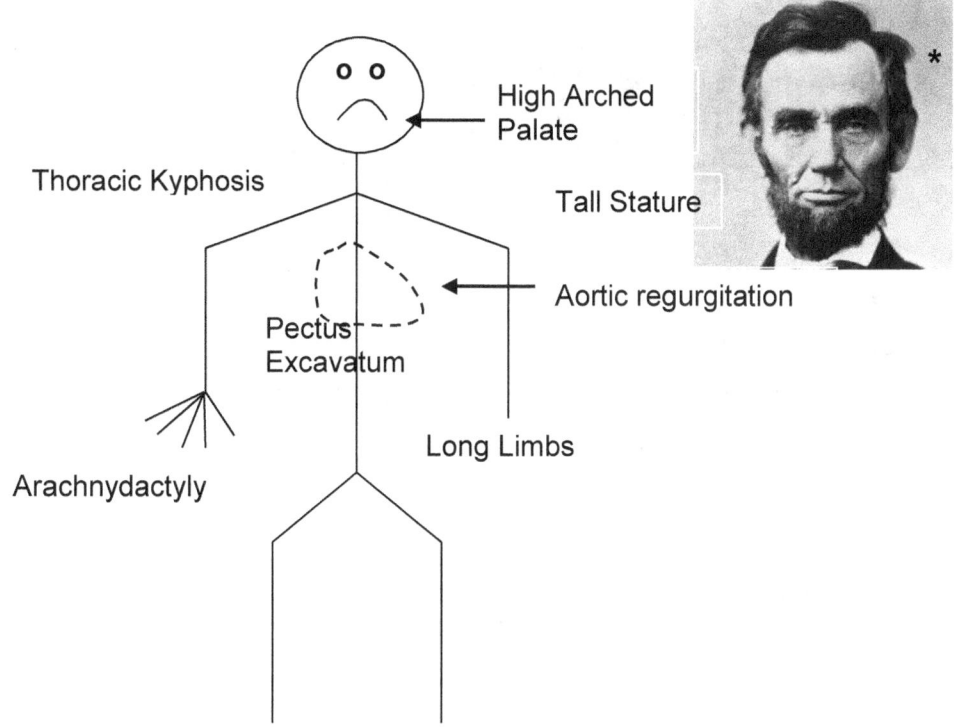

Adapted from: Talley NJ, et al. *Maclennan & Petty Pty Limited* 2003, page 35.

* President Lincoln (USA) may have Marfan syndrome

- Perform a physical examination to determine the severity of aortic regurgitation.

  - Wide pulse pressure
  - Soft S2
  - Duration of the decrescendo diastolic murmur
  - Austin Flint murmur (an apical, low pitched, diastolic murmur caused by vibration of the anterior mitral cusp in the regurgitation jet, and is heard at the apex)
  - Signs of left ventricular failure
  - Hill sign

Adapted from: Baliga RR. *Saunders/Elsevier* 2007, page 1; Burton JL. *Churchill Livingstone* 1971, page 9.

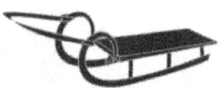

- Perform a focused physical examination for aortic regurgitation.

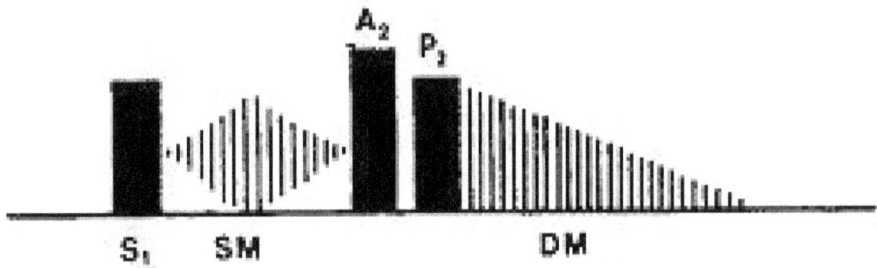

- o Often associated with Marfan's syndrome, rheumatoid spondylitis.
- o Precordium – Apex displaced laterally and anteriorly
- o Thrill often plapable along left sterna border and in the jugular notch.
- o Carotids – Double systolic wave
- o Auscultation – Decrescendo diastolic murmur along left sternal border
- o M_1 and A_2 are increased

Adapted from: Mangione S. *Hanley & Belfus* 2000, page 251.
Performance characteristics for aortic regurgitation (AR)

Finding	PLR
o Characteristic diastolic murmur	
- Detecting mild aortic regurgitation or worse	9.9
- Detecting moderate-to-severe aortic regurgitation	4.3
o Early diastolic murmur loudest on right side of sternum	
- Detecting dilated aortic root or endocarditis	8.2
o The finding of an early diastolic murmur which becomes softer with amyl nitrite inhalation is not of significant use to distinguish AR versus Graham Steell murmur	NS

Adapted from: McGee SR. *Saunders/Elsevier* 2007, Box 41-1, page 486.

o   Characteristics of moderate-to-severe AR

Finding	Sensitivity (%)	Specificity (%)	PLR	NLR
- Diastolic murmur • Murmur grade 3 or louder	30-61	86-98	8.2	0.6

- Only when the diastolic blood pressure is ≤ 50 mm Hg, the pulse pessure is ≥ 80 mm Hg, or Hill test is ≥ 60 mm Hg are these findings have a positive likelihood ratio (PLR) which makes then clinically useful (PLR, 19.3, 10.9 and 17.3 , respectively).

- Duroziez sign, femeral pistol shot bruit, and the water hammer pulse do not signify sevee AR. Modest PLRs are associated with S3 gallop (5.9), and enlarged or sustained apical impulse (2.4).

Source: McGee SR. *Saunders/Elsevier* 2007, Box 41-2, page 488.

➢ The murmur of AR is diastolic

- Give causes of a systolic murmur which may occur of AR.

  o   AR plus AS
  o   AR plus MR
  o   Aneurysm
  o   Systolic hypertension

- Give the clinical findings which help to distinguish PDA (patent ductus arteriosis) from the murmur of AR.

  o   Diastolic murmur in PDA is
    -   Late (rather than early as in AR)
    -   Loudest anteriorly, left side
    -   May be heard posteriorly
  o   Associated with a thrill

Adapted from: Mangione S. *Hanley & Belfus* 2000. page 271 and 272.

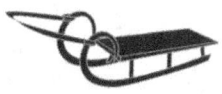

SO YOU WANT TO BE A WHIZ-KID CARDIOLOGY RESIDENT!

The sensitivity of the Duroziez maneuver for aortic regurgitation (AR) is 58 to 100%.

- Give causes of false-negative Duroziez maneuver.

  o Mild AR
  o AR plus AS
  o AS plus MS (↓ LV filling from mitral stenosis [MS])
  o AS plus MR (↓ LV emptying from mitral regurgitation [MR])
  o Coarctation of the aorta

- Perform a focused physical examination to distinguish between the Duroziez double murmur of AR, and the "false positive" Duroziez sign, which is not due to AR.

  o This sign in AR is due to one murmur from forward flow, and one from reverse flow
  o Any high – output state may cause a pulsus bisferiens as well as the Duroziez double murmur.
  o The double murmur in high- outflow states one both due to forward flow
    - Auscultate over the femoral artery, and hear the to – and –fro murmur
    - Pressure over the cephalad edge of the compression stethoscope diaphragm increases both murmurs in high- output states
    - Pressure over the caudad edge of the diaphragm increases only the murmur from the reverse flow, as occurs in AR

  o Distinction method

    - Cephalad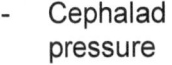
      pressure

      ↑ forward flow of
      both murmurs in
      high-output states

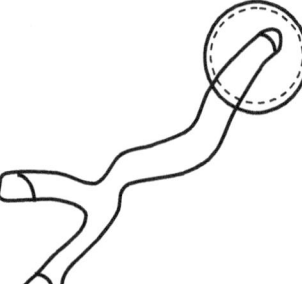

- Caudad pressure

↑ reverse flow
murmur portion of
the double murmur
of AR

This information regarding the Duroziez maneuver is used in the clinical examination of the murmur of aortic regurgitation (AR)

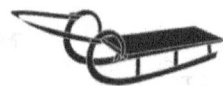

Trick Questions!

Aortic regurgitation (AR) has both a forward flow and a reverse flow component leading to the pulsus bisferiens to the "pistol shot" femoral bruit as well as the Duroziez' double murmur over the femoral artery.

- You auscultate a double murmur over the femoral artery, and pressure over the caudad portion of the compressing diaphragm of the stethoscope enhances the reverse flow murmur. But the patient does not have AR. What condition do they have?
  - PDA (patent ductus arteriosus)

A patient with AR was admitted and you discovered that she he had pulsus bisferiens. A week later the consultant cannot palpate this abnormal pulse.

- Did you overcall the presence of this abnormal pulse, because you knew they had AR and you thought they "should" have this kind of pulse?
  - Not necessarily. The pulsus bisferiens lessens and then disappears when L-CHF develops.

- The early diastolic murmur of AR is usually heard best with the diaphragm and at the left sternal edge. Give the significance of this murmur being auscultated at both the right and the left sterna edge?
  - As a result of the AR, the ascending aorta becomes dilated and displaced, so that this high pitched early diastolic murmur becomes audible on both sides of the sternum.

SO YOU WANT TO BE A CARDIOLOGIST!

- In which cardiac phases are the diagnosis and severity of AR and MR made.

  - Curious comparison
    - AR is diagnosed in diastole, but its severity assessed in systole
    - MR is diagnosed in systole, but its severity is assessed in diastole

- In the context of aortic regurgitation (AR), give what is the Landolfi sign.

  - The pupil contracts in systole, and dilates in diastole

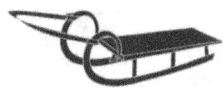

➤ Causes of collapsing pulse: Hyperdynamic circulation due to
  o Aortic regurgitation
  o Thyrotoxicosis
  o Severe anaemia
  o Paget's disease
  o Complete heart block

Source: Baliga RR. *Saunders/Elsevier*, 2007, page 78.

➤ Treatment

• Give the treatment of AR (aortic regurgitation)

o Acute AR (→ hypotension)	- IV diuretic - Nitroprusside - Dobutamine, or milrinone - As a bridge to urgent AV replacement
o Chronic AR - Pharmaceuticals	▪ ACEI ▪ CCB (nifedipine) ▪ Hydralazine ▪ Vasodilators
- AV replacement	▪ Symptomatic AR (regardless of value of LVEF) ▪ Planned CABG ▪ Planned surgery on other valves ▪ LV dilation worsenin ▪ LVEF < 50% ▪ ↓ exercise tolerance / performance

Abbreviations: BB, beta-blocker; CABG, coronary artery bypass graft; IABP, intra-aortic balloon pump; LVEF, left ventricle ejection fraction

---

  o Do **not** use BB in AR

  o Do **not** use intra-aortic balloon pump (IABP) for AR

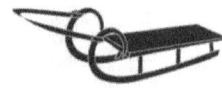

Mastering the Boards: Cardiology   A.B.R. Thomson

Useful background: Aortic regurgitation

○ If the examiner does NOT hear an AR murmur, the likelihood that the patient has AR is diminished as follows:
- NLR 0.1 for moderate or greater AR
- NLR 0.2 to 0.3 for mild or greater AR

○ If the examiner DOES hear an AR murmur, the likelihood that the patient has AR is increased as follows:
- PLR 4.0 to 8.3 for moderate or greater AR
- PLR 8.8 to 32.0 for mild or greater AR

Abbreviations: AR, aortic regurgitation; PLR, positive likelihood ratio; NLR, negative likelihood ratio

Source: Choudhry NK, et al. *JAMA* 1999; 281:2231-38.

• Give the positive and negative likelihood ratios of the physical examination for detecting aortic regurgitation.

		Patient Population	PLR	NLR
○	Overall cardiac examination	- Referred for evaluation of systolic murmur	5.1	0.82
○	Third heart sound (to identify severe AR)	- Patients with isolated aortic insufficiency, referred for echocardiography	5.9	0.83

Abbreviations: AR, aortic regurgitation; CI, confidence interval; PLR, positive likelihood ratio; NLR, negative likelihood ratio.

Source: Simel DL, et al. *JAMA* 2009, Table 32-4, page 429.

CLINICAL GEM AND PEARL

• In chronic AR, the systolic flow murmur is due to volume overload associated aortic stenosis (AS): AR plus AS
• In chronic AR, give the finding on auscultation, which best correlated with the severity of AR.
  ○ The severity of AR is reflected by the duration of the diastolic decrescendo murmur.

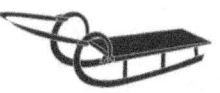

Mastering the Boards: Cardiology   A.B.R. Thomson

- Give the likelihood ratios for the typical murmur to predict aortic regurgitation (AR), or an S_3 to predict severe AR.

Finding		PLR	NLR
o Typical murmur	Mild or greater	8.8-32	0.2-0.3
- Cardiologist	Moderate or greater	4.0-8.3	0-0.1
- Murmur intensity (generalist or cardiologist)	Grade 3	4.5	
	Grade 2	1.1	
	Grade 1	0	
	No murmur	0	
o Third heart sound (S_3) (cardiologist)	Severe	5.9	0.83

Abbreviations: PLR, positive likelihood ratio; NLR, negative likelihood ratio

Source: Simel DL, et al. *JAMA* 2009, Table 32-5, page 430.

- Give the mechanism for the loss of the ↑ (wide) pulse pressure (PP) in some persons with AR.
  - o ↓ SR develops → ↓ SBP → ↑ PP

The typical murmur of AR is a short, soft diastolic murmur, heard best in the 3rd ICS. This diastolic murmur is often not audible, but a systolic murmur is auscultated.

- Give the mechanism of production of the systolic flow murmur in AR.

  - o The systolic flow murmur in AR is caused by
    - ↑ HR / hydrodynamic LV
    - ↑ volume (volume overload)

➢ Diagnostic testing
  - o Chest X-ray
    - Signs of HF
      - Pulmonary edema
      - Cardiomegaly
      - Wide mediastinum
  - o ECG
    - ↑ HR (tachycardia)
    - LAE (left atrial enlargement)
    - LVH (left ventricular hypertrophy)

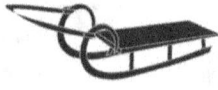

- o Transthoracic echocardiogram (TTE)
  - Structure
  - Function
    - LV systolic function
    - Severity of AR
- o Transesophageal echocardiogram (TEE)
  - Better detail of features seen on TTE, especially for
    - Bicuspid valve
    - Endocarditis
    - Aortic abscess
    - Aortic dissection
    - Prosthetic valve
- o Catheterization
  - Structure
    - LV pressure
    - LV function
    - Severity

  - CT angiography
    - Coronary arteries

  - MRI
    - Aortic dissection
    - Aortic size
    - Severity of AR

➤ Treatment

- o Associated
  - Hypertension (SBP)
    - Vasodilators*
  - Endocarditis
    - Antibiotics
- o Symptoms
  - Vasodilators

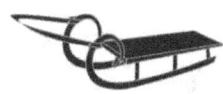

> Prevention

- Asymptomatic
  - Severe AS
  - LVE ⎤
  - Normal LV ⎬ Vasodilators
  - Systolic function ⎦

- ↓ mortality
  - B-blockers

*Vasodilators
- Nifedipine, ACE inhibitors, hydralazine

> Surgery

- Give the ACC / AHA guidelines – class I indications for aortic valve replacement (AVR) in severe aortic regurgitation (AR).
  - Acute AR
  - Chronic
    - Asymptomatic EF ≤ 50%
    - AVR at time of heart surgery
    - On other valves
    - On aorta (if aortic root / ascending aorta > 4.5 cm, repair / replace with surgery for AVR

> Prognosis
  - ↑ operative
    - NYHA functional class
    - EF (LV dysfunction)
    - Chronically
  - Asymptomatic
    - No symptoms plus LV function normal → Abnormal (< 4% / yr)
    - No symptoms → symptoms (< 6% / yr) ± ↓ EF
    - SCD < 0.2% / yr
    - No symptoms plus LV dysfunction → symptoms (> 25% / yr)
  - Symptoms
    - MR > 10% / yr

Abbreviations: AR, aortic regurgitation; AVR, aortic valve replacement; CABG, coronary artery bypass graft; EF, ejection fraction; LV, left ventricle; MR, mortality rate; NYHA, New York Heart Association; SCD, sudden cardiac death

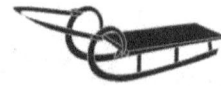

BICUSPID AORTIC VALVE

- o Murmur may be that of AS or AR (aortic stenosis > aortic regurgitation)
- o Associations
  - Ascending aortic dilation (aortopathy)
  - Aortic coarctation
  - Turner syndrome
- o ↑ risk of infective endocarditis
- o Treatment
  - Balloon valvotomy
  - Aortic valve replacement
  - Replace ascending aorta if > 4.5 cm

➤ Diagnosis
  - o Chest X-ray
    - Rib notching (from collateral vessels)
    - "figure 3 sign" (narrowing from coarctation with dilation of the aorta above and below)
  - o ECG LV hypertrophy
    - ST-T wave abnormalities
  - o CT, CMR, cardiac catheterization (before secondary intervention percutaneous repair)

➤ Treatment

Collateral flow	Peak-to-peak coarctation gradient, mm Hg
No	≥ 20
Yes	< 20

- o Primary surgery
- o Secondary (recurrence after surgery) percutaneous
- o Treatment of associated cardiac defects, as needed and appropriate

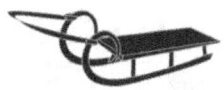

MITRAL VALVE PROLAPSE (MVP)

- o Mitral valve prolapse "…. diagnosed by echocardiography with visualization of a displaced coaptation level of the anterior and posterior mitral leaflet 2 mm or more above mitral annulus" (MKSAP 16 2012, Cardiology, page 80).

SO YOU WANT TO BE A CARDIOLOGIST!

- Distinguish between the murmur of MR due to RHD, from LV dilation and reduced contractility.

  - o MR from RHD: pansystolic murmur
  - o MR from LV dilation: mid, late or pansystolic

- Distinguish between the murmur of MR and AS with calcification.

  - o If there is a premature beat, or if there is associated AF, listen after the pause, when there is ↑ loudness of murmur in AS, but not in MR.

Abbreviation: AF, atrial fibrillation; AS, aortic stenosis; ASD, atrial septal defect; AV, atrioventricular; BV, blood volume; FP, filling pressure; LV, left ventricle; MR, mitral regurgitation; OS, opening snap; RHD, rheumatic heart disease; TR, tricuspid regurgitation; VSD, ventricular septal defect

- In the context of MR, why does the peripheral pulse have rapid upstroke of short duration?

  - o ↑ BV regurgitating into LA causes ↓ LV ejection time.

- In the patient with MR, give the meaning of a diastolic rumble?

  - o MR+ MS (combined mitral disease)
  - o ↑ BV flow across the mitral valve during diastole

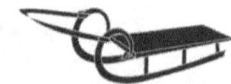

YOU HAVE DECIDED NOT TO BE A PEDIATRIC BUT RATHER AN ADULT CARDIOLOGIST!

- In the context of an ejection systolic murmur, give the 'Gallavardin phenomenon'.

    o The high-frequency components of the ejection systolic murmur may radiate to the apex, falsely suggesting mitral regurgitation

Source: Baliga RR. *Saunders/Elsevier* 2007, pages 32 and 33.

Trick Questions

- The murmur of MR is usually associated with the apex beat displaced down and out, give the mechanism by which the murmur of MR may radiate to the neck.

    o If a stream of blood regurgitates from the LV into the LA near the aortic root, the murmur may radiate into the neck.
    o This get of blood regurgitating to the aortic root may be seen with a ruptured cord as tendinae, or with disease involvement of the posterior leaflet of the mitral valve leaflet.

- From the examination of the heart, how do you access the severity of MR?
    o An S_3 suggests ↑ MR severity
    o A diastolic rumble (in the absence of associated MS) indicates ↑ BV flow across the mitral valve during diastole.

- When does the absence of a mitral area murmur or a late systolic/ holosystolic murmur significantly reduce the likelihood of mitral regurgitation?

    o In the setting of an acute myocardial infarction.

Source: Simel DL, et al. The Rational Clinical Examination: Evidence-based clinical diagnosis. *JAMA* 2009, page 439.

 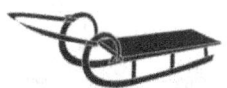

SO YOU WANT TO BE A CARDIOLOGIST!

- During the strain phase of the Valsalva maneuver, there is increased intrathoracic pressure, which leads to a decrease in venous return and therefore a reduction of the blood volume moving into the LV. Thus, straining reduces the loudness of heart sounds and murmurs, because of the decrease in cross-Valvular gradients. So what is the question? What are the two exceptions to the Valsalva maneuver softening heart sounds/murmurs during the held phase?

  - HOCM (hypertrophic obstructive cardiomyopathy)
  - MVP (mitral valve prolapse)

Source: Mangione S. *Hanley & Belfus* 2000, page 257 and 268.

SO YOU WANT TO BE A CARDIOLOGIST!

- How do you make the diagnosis of MR, in the absence of a murmur? (In the patient with a thick chest, well aerated lung tissue and a large RV, even severe MR may not have an audible murmur of MR)

  - Large L-atrium and L-ventricle
  - S2 widely split

Trick Questions

- What is the significance of an S3 associated with MR?

  - In the patient with MR and S_3, the S_3 arises from rapid LV filling, and the S_3 in MR does not suggest ↑ FP of LV or LV dysfunction.

- In the patient with combined MR and MS, (usually due to RHD), what is the significance of the presence of an S_3 or a large LA?

  - MR + MS + S_3 – indicates the MS is mild, and the dominant murmur is the MR.

  MR + MS + large LA – samething: MS is not clinically significant, and the main problem is the MS.

Source: Baliga RR. *Saunders/Elsevier* 2007, page 12.

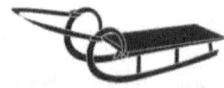

SO YOU WANT TO BE A CARDIOLOGIST!

- You auscultate a systolic murmur which is suggestive of MR (mitral regurgitation). From the auscultation, give how you would distinguish a MR murmur caused by (rheumatic heart disease [RHD]), versus MVP (mitral valve prolapse) or PMA (papillary muscle dysfunction)?

  - RHD
    - Platform murmur
  - MVP or PMA
    - Systolic murmur of MR begins in mid-systole, and extends to A_2
    - Soft murmur, heard best at apex
    - Crescends pattern towards S_2
    - "Cooing" sound
    - "Honking" sound (like Canada geese)
    - Myxomatous degeneration of posterior leaflet
    - MVP syndrome:
      - Atypical chest pain
      - Arrhythmias
      - Abnormal ECG
  - Mimics PMD from MI or HOCM
  - Sharp systolic click (chordal snap) in either mid or late systole, followed by murmur is typical of MVP, and can be made buder by exercise.

Adapted from: Mangione S. *Hanley & Belfus* 2000, pages 261 and 263.

SO YOU WANT TO BE A CARDIOLOGIST!

- When does the absence of a mitral area murmur or a late systolic/ holosystolic murmur significantly reduce the likelihood of mitral regurgitation?

  - In the setting of an acute myocardial infarction.

Source: Simel DL, et al. *JAMA* 2009, page 439.

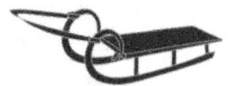

```
SO YOU WANT TO BE A CARDIOLOGIST!

•  In persons with mitral regurgitation (MR), what is the meaning of a
   diastolic rumble?

   o  Coexistent mitral stenosis (MS)


•  OK. In persons with MR, a diastolic rumble and a large left atrium,
   what is the interpretation?

   o  No MS

Source: Baliga RR. Saunders/Elsevier, 2007, page 13.


•  Give the causes of a precordial pansystolic murmur.

      o  Mitral regurgitation (MR)
      o  Tricuspid regurgitation (TR)
      o  Ventricular septal defect (VSD)
```

➤ Studies   o Echocardiogram for diagnosis
                    o Ambulatory ECG monitoring if MVP causes
                       symptoms of arrhythmia

➤ Treatment   o ASA
                       - Unexpected TIA
                       - Sinus rhythm
                       - No thrombi in atrium
                    o Warfarin
                       - Recurrent TIA despite ASA
                       - History of CVA
                       - AF in person > 65
                       - Hypertension
                       - MR
                       - HF
                    o Surgery
                       - Significant AF
                       - Ruptured chordae
                       - Chordal elongation

Abbreviations: TIA, transient ischemic attack; CVA, cerebrovascular accident;
AF, atrial fibrillation; MR, mitral regurgitation; HF, heart failure; ASA, aspirin

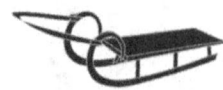

- ➢ Causes / associations
  - o Hereditary
    - Marfan syndrome
    - ASD, secundum (atrial septal defect)
    - Ehlers – Danlos syndrome
    - Ebstein's anomaly
  - o Rheumatic
    - Rheumatic heart disease
    - Systemic lupus erythematosis
  - o Ischemic heart disease
  - o Idiopathic – cardiomyopathics

Adapted from: Baliga RR. *Saunders/Elsevier*, 2007, page 66.

- Take a direct history and perform a focused physical examination for mitral valve prolapse (MVP).
  - o History
    - Palpitations associated with mild tachyarrhythmias
    - Adrenergic symptoms
    - Chest pain
    - Anxiety or fatigue
  - o Physical Examination

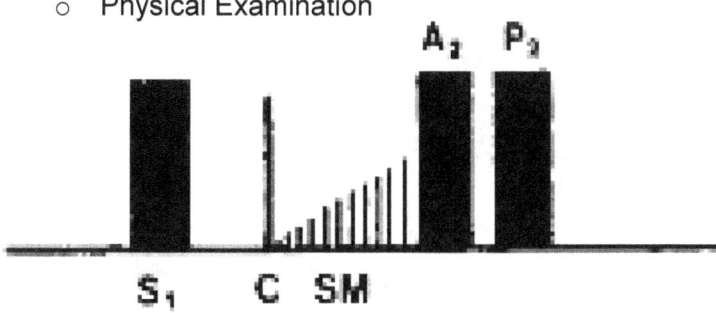

Abbreviations: A_2, aortic component of second heart sound; C, click; P_2, pulmonary component of second heart sound; S_1, first heart sound; SM, systolic murmur

- o Click is followed by late or mid-systolic high pitched crescendo murmur
    - Mid-systolic click, best heard at the apex in the left deculsitus postion
    - Late systolic murmur, loudest at apex
    - MVP may / may not be associated with MR

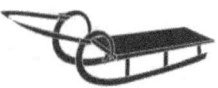

- o Click varies from cycle to cycle

- o Click is legthened by valsalva maneuver

- o Squatting will bring the click closer to the second heart sound and decrease the duration of the murmur
  - Squatting ↓ duration of systolic murmur
  - Standing, valsalva
    - ↑ MSC and S2
    - ↑ duration of systolic murmur

➢ Mechanism

- o Backward snapping of prolapsed mitral leaflet, and sudden distention of chordal apparatus, from mitral or tricuspid valve prolapse.

- o Which two and only two murmurs are enhanced by Valsalva maneuver? – mitral valve prolapse) and HOCM (idiopathic hypertrophic subaortic stenosis)

- o Mid-to-late systolic click plus late systolic murmur suggests mitral valve prolapse plus mitral regurgitation (MVP + MR).

Source: McGee SR. *Saunders/Elsevier* 2007, page 498 to 501; Mangione S. *Hanley & Belfus* 2000, page 251; Baliga RR. *Saunders/Elsevier* 2007, page 65; and Ghosh AK. *Mayo Clinic Scientific Press* 2008, Figure 3-9, page 49.

➢ Complications

- o Murmurs
  - Associated MR
  - SBE

- o Arrhythmias
  - VPC (ventricular premature contractions)
  - VT (Ventricular tachycardia)
  - PST (paroxysmal supraventricular tachycardia)

- o CNS
  - TIA (transient ischemic attack)
  - CVA (cerebrovascular accident)

- o Atypical chest pain

- o Sudden cardiac death

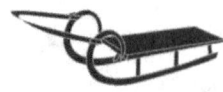

SO YOU WANT TO BE A CARDIOLOGIST!

- Give the complications of hypertrophic cardiomyopathy.

    o Sudden death
    o Atrial fibrillation
    o Infective endocarditis
    o Systemic embolization

- Give the most characteristic pathophysiological abnormality in hypertrophic cardiomyopathy.

    o Diastolic dysfunction

Source: Baliga RR. *Saunders/Elsevier* 2007, page 76.

SO YOU WANT TO BE A CARDIOLOGIST!

- Give the mechanism of the click in MVP.

    o Clicks result from sudden tensing of the mitral valve apparatus as the leaflets prolapse into the left atrium during systole.

    o Your morning smile: Mitral valve prolapse (MVP, not to be confused with most valuable [Sports] player)

"Play a crucial and critical role in finding your own humility and humanity."

Grandad

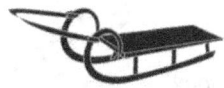

TRICUSPID REGURGITATION (TR)

➤ Clinical

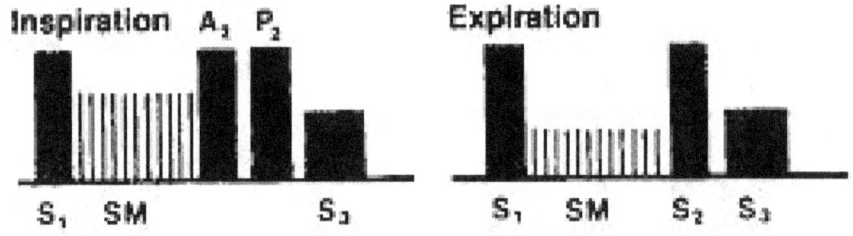

o Precordium – Right ventricular papasternal lift:
o Auscultation – Holosystolic murmur increasing with inspiration

Adapted from: Mangione S. *Hanley & Belfus* 2000, page 251.

- Perform a focused physical examination for TR.
    - o General   - Peripheral cyanosis
                        - Ankle edema
    - o Pulse   - May have associated atrial fibrillation (AF)
    - o JVP   - ↑ 'v' waves
    - o Precordium   - L. parasternal heave
                        - Heave systolic thrill at tricuspid area
                        - Heart sounds
        - ↑ P_2 (may be palpable)
        - S_3
                        - Murmur
        - Pansystolic murmur
          - L. lower SE
          - Carvallo's sign
          - ↑ with inspiration (Carvallo sign)
          - May be associated mid-diastolic murmur of associated MS
    - o Liver   - Systolic-pulsations/ bruit
                        - Hepatomegaly

| o Causes / complications | - Usually secondary to pathology elsewhere in heart. |

- o Causes / complications
  - Usually secondary to pathology elsewhere in heart.
  - Don't be tricked: mild TR is normal
  - Functional
    - HF
    - PHT (cor pulmonale)
  - Rheumatic – mitral and/ or aortic valve disease
  - Infection – R.heart endocarditis
  - Endocrine – carcinoid syndrome
  - Hereditary
    - Ebstein anomaly
    - Endomyocardial fibrosis
  - Infarction
    - RV papillary muscles
  - Miscellaneous
    - Tricuspid valve prolapse
    - Blunt trauma
  - Without pulmonary hypertension (PHT)
    - Congenital
    - Trauma
    - Endocarditis, R. side of heart
  - With (secondary to) PHT
    - Mitral stenosis plus PHT
    - ASD / R-HF plus PHT
    - R-HF plus PHT, plus L-HF

Abbreviation: ASD, atrial septal defect; HF, heart failure; LLSB, left lower sterna border; LSE, left sterna edge; PHT, pulmonary hypertension; R-HF, right-side heart failure; RV, right ventricle

Adapted from: Baliga RR. *Saunders/Elsevier* 2007, pages 64 and 65.

SO YOU WANT TO BE A CARDIOLOGIST!

- Under what circumstances is the blood pressure lower in the legs than arms (normal difference: 10-15 mm Hg higher in legs than arms)?

  - o Abnormal difference (Hill sign, > 20 mm Hg; exaggeration of normal, indicating ↑ SV (stroke volume)' such as from tachycardia
  - o Atherosclerosis in the elderly
  - o Aortic dissection
  - o Aortic regurgitation (severe)

Adapted from: Baliga RR. *Saunders/Elsevier* 2007, page 15.

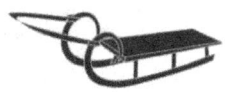

Mastering the Boards: Cardiology A.B.R. Thomson

- Give the commonest causes of a palpable pulsation in the liver.

  - ○ Tricuspid regurgitation (TR)
  - ○ Large angioma
  - ○ Hepatocellular cancer (HCC)

SO YOU WANT TO BE A CARDIOLOGIST!

- In the context of a systolic murmur, what is the significance if after a long diastole (such as following a premature beat), the intensity of the murmur becomes louder at the base but not at the apex?

  - ○ The systolic murmur is likely comprised of both a regurgitation murmur plus an ejection murmur.

- Give the exception to this general rule.

  - ○ The exception is mitral valve prolapse (MVP), in which, the murmur becomes softer after a long diastole.

- Give the explanation for the murmur of TR (tricuspid regurgitation) not being auscultated loudest at the left lower sternal border or epigastric area.

  - ○ When the RV enlarges from TR and displaces the LV laterally and postoriorly, the murmur of TR will then be heard best at the right sternal border or apex
  - ○ If the person with TR has COPD and air trapping, the murmur will be heard over the free edge of the liver.

Source: Mangione S. *Hanley & Belfus* 2000, page 264.

- In the context of tricuspid regurgitation, what is the Carvallo sign?

  - ○ The Carvallo sign is the pansystolic murmur of TR which increases with inspiration.

- In the context of inspiration and its effect on cardiac murmurs, give what is the Rivera-Carvallo (RC) maneuver, and how it differs from the Carvallo sign.

  - ○ R-C maneuver
    - Inspiration causes a louder murmur across the pulmonic valve
  - ○ Inspiration causes a louder pansystolic murmur of TR (tricuspid regurgitation, during or at the end of inspiration)
  - ○ Carvallo sign has high specificity but only 61% sensitivity to distinguish TR from MR (mitral regurgitation), in which inspiration does not cause a louder murmur.

Source: Mangione S. *Hanley & Belfus* 2000, page 218 and 258.

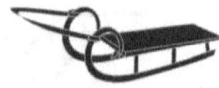

MITRAL STENOSIS (MS)

➤ Pathophysiology

- o Progressive stenosis → ↑ pressure in LA (left atrium), PA (pulmonary artery), PV (pulmonary vein) → ↓ LV diastolic filing time)

- o Sudden ↑ PA pressure (development of AF, pregnancy)
  - SOBOE (shortness of breath an exertion, i.e. exertion dyspnea)
  - Acute pulmonary edema

- o The normal area of the mitral valve is 4 to 6 cm^2.
  - The flow across the valve becomes turbulent when the cross sectional area is < 2 cm^2
  - MS is said to be "tight" when this area is < 1 cm^2.

Source: Burton JL. *Churchill Livingstone* 1971, page 7.

- o ↓ mitral valve area → ↓ LA (left atrial) filling in diastole → ↑ LAP → ↑ LAE

  ↑ LAR

  ↓   ↓

  ↑ diastolic pressure gradient between LA and LV   ↑ PVR → P-HTH

                     ↓   ↓

  RVH

                      RV dilation may cause mitral regurgitation

➤ Causes / associations
- o Rheumatic heart disease
- o Rheumatoid arthritis
- o Systemic lupus erythematosis (SLE)
- o Malignant carcinoid (carcinoid syndrome)
- o Congenital
  - Parachute mitral valve with one papillary muscle having chordate attached to both leaflets of mitral valve
- o Myxoma of left atrium
- o Calcified bacterial vegetation of mitral valve annulus and leaflets

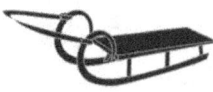

- o Mimics of MS (conditions that may simulate MS)
    - Severe MR
    - VSD
    - Austin Flint murmur of severe AR
    - Carry Coombs murmur of active rheumatic carditis (may cause MS- or TS-like murmur)
    - Ball valve thrombus in LA
    - Cor triatriatum (a rare congenital heart condition where a thin membrane across the left atrium obstructs pulmonary venous flow)

Abbreviations: MR, mitral regurgitation; VSD, ventricular septal defect; AL, left atrium

Adapted from: Mangione S. *Hanley & Belfus* 2000. page 266 to 269; and Baliga RR. *Saunders/Elsevier* 2007, pages 4 and 7.

- Give the commonest cause of mitral stenosis.

    - o Rheumatic heart disease.

- Give rare causes of MS.

    - o Congenital
    - o Rheumatoid arthritis
    - o SLE
    - o Malignant carcinoid
    - o Mitral valve calcification

Abbreviation: SLE, systemic lupus erythematosis; MS, mitral stenosis

- ➢ Etiology: ↓ mitral valve area

    - o Inherited   - Congenital

    - o Infection   - Rheumatic fever → mitral valve ⎤ Fusion of
                 Thick   Chordae
                 Fibrotic   Papillary muscles
                 Calcified   Leaflets
                       Commission

             - SLE (systemic lupus erythematous)

    - o Surgery   - Patient prosthesis mismatch
                    - Annuloplasty ring too small overseen

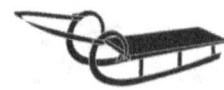

- o Obstruction of outflow from left atrium
  - Tumor
  - Thrombus
  - Endocarditis
  - Congenital membrane LA (Cor triatriatum)

- ➢ Clinical

  - o ↑ symptoms
    - Exercise
    - Fever
    - Pregnancy ⎤ ↓ diastolic filling
    - Hyperthyroidism ⎦ ↓ LV-CO
    - Atrial fibrillation with
    - ↑ ventricular response

  - o Signs
    - Characteristics features of the murmur, and their significance
      - ↑ S1   Only when leaflets of mitral valve are flexible
      - OS   Sudden tensing of valve leaflets
        ↑ A2 – OS interval less severe stenosis
        More severe MS ↓ A2-OS internal (inverse proportionality)
      - Diastole   Low-pitch, mid-diastolic rumble, heard best with bell at apex
    - Signs of pulmonary hypertension
      - ↑ P2
      - PA tap
      - PV heave
      - TR (tricuspid regurgitation)
    - Signs of right-sided heart failure (R-HF)
      - ↑ JVP
      - Hepatomegaly
      - Ascites
      - Peripheral edema

  - o Mitral stenosis- use bell, lightly applied at apex with patient on L side after exercise. Presystolic accentuation is often a sign of pure stenosis, but is absent in atrial fibrillation

  - o Head/ neck
    - Malar flush
    - ↑ JVP

  - o Peripheral pulse – sinus or AF

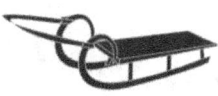

- o Apex
    - Tapping (5th ICS, MCL)
    - Diastolic thrill
    - Left parasternal heave (RV large)

- o Heart sounds
    - ↑ S_1
    - OS (apex, left decubitus position)
    - ↑ S_2 (from ↑P_2)
    - ↑ S_3 (rapid LV filling)

CLINICAL GEM

Pathophysiologically, the murmuring of mitral stenosis is more severe with

- o ↓ mitral valve area (< 1.0 cm²)
- o ↑ LAP
- o ↑ LAE
  Diastolic pressure
  ↑ gradient > 10 mmHg (LA and LV)
- o ↑ PVR
- o ↑ P-HTN
- o ↑ RV-overload
- o ↓ CO
- o LA – LV mean gradient > 10 mmHg
- o PASP > 50 mmHg

- Give the auscultated characteristics of the murmur of MS which that it is hemodynamically more severe.

    - o Short A2 – OS internal
    - o ↑ duration of diastolic murmur
    - o Point deduction for saying that a louder murmur of MS is more severe

Abbreviations: A2 – OS interval, interval between aortic component of second heart sound, and opening snap of mitral valve leaflet; LA, left atrium; LV, left ventricle; MS, mitral stenosis

---

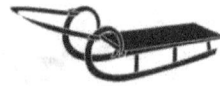

o Selected features of diastolic murmurs

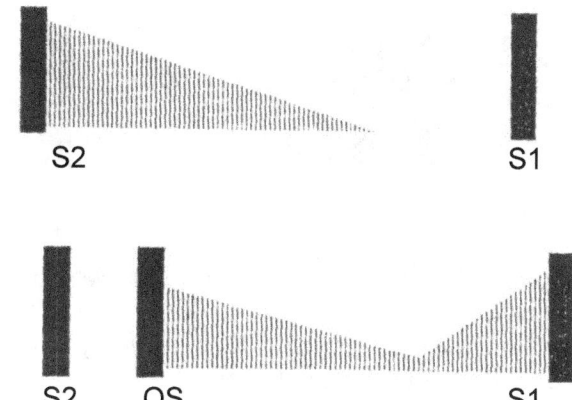

Adapted from: Simel DL, et al. *JAMA* 2009, Figure 32-2, page 421.

o Teaching point

- Presystolic accentuation is present only if the patient is in sinus rhythm

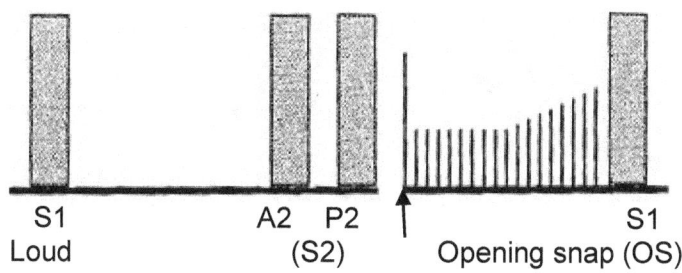

o Teaching point
- This distance between S2 (A2, P2) and OS is inversely proportional to the severity of the stenosis

Source: Talley NJ, et al. *Maclennan & Petty Pty Limited* 2003, Figure 3.28, page 74

Systole   Diastole

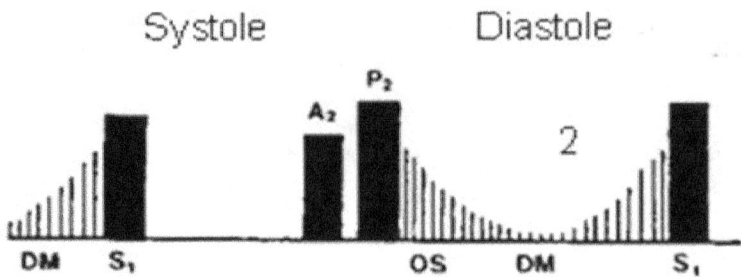

Auscultation-loud S1, P2 diastolic opening snap followed by rumble with presystolic accentuation. Atrial fibrillation may be pulse pattern. Cold extremities. 1) This distance is inversely proportional to the severity of the stenosis; 2) Presystolic accentuation is present only if patient is in sinus rhythm

- o Murmur
  - - Rumbling
  - - Low-pitched
  - - Mid-diastolic
  - - Left lateral position
  - - During expiration
  - - Presystolic accentuation
  - - Louder after sit-ups or hopping

- o Periphery
  - - Cold

➢ Assessment of severity

- o The louder the murmur and the thrill, the more severe the MS

- o Conditions making murmur louder without necessarily a greater pressure gradient(false positive), unless there is associated pulmonary hypertension which softens the murmur of severe MS, and unless there is associated mitral regurgitation (which increases diastolic flow across the mitral valve making a louder murmur of MS)

- o Conditions making murmur softer, causing overestimation of severity (false negative)
  - - Emphysema
  - - Very severe stenosis mitral or tricuspid valve
  - - Severe pulmonary hypertension
  - - Atrial fibrillation

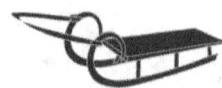

Clinical Gem

- Give what is the effect of the development of atrial fibrillation on the murmur of MS.

    o The usual presystolic accentuation disappears.

- Give what is "mitral facies".

    o Dilated capillaries and venules on face
    o Is not pathognomonic for MS

- In MS, there is right ventricular hypertrophy, without LV enlargement. In the patient with MS who has a displaced apex beat suggesting left ventricular hypertrophy, give what are the explanations (murmur of MS, plus displaces apex beat).

    o A second disease valve (eg aortic regurgitation)
    o Systemic hypertension
    o Pericardial adhesions

Note: MS plus HF does not by itself give a displaced apex beat.

- Give features obtained from auscullation which suggest that the murmur of MS is severe.

    o Long murmur of MS
    o S_1 loud
    o Opening snap close to S_2

SO YOU WANT TO BE A CARDIOLOGIST!

- Give the definition of the Austin Flint murmur.

    o Diastolic murmur (rumble) caused by functional closure of the anterior leaflet of mitral valve when there is moderate-to-severe aortic regurgitation,
    o Distinguish from MS by the absence of an opening snap in a non-calcified valve, and the presence of S3 (rare in mitral stenosis).

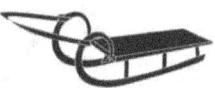

- Give the performance characteristics of other cardiac findings in mitral stenosis.

Finding (Ref)	PLR
o Graham Steell murmur	
- Detecting pulmonary hypertension	4.2
o Hyperkinetic apical movement	
- Detecting associated mitral regurgitation or aortic valve disease	11.2
o Hyperkinetic arterial pulse	
- Detecting associated mitral regurgitation	14.2

Source: McGee SR. *Saunders/Elsevier* 2007, page 506.

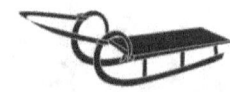

SO YOU WANT TO BE A CARDIOLOGIST!

- A mid-diastolic murmur is auscultated, and MS is suspected. Give the differential of the causes of a murmur which simulates MS.
  - LA myxoma
  - Ball valve thrombus of LA
  - ASD
  - Cor tri atriatum (a membrane across the LA which partially blocks the pulmonary venous flow)

- In the context of a mid-diastolic murmur, which must be differentiated from MS, what is Lutembacher syndrome, and Ortner's syndrome?
  - Lutembacher syndrome: ASD + MS
  - Ortner syndrome: Large LA in MS causing paralysis of left vocal cord, leading to hoarsensess.

Source: Baliga RR. *Saunders/Elsevier* 2007, page 7.

Trick Question

- Give what the clinical significance of the diastolic murmur of MS becoming softer
  - When the stenosis across the mitral valve becomes tighter, the murmur becomes less prominent, even to the point of disappearing.

- Give effect of pregnancy on MS.
  - Patients usually become symptomatic in T_2
  - Blood volume increases

- In the context of MS, give the meaning of Ortner syndrome.
  - Hoarseness of voice cause by keft vocal cord paralysis associated with enlarged left atrium in mitral stenosis

Source: Baliga RR. *Saunders/Elsevier* 2007, pages 4 and 7.

- Give two circumstances when an opening snap (OS) does not occur with mitral stenosis (MS)
  - Combined MS and MR (mitral regurgitation)
  - Calcified mitral stenosis

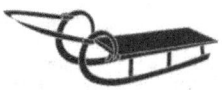

➤ Complications

- Give complications of MS.
  - LA enlargement
  - AF
  - Embolization (eg CVA)
  - PHT
  - TR
  - R-HF

Abbreviation: AF, atrial fibrillation; LA, left atrium; PHT, pulmonary hypertension; R-HF, right-sided heart failure; TR, tricuspid regurgitation.

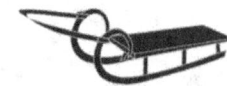

➤ Diagnostic tests
- GCG
  - P mitrale (P wave in lead II ≥ 0.12 sec, indicating left atrial enlargement [LAE])
  - RVH (right ventricular hypertrophy)
  - AF (atrial fibrillation)
- Chest X-ray
  - Enlarged
    - LA (LAE)
    - RV
    - RA
    - Pulmonary arteries
  - Calcified mitral
    - Valve
    - Annulus
- Transthoracic echocardiogram (TTG)
  - Morphology of MV
    - Mitral valve area
    - Mean transmitral gradient (LA-LV)
    - RV size and function
    - PASP (pulmonary artery systolic pressure)
    - Hemodynamics
- TTE or RHC (right heart catheterization) exercise testing
  - Mean transmitral gradient
  - PASP with exercise (function capacity)
- Transesophageal echocardiogram (TEE)
  - MV morphology / hemodynamics not optimally clarified by TTG
  - LA clot diagnosis
  - Assessment of morphology for possible percutaneous mitral balloon (PMBV)
- Cardiac catheterization
  - Clarify any discrepancy in clinical vs. echo assessment of MS severity
  - Access cause / reversibility of pulmonary hypertension

• Give the typical findings on chest X-ray (CHX) and ECG of the patient with MS (mitral stenosis).
- CHX   - ↑ LA, ↑ RV, ↑ RA, ↑ PA
- ECG   - RVH (right ventricular hypertrophy)
                   - P pulmonale: P wave
    - Notched
    - > 0.12 sec in lead II

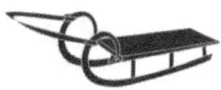

Trick Question

- In the patient with known MS, give the meaning of the loss of the opening snap (OS)?
    - The OS is caused by the opening of the stenosed valve when the leaflets are pliable. Once the leaflets become calcified, the OS disappears.

The high-pitched OS occurs shortly after S_2, and the shorter the interval between S_2 and OS, the higher the LA pressure.

- Give the clinical significance of a short interval between S_2 and OS?
    - A short interval between S2 and OS signifies ↑ LA pressure, and greater severity of MS.

- The rumbling, low-pitched, mid-diastolic murmur of MS may be associated with presystolic accentuation give the cause of the presystolic accentuation, first when the patient is in sinus arythm, and secondly in atrial fibrillation (AF).
    - Sinus rhythm: increased flow during atrial systole across the narrowed.
    - AF: turbulent flow across the mitral valve at the start of ventricular systole

- Give 3 findings suggesting that the MS is severe.
    - Short distance between S_2 and OS
    - Long duration of MS murmur
    - Murmur of MS becoming softer
    - Signs of pulmonary hypertension (PHT)

- Give the indications for **TEE** (transesophageal echocardiogram) **in** MS.

    - Confirm MS diagnosis.

    - Detect a thrombus

    - Evaluate source of thrombus in patient suffering from thromboembolic event

➢ Treatment

    - β-blockers will be help to increase the ↓ LV diastolic filling time

    - Anti-coagulation for AF (atrial fibrillation), paroxysmal or chronic

    - Percutaneous balloon Valvulotomy

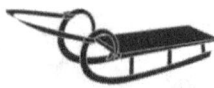

- o Surgical valve replacement
  - Symptoms
  - Pulmonary artery systolic pressure
    - At rest ≥ 50 mm Hg
    - With exercise ≥ 60 mm Hg

- Give the treatment of mitral stenosis.
  - o Pharmacological   - If sinus tachycardia
    - BB or CCB
    - New onset AF
      - BB or CCB, plus heparin → warfarin → long-term A/C :
    - Rhythm
      - AF, paroxysmal or transient
      - Sinus rhythm plus LA diameter > 5 cm
    - Thrombus
      - Previous thromboembolic event
      - LA thrombus
    - Treat all patients with MS and AF, with warfarin, regardless of CHADS2 score

  - o Surgery (commissurotomy, or MV replacement) when percutaneous valvulotomy less likely to be successful
    - Leaflets of MV stiff
    - Calcification: valvular or subvalvular
    - Fusion of commissure

  - o Electrical cardioversion - New onset AF

  - o Percutaneous valvulotomy
    - Symptoms from MS, plus
    - MV area < 1 cm^2, or
    - MV area < 1.5 cm^2 plus limitations on ability to exercise
    - Clinical caution: do not perform percutaneous valvulotomy for MS if there is associated MR

Abbreviations: A/C, anticoagulation; AF, atrial fibrillation; BB, beta blocker; CCB, calcium channel blocker; LA, left atrium, MS, mitral stenosis; MR, mitral regurgitation; MV

- o Treat associated conditions
  - Rheumatic fever
  - HF (heart failure)
  - AF (atrial fibrillation)
    - Occurs in ~ 1/3 MS patients
    - Treat with B-blockers, diltiazem or

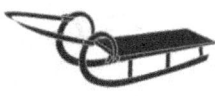

- - Risk of thromboembolism
    - Anticoagulation, when verapamil indicated (please see below)
  - o Exercise-induced symptoms
    - B-blockers
    - Non-dihydropyridine CCBs
      - Diltiazem
      - Verapamil
    - Digoxin less effective for control of tachycardia with exercise
  - o Anti-coagulation (INR 2.0 – 3.0) in MS
    - Prior embolic event
    - LA thrombus
    - Associated atrial fibrillation
  - o Note – the American College of Cardiology (ACC) and the American Heart Association (AHA) do not recommend antibiotic prophylaxis for rheumatic MS

- Percutaneous Mitral Balloon Valvotomy (PMBV)
  - o Indications (ACC / AHA guidelines)
    - Symptoms NYHA II to IV; moderate / severe MS; acceptable morphology of MV
      - No LA thrombus
    - Asymptomatic
      - Moderate / severe MS, acceptable morphology of MV: no LA thrombus
      - PASP
        - 50 mmHg at rest
        - > 60 mmHg with exercise
  - o Benefits
    - Transmitral gradient ~ 50%
    - Cardiac out ↑ 10% to 20%
    - Mitral valve area ↑ 1.0 to 2.0 cm^2
  - o Prognosis
    - "event" free survival (is repeat PMBV, MV surgical replacement or death) at 3-7 yr
      - 80% to 90%
  - o Complications
    - CNS
    - Heart
      - Mitral regurgitation (MR) requiring surgical connection
    - ASD (atrial septal defect)
    - Death (1%)

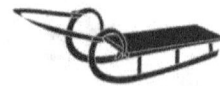

Surgical Valve Replacement

- o Failed / unavailable / contraindicated PMBV (percutaneous mitral balloon valvotomy) in symptomatic NYHA III/IV with moderate / severe MS with acceptable operative risk

- o Open or closed surgical mitral commissurotomy

➢ Prognosis

- o Asymptomatic or minimal symptoms at presentation of MS ~ 10 yr survival 80%

- o Symptomatic

- o Severe pulmonary hypertension
  - - 10 yr, survival ~ 10%
  - - Mean survival yr

Tricuspid Stenosis (TS)

➢ Causes
  - o Associated with
    - - TR
    - - MS
  - o SLE
  - o Carcinoid tumor

- Perform a focused physical examination to distinguish between the diastolic murmurs of mitral stenosis (MS) versus tricuspid stenosis (TS).

Physical finding	TS	MS
o Location	Epigastric and R/L parastenal area Over apex if RV is very large	
o Effect on murmur of inspiration	Louder	Softer
o Position to best hear murmur	R lateral decubitus	L lateral decubitus
o Quality	"scratchy"	Low pitch
o Presystolic accentuation	Absent	Present

Source: Mangione S. *Hanley & Belfus* 2000, pages 266 to 269.

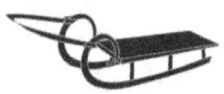

RHEUMATIC FEVER AND RHEUMATIC HEART DISEASE

➢ Clinical

- Take a directed history and perform a focused physical examination for rheumatic fever and rheumatic heart disease (RHD).

- o Heart
  - Endocarditis
  - Pericarditis
  - Valvulitis
  - yocarditis (MV > AV)
- o CNS
  - Chorea
- o Systemic
  - Weight loss, fever
- o Joints
  - Polyarthritis

- o Skin
  - Rheumatic nodules
  - Non-tender, painless, subcutaneous lesions along tendons and over bony prominences on back of hands, elbows, knees, spine)
  - Erythema multiforme
- o Blood
  - Anemia
- o Lung
  - Pleursy, pneumonia
- o GI
  - Peritonitis

Abbreviations: AV, aortic valve; CNS, central nervous system; GI, gastrointestinal; MV, mitral valve; RHD, rheumatic heart disease;

Adapted from: Davey P. *Wiley-Blackwell* 2006, pages 30 and 31.

- Give the **Ducket Jones diagnostic criteria** for the diagnosis of rheumatic fever (RF).

- Major
  - o CNS – chorea
  - o Heart – carditis
  - o Skin
    - Subcutaneous nodules
    - Erythema marginatum
  - o MSK
    - Polyarthitis

- Minor
  - o Clinical
    - Arrthralgias
    - Fever
  - o Bacteriology – throat culture evidence for group A hemolytic streptococcal infection
  - o Laboratory
    - ↑ acute phase reactants (erythrocyte sedimentation rate [ESR], C-reactive protein)
    - Prolonged PR interval
    - Supporting evidence of antecedent group A streptococcal infection
      - Positive throat culture or rapid diagnostic test
      - Elevated or rising streptococcal antibody titer

Diagnosis of RF = 2 major, or 1 major plus 2 minor criteria
Usual affected valves: mitral > aortic

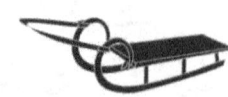

➢ Ducket Jones diagnostic criteria for Rheumatic Fever

Rheumatic fever= 2 major or 1 major+ 2 minor + evidence of recent streptococcal infection (Group A streptococcal (throat) infection can → immune reaction → acute rheumatic fever).

Abbreviations: CRP, C reactive protein; ESR, erythrocyte sedimentation rate.

Adapted from: Davies IJT. *Lloyd-Luke LTD* 1972, page 30, 31; Davey P. *Wiley-Blackwell* 2006, page 166; Burton JL. *Churchill Livingstone* 1971, page 9.

Major Criteria for the Diagnosis of Rheumatic Fever (Ducket Jones)

- o Carditis
  - Murmurs, often mitral stenosis (MS), may take years for the murmur to appear
- o HF
  - Cardiomegaly
  - Pericarditis
  - Arrhythmia

- o Polyarthritis
  - Large joints
  - Severity may be inversely proportional to severity of chorea

- o Rheumatic nodules
  - Usually seen in children, not adults
  - Seen in severe infection
  - Usually indicates cardiac involvement
  - Attatched to tendons, ligaments (not to skin)
  - Painless
  - No inflammation

- o Erythema marginatum
  - Tender red, nodules on legs, thighs
  - Distinguish from rheumatic nodules, or rash due to sweating or salicylates.

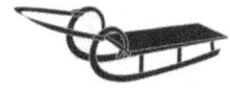

- o Sydenham chorea (chorei form movement)
  - Usually face & upper limbs affected
  - Bilateral
  - ↑ by emotion or observation
  - ↓ by sleep
  - Ataxia
  - Weakness
  - Choreiform movements often inversely proportional to severity of the arthritis

Curiosity: pregnant women with rheumatic fever often develop mania.

CLINICAL CHALLENGE

- In the patient with 2 murmurs, and using just the vital signs, determine which is likely the prominent murmur.

  - o MS + AR
    - If there is atrial fibrillation, MS is the main murmur
    - If there is ↑ pulse pressure, AR is the main murmur

  - o AS + AR
    - Determine which is the main murmur from the character of the pulse (collapsing → AI, plateau → AS)

Caution: in the older person with onset of a diastolic murmur suggestive of MS, consider the possibility of an atrial myxoma.

- Give the features seen on a chest X-ray which suggest the presence of MS?
  - o Enlarged hilar vessels, usually large pulmonary artery and left main branch
  - o Enlarged RA, but not LV

- ➤ Radiation of murmurs
  - o Apical murmur to base of heart
  - o Basal murmur to axilla

- Give the two diseases which are the usual causes of combined AS plus AR.
  - o Atherosclerosis
  - o Rheumatic heart disease
  - o Rheumatic heart disease or combined AS plus MS/MR?

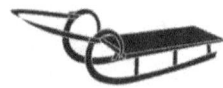

➢ Treatment

- Give the treatment for rheumatic fever (RF).

  o ASA (aspirin)
  o Antibiotic (penicillin, erythromycin allergy) long-term for both
     - Rheumatic heart disease for 16 year after last attack of RF, or
       until age 40 year (whichever is longer)

> A Trick Question:
>
> ASA (aspirin) plus antibiotics are the drugs of choice for rheumatic fever
> (RF).
>
> - Give the second-line drug if there is a poor response to ASA.
>
>   o None: the trick is, if "RF" does not respond to ASA, then it's
>   probably not "RF" → look for another diagnosis

- Give the **rheumatological disorders**, which are assorted with 8 of the
  following cardiac conditions.

o Pericarditis disease	-	SLE (25%-50%)
	-	RA (~30%)
	-	SSC
	-	BS
o Myocardial disease	-	SSC
	-	BS
	-	PN
	-	SAR
o Aortitis, arteritis	-	SAR
	-	AS (25%-60%)
	-	TA
o Endocarditis	-	SLE (~20%-60%)
o Premature CAD	-	SLE (↑ risk 50x!)
	-	RA
	-	KD

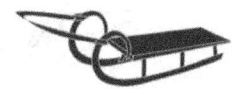

o   Valve disease
- AR SLE (~20%), AS (~40%), BS
- Leaflet fibrosis
- RA (~15%)

o   LV diastolic dysfunction
- AS

o   Conduction defects,
arrhythmias
- AS (~10%)
- BS
- SAR

o   Systemic hypertension
- SSC
- SSC renal crisis
- TA

o   Pulmonary artery
hypertension
- SSC

o   Peripheral artery disease
- GCA

Note: All of these systemic inflammation disorders are MSK (musculoskeletal) disorders, also considered in the Chapter on Rheumatological disorders

Abbreviations: AR, aortic regurgitation; AS, ankylosing spondylitis; BS, Behcet syndrome; GCA, giant cell arthritis; KD, Kawasaki disease; PW, polyarteritis nodosa; RA, rheumatoid arthritis; SAR, sarcoidosis; SLE, systemic lupus erythematosus; SSC, systemic sclerosis; TA, Takayasu arteritis

American Heart Associated:http://www.my.americanheart.org/professional/guidelines.jsp

Framingham Risk Calculation: http://www.hp2010.nhlbihin.net/atpiii/calculator.asp?usertype=prof.

Cardiology / American Heart Association Task Force on Practice Guidelines: www.cardiosource.org/~/media/Images?ACC/Science%20and%20Quality/Practice%20Quality/Practice%20guidelines/s/stable_clean.ashx

"Science, like good diagnosis, represents incremental progress of small steps taken slowly on solid ground."
Grandad

 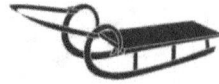

CARDIOGENIC SHOCK

➤ Definition

- o SBP < 80-90 mm Hg
- o MAP ↓ 30 mm Hg from baseline
- o CI (cardiac index)

Hemodynamic support	CI (L/min per m^2)
No	< 2.0-2.2
Yes	< 1.8

➤ Pathogenesis

↓ CO → ↓ SBP → ↓ tissue perfusion → end organ damage

- o CNS   Confusion
- o Liver   ↑ AST, ALT, bilirubin
- o Kidney   Acute kidney injury (AKI)
- o Extremities   Cool

➤ Diagnosis

- o Emergency echocardiogram ± PA (pulmonary artery) catheter
- o Diagnose (echocardiogram) and treat under lying causes
  - LV   Free wall rupture
               Infarction (↓ RV function → ↓ LV function)
  - RV
  - VSD (ventricular septal defect)
  - MR (mitral regurgitation)

Abbreviations: CO, cardiac output; LV, left ventricle; MR, mitral regurgitation; RV, right ventricle; SBP, systolic blood pressure; VSD, ventricular septal defect

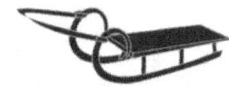

➤ Treatment

    ◦ Vasopressors by central venous catheter
        - First-line
          Dopamine
        - Second-line
          Epinephrine
          ↓

Cardiogenic
◦ ↓ CO, SV

↓ tissue perfusion
tissue ischemia
SBP < 90 mm Hg
acute ↓ SBP by > 40 mm Hg

No initial MAP response to IV fluids
MAP < 60 mm Hg

Hypovolemic		Distribution
◦ ↓ preload		◦ ↓ systemic vascular resistance

↑   ↑   ↑

◦ IV crystalloid, with CVP monitoring

◦ RBC transfusion
  Target hemoglobin concentration ≤ 70 g/L (7.0 g/dL), unless
  - Active bleeding
  - Acute coronary syndrome
  - Active bleeding
  - Acute coronary syndrome

◦ CNS
  - ↓ LOC (level of consciousness)

◦ Kidney
  - ↓ UO (urine output)

◦ General
  - ↑ serum LA (lactic acidosis)

◦ Vassopressors
  - First-line
    Norepinephrine
    Dopamine
  - Second-line
    Epinephrine

◦ Low dose corticosteroids for lack of response to vasopressors

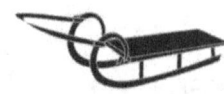

➢ Treatment of cardiogenic shock

- Pharmaceutical
  - ○ Vasoactive inotropic agents (↑ CO)

    | -++ | Dobutamine | β1, β2 receptors |
    | | Milrinone | Phosphodiesterase inhibitor |
    | -+ | Norepinephrine | α1, α2, β receptors |
    | + | Dopamine | D receptor |
    | | | β1 receptor (↑↑ dose) |
    | | | α1 receptor (↑↑↑ dose) |

  - ○ Peripheral vasoconstriction vasopressors (↑ SBP)
  - ○ Vasodilation (↓ afterload)
    - Arterial
      - NO (nitric oxide)
      - Nesiritide (natriuretic peptide receptors)
    - Venous
      - Nitroglycerine (NO)

- Mechanical circulatory support (aka VASs [ventricular assist devices])
  - ○ Intra-aortic balloon pump
    - Percutaneous placed
    - Surgically placed

- Cardiac transplantation

SO YOU WANT TO BE A CARDIOGRAHER!

Vassopressors used in shock act on a variety of smooth muscle receptors, and for some vasopressors their dose influences their main effect.

- For epinephrine, norepinephrine dopamine and phenylephrine, give their relative effects on the adrenergic receptors α1, β1 and β2 and the DA (dopaminergic receptor).

    | α1 = β1 | - Phenylephrine | |
    | | - Epinephrine (high dose) | Septic shock |
    | α1 > β1 | - Norepinephrine | |
    | | - Dopamine (high dose) | |
    | DA > β1 | - Dopamine (low dose) | Septic shock |
    | β1 > β2 | - Dopamine (medium) | |
    | | - Epinephrine (low) | Cardiogenic shock |

DISEASES OF THE AORTA

- ➤ Types
  - o Aneurysm
  - o Dissection
  - o Intramural hematoma
  - o Ulcer

- ➤ High risk groups
  - o Genetic syndrome
    - Marfan
    - Ehler-Danlos
    - Loeys-Dietz
    - Aortopathy associated with congenital heart disease (often ↓ bicuspid aortic valves)
    - Family history (familial thoracic aorta aneurysm / dissection)
    - GCA (giant cell arteritis)
  - o Atherosclerosis
    - Hypertension
    - Smoking
  - o Inflammation / infection
    - Syphilis
    - Takayasu arteritis

- ➤ Diagnosic imaging
  - o Echocardiogram
    - Root and proximal ascending aorta
  - o CT, MRI
    - All parts of aorta and side branches

- ➤ Surveillance
  - o Rapid expansion > 0.5 cm / yr
  - o Absolute size > 5 cm by CT, MRI
  - o Etiology

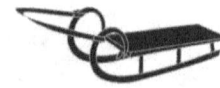

- Take a directed history and perform a focused physical examination for acute aortic syndromes (dissection, intramural hematoma, penetrating atherosclerotic ulcer)

  - History   -   Pain
    - Severe
    - "tearing" quality

  - Physical   -   BP
    - Differences between ARMS
    - PR
      - Differences between ARMS
    - Aortic valve
      - Murmur of aortic insufficiency

Abbreviations: BP, heart rate; PR, pulse rate

SO YOU WANT TO BE A CARDIOLOGIST!

- In the context of genetic disease of the aorta and Marfan syndrome, give the meaning of the Loeys-Dietz syndrome, and the reason why making this diagnosis is important.

  - The patient with Loeys-Dietz syndrome has the body phenotype of Marfan syndrome, plus
    - Palate   • Cleft
    - Uvular   • Bifid
    - Skull   • Craniosynostosis
    - Skin   • ↑ telorism
      - Thin skin

  - Surveillance for aortic disease
    - Marfan syndrome
      TTE at diagnosis
    - Loeys-Dietz syndrome
      MRI from head to pelvis every year

  - Endovascular stent grafts

  - Surgical repair (CT, MRI; external diameter)
    - Marfan syndrome   ≥ 5 cm
    - Loey-Dietz syndrome   4.4-4.6 cm

Abbreviations: TTE, transthoracic echocardiography

 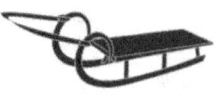

➢ Treatment
- o Treat associated
  - - Conditions
  - - Complications (e.g. hypertension, risk factors associated with atherosclerosis)
- o Follow literature for further evidence of use of ARBs (angiotensin receptor blockers)
- o When not in shock
  - - β-blocker to ↓ heart rate to 60-80 bpm; then
  - - IV sodium nitroprusside or fenoldopam to ↓ MAP (mean arterial pressure)
  - - Atheroma in ascending aorta or arch plus otherwise unexplained CVA
    - ▪ Statin
    - ▪ Warfarin (INR 2.0-3.0)

- o Endovascular stent grafts
  - - Type A aortic dissection, descending thoracic aorta
  - - Major complication (~5%)
    - ▪ CVA
  - - Techniques

▪ Dissection	- Continuing despite medical therapy
	- Visceral or limb ischemia
▪ Hematoma	(Contained rupture)
▪ Ulcer	- Diameter ≥ 20 mm
	- Depth > 10 mm

  - - ▪ Ulcer plus intramural hematoma

- o Surgery, including associated defects in aortic valves
  - - Major complications
    - ▪ Spinal cord injury
  - - Indications
    - ▪ Type A aortic dissection (proximal left subclavian artery)

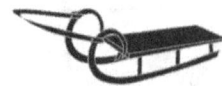

Coarctation of the Aorta (adult type)

➢ Definition
   o Narrowing of descending aorta, usually below left subclavian artery

➢ Clinical

• Take a directed history and perform a focused physical examination for coarctation of the aorta.

• History

- Exertional	▪	Fatigue
	▪	Headaches
	▪	Claudication

   - Hypertension
   - HF (heart failure)

- Early onset	▪	Aortic dissection
	▪	Recoarctation
	▪	Aneurysm after repair
	▪	CAD (coronary artery disease)
	▪	CVA (cerebrovascular accident)
	▪	AF (atrial fibrillation)

• Perform a **physical examination** for coarctation of the aorta.

o Precordium	-	AS (aortic stenosis) murmur
		▪ Over left infraclavicular area back
		▪ Collateral intercostal arteries
	-	Continuous murmur over back
o Brachial artery	-	Systolic hypertension
o Radial artery	-	Delay in pulse between radial and femoral arteries (radial-to-femoral delay)
o Femoral pulse	-	Delayed, as compared to radial

   o Physical
      - Murmur systolic
      - BP upper extremities > lower (radial artery-to-femoral artery pulse delay)
      - Signs of Turner syndrome, or associated cardiac abnormalities

   o Associated findings
      - Aortic valve bicuspid (> 50% of patients)
      - Subaortic stenosis
      - VSD (ventricular septal defect)
      - Mitral valve "parachute"

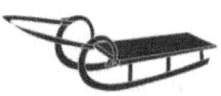

- Cerebral artery aneurysms
- Turner syndrome
  - Short women
  - Neck webbed
  - Wide chest
  - Nipples widely spaced
  - Heart defects, including
  - Aortic coarctation

You are given the stem of a patient with the above changes in the precordium as well as the brachial, radial and femoral arteries. You suspect coarctation of the aorta. You are also given a chest X-ray.

- Give the findings on **chest X-ray** which suggest coarctation of the aorta.

  o Notching of inferior surface of posterior portion of ribs
  o "figure 3" sign, arising from pressure on and indentation if the wall of the aorta, at the site of the coarctation, with dilation above and below this indentation.

- In the patient with coarctation of the aorta and notching of the ribs, give which ribs are not affected.

  o Ribs 1 & 2: intercostals arteries arise from the subclavian artery,
  o Remainder of ribs: intercostal arteries arise from the aorta belo/ abuse (?) the coarctation.

- In the patient with unrepaired coarctation of the aorta, give the circumstances when
  - The radial artery-to-femoral artery pulse delay is small, or non-existent
  - A new murmur heard over anterior or posterior chest

  o The development of collateral flow in intercostal arteries will lessen the gradient and lead to a second and new murmur

  In childhood type coarctation, there is
  - The narrowing is above the ductus arteriosus (PDA)
  - Cyanosis of the legs and clubbing of the toes
  - Cyanosis of the left, but not the right hand and arm.

- Give the explanation for these findings.
  o As a result of the associated pulmonary hypertension, unsaturated blood flows from the pulmonary artery, and is shunted through the ductus arteriosis to the lower aorta.
  o The left subclavian artery arising below the patent ductus arteriosus.

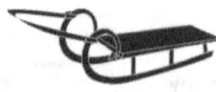

A systolic bruit heard best in the left scapular region, or the post – axillary region may be caused by either coarctation of the aorta or by a pulmonary AV aneurysm

- Give the clinical way to differentiate the two

    o With pulmonary AV aneurysm, there is associated cyanosis, whereas in adulti-type coarctation, there is no cyanosis (please not differences between adult- and childhood types of coarctation).

Systemic hypertension is commonly associated with coarctation of the aorta.

- Give in which arteries do they develop thrombosis.

    o Not in brain, heart or kidney
    o Why – no associated 'atherosclerosis (ie, while the cause of the hypertension in coarctation is not clear, it is not due to atherosclerosis)

- Give the commonest causes of death in the patient with coarctation of the aorta.

    o Brain – ruptured cerebral aneurysm
    o Heart
        - SBE
        - HF
        - Rupture of aorta

- Give the performance characteristics of aortic dissection.

Finding	Sensitivity (%)	Specificity (%)	PLR	NLR
o Individual findings				
– Pulse deficit	12-49	82-99	6.0	NS
– Aortic regurgitation murmur	15-49	45-95	NS	NS
– Focal neurologic signs	14	100	33.4	NS
o Combined findings				
– 0 predictors	4	47	0.1	...
– 1 predictor	20	...	0.5	...
– 2 predictors	49	...	5.3	...
– 3 predictors	27	100	65.8	..

Source: McGee SR. *Saunders/Elsevier* 2007, Box 14.1, page 149.

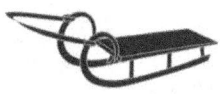

SO YOU WANT TO BE A PEDIATRIC CARDIOLOGIST!

- Give the causes rib notching.
    - Coarctation of the aorta
    - Pulmonary oligemia
    - Blalock-Taussig shunt
    - Subclavian artery obstruction
    - Superior vena caval syndrome
    - Neurofibromatosis
    - Arteriovenous malformations of the lung or the chest wall

Source: Baliga RR. *Saunders/Elsevier* 2007, page 86.

- Give the types of aortic coarctation.

➢ Common:
  - Infantile or preductal where the aorta between the left subclavian artery and patent ductus arteriosus is narrowed. Its manifests in infancy with heart failure. Associated lesion include patent ductus arteriosus, aortic arch anomalies, transposition of the great arteries, ventricular septal defect.
  - Adult type: the coarctation in the descending aorta is juxtaductal or slightly postductal. It may be associated with bicuspid aortic valve or patent ductus arteriosus. It commonly between the age of 15 and 30 years.

➢ Rare
  - Localized juxtaductal corctation
  - Coarctation of the ascending thoracic aorta

Source: Baliga RR. *Saunders/Elsevier* 2007, page 85.

- Give the fundal findings in coarctation of aorta.
  - Hypertension due to coarctation of aorta causes retinal arteries to be tortuous with frequent 'U' turns; curiously, the classical signs of hypertensive retinopathy are rarely seen.

- Young persons may be diagnosed with coarctation of the aorta, whereas in older persons aortic disease may be from dissection or obstruction from atherosclerosis. Give what abnormalities found on physical examination will suggest these diseases of the aorta?

    - Asymmetry   - R. vs L. arm   ⎤   ▪ Pulse strength, timing

                           ▪ Systolic blood
               - Arm vs Leg   ⎦   pressure

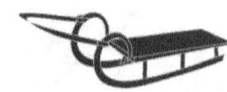

ANEURYSM AND DILATION OF THORACIC ANEURYSM

➢ Clinical

- Give the symptoms and signs which suggest aortic aneurysm with dissection.

    o Symptoms
    - Hoarseness, dysphagia
    - Pain-chest, back, abdomen, flank
    - Recurrent pneumonia
    - Cocaine abuse

    o Signs
    - SBP (systolic hypertension)
      - ↑ SPB (systolic hypertension)
      - SPB R ≠ L arms
    - Thromboembolism / dissection
      - CVA (cerebrovascular accident)
      - MI (myocardial infection)
    - Heart
      - New murmur of AR (aortic regurgitation)
      - HF (heart failure)
      - Pericardial tamponade

- Give the clinical findings which help to distinguish the murmur from an aortic aneurysm from the similar murmur of AS? In aortic aneurysm,

    o No thrill
    o No plateau pulse
    o ↑ A_2 (not ↓, as with AS)

- Give the clinical findings in aorta aneurysm which suggest the murmur is due to dissecting aortic aneurysm?

    o Expansile pulsation in right 2nd, 3rd intercostals spaces
    o Right-sternal dullness
    o Expansile pulsation on right side of neck
    o Tracheal tug in suprasternal notch

All other symptoms/signs (including pulse deficit, murmur of aortic induffiency and widened mediasternum on chest X-ray have low sensitivity – [Simel David L, Rennie Drummond, Keitz Sheri A. The Rational Clinical Examination: Evidence- based clinical diagnosis. *JAMA* 2009, Table 50-8, page 672.])

Source: Simel DL, et al. *JAMA* 2009, Chapter 50, Table 50-9, page 673.

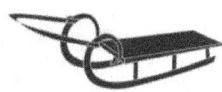

╔══╗

SO YOU WANT TO BE A CARDIOLOGIST!

- The pulse rate assessed in the right radial artery is slower than on the left side (R < L). Give the likely explanation.
  - An aneurysm of the ascending aorta, or common carotid artery.

- A patient has a higher blood pressure taken from the right as compared with the left arm, give the likely explanations.

  - R. brachial artery   - Occlusion/ stenosis

  - Aorta   - Coarctation
    - Dissection

  - Thoracic outlet syndrome

  - Heart   - Aortic stenosis (supraventricular)
    - Patent ductus arteriosus

╚══╝

➤ Differential

- Take a directed history and perform a focused physical examination to distinguish between aortic dissection (AD) and valvular aortic regurgitation.

Finding	PLR	NLR
o Chest pain		
o Pulse pressure deficit between arms (SBP > 20 mmHg between right and left arms)	6.0	NS
o Focal neurological signs (obstruction of cranial or vertebral arteries)	33.4	NS
o 2 of above findings	5.3 (> 30% ↑ probablility of AD)	-
o 3 of above findings	65.8 (> 50% ↑ probablility of AD)	
o Differences in SBP > 20 mmHg between right and left arms		

Note: The presence of aortic regurgitation is not mentioned here, since its PLR is < 2.

Abbreviation: AD, aortic dissection; PLR, positive likelihood ratio; NLR, negative likelihood ratio; NS, not significant; SBP, systolic blood pressure

Adapted from: McGee SR. *Saunders/Elsevier* 2007, Box 15.2, page 163.

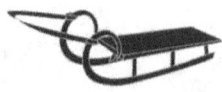

- Give the performance characteristics of the physical examination for **abdominal aortic aneurysm**.

Width of aorta by palpation	Sensitivity (%)	PLR	NLR
o ≥3.0 cm (all)	39	12.0	0.72
o 3.0 cm –3.9 cm	29		
o ≥4.0 cm		15.6	0.51
o 4.0 cm-4.9cm	50		
o ≥5.0 cm	76		

Physical sign	Sensitivity (%)	Specificity (%)
o Definite pulsatile mass	28	97
o Definite or suggestive pulsatile mass	50	91
o Abdominal bruit	11	95
o Femoral bruit	17	87
o Femoral pulse deficit	22	91

➢ Treatment

- Give the treatment of thoracic aneurysm.
  - o Surveillance — Echocardiography every 1 hour until 4.5 cm aortic root, thereafter every 6 months
  - o Prevention of enlargement
    - BB (beta-blockers) to slow growth of thoracic aneurysm
    - Treat associated hypertension
    - Advise female patient from become pregnant
  - o Surgery
    - Prophylactic
    - Hoarseness, dysphagia, back pain
    - Size of aorta aneurysm
      - Ascending (type A) > 5 cm
      - Descending (type B) > 6 cm
      - Rapid annual growth > 1 cm
    - Urgent
      - For type A (ascending aorta) dissection
      - For type B dissections (descending thoracic aorta)
        - Medical therapy, unless
        - Renal arteries involved
          - Do **not** use hydralazine to treat hypertension associated with acute aortic dissection

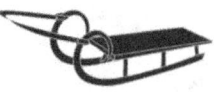

o Sensitivity of findings for thoracic aortic dissection (TAD)

Finding	Sensitivity
- History	
• Hypertension	65%
• Hypertension, age <40 y	34%
- Symptoms	
• Abrupt onset	84%
• Abrupt onset < 40 y	96%
• Chest pain	71%
• Chest pain, age <40 y	100%

Symptom or sign	PLR	NLR
o Focal neurologic deficit	6.6-33	0.7-0.9
o Pulse deficit	5.7	0.7
o Enlarged aorta or wide mediastinum	2.0	0.3
o Chest radiograph		
- Widened mediastinum	0.63	

- Note: Some possible findings in TAD are not included because the sensitivity is < 66%. These would include
  - Age < 40 y (0.05)
  - Marfan syndrome (0.04)
  - Pulse deficit (0.32)
  - Murmur of aortic insufficiency (0.28)
  - Back pain (0.30).

Source: Simel DL, et al. *JAMA* 2009, Table 50-8, page 672.

- Give the **treatment** of Abdominal Aortic Aneurysm (AAA).

  o Surveillance
    - Abdominal utrasound (AUS)
    - AAA < 4 cm q 2-3 yr
    - AAA 4 to 5.4 cm q 6-12 mon

  o Prevention of enlargement
    - Treat associated hypertension

  o Surgery urgent for ruptured AAA
    - Elective AAA ≥ 5.5 cm diameter, or rapid annual growth > 0.5 cm

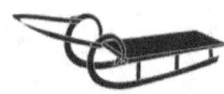

- o   Unproven use   -   Statins (except for associated hyperlipidemia)
  -   ACE inhibitors (except for associated hypertension)
  -   Antibiotics (macrolides) for Chlamydia pneumonia positive serology
- o   EVAR (endovascular aneurysm repair, useful in high-risk surgical candidates)
- o   Open surgery repair

Aortic Cholesterol Atheroemboli

- Perform a focused physical examination for **aortic cholesterol atheroemboli**.
  - o   Eye   -   Yellow body in arteries (Hollenhorst plaque)
  - o   Skin   -   Livedo reticularis (purplish discolouration)
  - o   Kidney   -   Gangrene of digits
    -   Cholesterol embolization
  - o   CNS   -   ↑ risk of CVA
  - o   Risk factors   -   Recent cardiac or aortic
    - Catheterization
    - Surgery

Syphilitic Aortitis

- Perform a focused physical examination for syphilitic aortitis with saccular aneurysm of aorta.

  - o   Nerves
    - L. recurrent laryngeal nerve
      - Hoarseness or aphonia
    - Cervical sympathetic nerve
      - Unequal pupils (Horner's syndrome)

  - o   Trachea
    - Tug
    - Displacement
    - Stridor

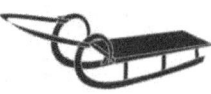

- o Bronchi
  - Cough
  - Atelectasis
- o Brachial artery
  - Difference in BP in arms > 20 mmHg
- o Heart
  - Aortic dilation
  - AR
  - Signs of MI, from obstruction of coronary arteries
  - Signs of myocarditis
  - Conduction defects (syphilitic gamma)
- o Bone
  - Erosion of spine, pulsation in region of L. scapula
  - Bulging of aortic area of chest wall

Abbreviations: AR, aortic regurgitation; BP, blood pressure; MI, myocardial infarction

Source: Davies IJT. *Lloyd-Luke LTD.*, 1972, page 38.

- Give clinical features that suggest that a patient's AR is not due to the commonest cause (rheumatic fever), but rather is due to syphilis.

  - o No murmurs other than just AR
  - o Angina, not relieved with nitrates
  - o Calcified ascending aorta

SO YOU WANT TO BE A CARDIOLOGIST!

- Give the circumstances when the blood pressure lower in the legs than arms (normal difference: 10-15 mm Hg higher in legs than arms).

  - o Abnormal difference (Hill sign, > 20 mm Hg; exaggeration of normal, indicating ↑ SV (stroke volume)' such as from tachycardia
  - o Atherosclerosis in the elderly
  - o Aortic dissection
  - o Aortic regurgitation (severe)

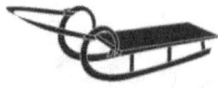

HEART FAILURE

➢ Causes

• Give causes of congestive heart failure (HF).

➢ LV failure (L-HF, systolic dysfunction)

- ○ *Inadequate LV filling*
  - Mitral stenosis
  - LV diastolic dysfunction (e.g. LVH)
  - Pericardial constriction

- ○ Pressure overload
  - Aortic stenosis
  - Systemic hypertension
  - Pulmonary hypertension

- ○ *Volume overload*
  - Aortic or mitral regurgitation
  - High output heart failure e.g. beri beri, thyrotoxicosis, Paget disease, AV fistula

- ○ LV muscle disease
  - Myocardial infarction
  - Cardiomyopathy – hypertrophic, dilated, restrictive
  - Myocarditis

➢ RV failure (R-HF, diastolic dysfunction)

- ○ Secondary to L-HF

- ○ Secondary to pulmonary hypertension ([cor pulmonate] e.g. PEs, chronic lung disease)

- ○ Mitral stenosis

- ○ Tricuspid regurgitation

- ○ Atrial myxoma

- ○ Congenital heart disease (atrial septal defect)

Abbreviation: AV, aortic valve; HF, heart failure; L-HF, left sided heart failure; LV, left ventricle; NSAIDs, nonsteroidal anti-inflammatory drugs; PE, pulmonary embolus; R-HF, right-sided heart failure; RV, right ventricle

Adapted from: Ghosh AK. *Mayo Clinic Scientific Press* 2008, Table 3-36; and Burton JL. *Churchill Livingstone*, 1971.

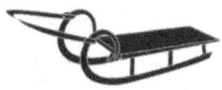

- Give factors that can precipitate / exacerbate heart failure (HF).

  - Patient-specific factors
    - Non-compliance with drug therapy inadequate dosing or dietary restrictions
    - Anemia
    - Arrhythmias (eg. Atrial fibrillation, bradycardia)
    - Infections (bacterial, viral)
    - Myocardial ischemia / infarction
    - Pulmonary embolism
    - Renal dysfunction
    - Uncontrolled hypertension
    - Valvular heart disease

  - Drugs
    - Drugs that cause sodium and fluid retention:
      - NSAIDs including selective COX-2 inhibitors and high-dose salicylates (Na+ retaining medications)
      - Corticosteroids
      - Minoxidil
      - Androgens
      - Thiazolidinediones (pioglitazone, rosiglitazone)
      - Drugs with high sodium content
      - Licorice-containing products

    - Negative inotropes:
      - Antiarrhythmic agents except amiodarone and dofetilide
      - Beta-blockers at maintenance doses
      - Calcium channel blockers: diltiazem, nifedipine, verapamil, but not amlodipine or felodipine
      - Itraconazole

    - Cardiotoxic drugs
      - Alcohol
      - Anthracyclines (doxorubicin)
      - Cocaine
      - Cyclophosphamide
      - Imatinib
      - Trastuzumab

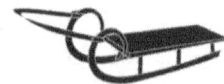

- Give conditions that commonly prompt hospitalization in heart failure (HF).

    o Social   –   Lack of outpatient care

    o CNS   –   Altered mentation

    o Heart   –   Hypotension
                    –   Dyspnea at rest
                    –   Significant arrhythmias

    o Kidney   –   Worsen renal function
                    –   Disturbed electrolytes

Adapted form: Ghosh AK. *Mayo Clinic Scientific Press* 2008, Table 3-31, page 112.

➢ Clinical

- Give the major and minor Framingham criteria for clinical diagnosis of heart failure.

Major	Minor
o PND	– Peripheral edema
o Orthopnea	– Night cough
o Increased JVP	– DOE
o Rales	– Hepatomegaly
o Third heart sound	– Pleural effusion
o Chest radiography	– Heart rate >120 beats per minute
- Cardiomegaly	– Weight loss $\geq$4.5 kg in 5 days with diuretic
- Pulmonary edema	

Abbreviations: DOE, dyspnea on exertion; JVP, jugular venous pressure; PND, paroxysmal nocturnal dyspnea

Source: Ghosh AK. *Mayo Clinic Scientific Press* 2008, Table 3-33, page 113.

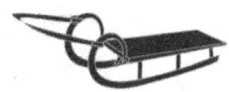

Mastering the Boards: Cardiology   A.B.R. Thomson

- Distinguish diastolic dysfunction from systolic dysfunction

Finding	LR for diastolic dysfunction	LR for systolic dysfunction (EF < 45%)
In favor of normal systolic function		
- Female sex	1.6	0.62
- Systolic blood pressure ≥160 mm Hg	1.8	0.55
In favor of systolic dysfunction		
- Heart rate ≥ 100/min		
- Left atrial ECG abnormality	0.42	2.4

Abbreviations: ECG, electrocardiogram; EF, ejection fraction; LR, likelihood ratio

Source: Simel DL, et al. *JAMA* 2009, Table 16-11, page 211; Hauser SC, et al. *Mayo Clinic Gastroenterology and Hepatology Board Review. 3rd Review,* Box 44-1, pages 522 and 523.

Left-sided Heart Failure (L-HF) **vs. Right-sided Heart Failure** (R-HF)

- Perform a focused physical examination to distinguish between the presence of left-sided congestive heart failure (L-HFand e.g. LV failure [LVF]), and right-sided congestive heart failure (R-HF and e.g. RV failure [RVF]).

	LVF (L-HF)	RVF (R-HF, PHT, cor pulmonale)
Inspection		
o Nourishment	- Cachexia	
o Breathing, RR	- ↑ - Dyspnea - Chgyne-Stokes respiration - Orthopnea	- ↑
o Skin	- Peripheral cyanosis	- Yes – "mitral facies": rosy cheeks with blue tinge
o Voice		- Hoarse (PHT: large PA compresses L. recurrent laryngeal nerve)

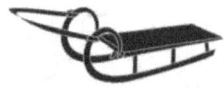

	LVF (L-HF)	RVF (R-HF, PHT, cor pulmonale)
Palpation		
○ Skin	- Cold extremities - Edema	- Cold extremities – Edema
○ Pulse	- ↑ PR - ↓ pulse pressure - Pulsus alternans - Irregular (e.g. AF)	
○ JVP		- ↑ JVP - ↑ a, v waves - HJR - Kussmaul sign
○ Apex	– Displaced – Dyskinetic – Gallop	- RV heave - Palpable P_2
○ BP	– May be ↓ or ↑	- May be ↓ (with LVF)
○ Liver		- Tender hepatomegaly
Auscalation		
○ Lungs	– Crackles, wheezes	- Tender hepatomegaly
○ Heart sounds	– LV-S_3	- RV-S_3 - ↑ P_2 (PHT) - Systolic ejection click (PHT)
○ Murmur	– Valvular disease	- PR (dilation of PA; PHT) - Systolic ejection murmur
○ Liver		- Bruit / thrill
Associations		
○ Anemia		
○ Hyperthyroidism		
○ Atherosclerosis		

Abbreviations: AF, atrial fibrillation; CHF, congestive heart failure; HJR, hepatojugular reflux; JVP, jugular venous pressure; L-HF, left side heart failure; LV, left ventricle; PA, pulmonary artery; PHT, pulmonary hypertension; PR, pulse rate; PR, pulmonary regurgitation; R-HF, right side heart failure; RR, respiratory rate; RV, right ventricle; TR, tricuspid regurgitation

Adapted from: Davey P. *Wiley-Blackwell* 2006, page 156.

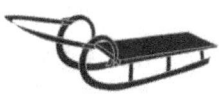

Mastering the Boards: Cardiology   A.B.R. Thomson

```
✗✗✗✗✗✗✗✗✗✗✗✗✗✗✗✗✗✗✗✗✗✗✗✗✗✗✗✗✗✗✗✗✗✗✗✗✗✗✗✗✗✗✗✗✗✗✗
```

SO YOU WANT TO BE A CARDIOLOGIST!

- In the context of wanting to pass the cardiology fellowship examination, give what is "cor bovinum?"

    o Slow and progressive left ventricular dilatation and hypertrophy in an attempt to normalize wall stress. The heart may thus become larger and heavier than in any other form of chronic heart disease – cor bovinum (bovine or ox heart)

Source: Baliga R.R. 250 Cases in Clinical Medicine. Saunders/Elsevier, Philadelphia 2007,page 15.

- Give when the person with chronic left sided (L) congestive heart failure lose their orthopnea (preferance to breathing in an upright position)?

    o Once the L-HF causes R-HF, the failure of the RV causes unloading of the LV, relieving the pulmonary congestion.

```
✗✗✗✗✗✗✗✗✗✗✗✗✗✗✗✗✗✗✗✗✗✗✗✗✗✗✗✗✗✗✗✗✗✗✗✗✗✗✗✗✗✗✗✗✗✗✗
```

- Give the performance characteristics of physical examination **Low Ejection Fraction.**

	PLR	NLR
➢ Vital signs		
o Heart rate >100 beats/min at rest	2.8	NS
o Abnormal Valsalva response	7.6	0.3
➢ Heart examination		
o Elevated neck veins	7.9	NS
o Supine apical impulse lateral to MCL	10.1	0.6
o S_3 gallop	3.4	0.7

Abbreviations: MCL, midclavicular line; NLR, negative likelihood ratio; PLR, positive likelihood ratio

Note: The findings of lung crackles, murmur of mitral regurgitation, hepatomegaly and peripheral edema are not shown since the valve of their PLR was < 2.

Adapted from: McGee SR. *Saunders/Elsevier* 2007, page 523.

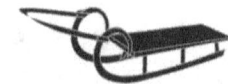

- Give the performance characteristics of physical examination for heart failure (HF).

Sign	PLR
o Vital signs	
– HR > 100/bpm at rest	5.5
– Abnormal Valsalva response	7.6
o Lung examination	
– Crackles	NS
o Heart examination	
– Elevated jugular venous pressure	3.9
– Positive abdominojugular test	8.0
– Supine, apical impulse lateral to MCL	5.8
– S_3 gallop	5.7
o Legs, sacrum	
– Edema	NS

*Diagnostic standard: For elevated left heart filling pressures, *pulmonary capillary wedge pressure > 12 mmHg or > 15 mmHg, or left ventricular end diastolic pressure > 15 mmHg*

Abbreviations: HF, heart failure; HJ, hepatojugular; HR, heart rate; PLR, positive likelihood ratio; NLR, negative likelihood ratio; MCL, midclavicular line

Adapted from: McGee SR. *Saunders/Elsevier* 2007, Table 44-1, page 522.

Systolic Heart Failure (↓ ejection fraction [EF])

Medical inpatients, including post myocardial infarction	PLR	NLR
o Clinical diagnosis		
- ECG abnormal	2.0-	0.41-
- *Outpatients*	3.1	0.62
- Clinical score with a BNP > 37 pg/mL	2.8	0.03
o The breathless ER patient's history		
- Patient history		
- Heart failure	5.8	0.45
- Myocardial infarction	3.1	0.69

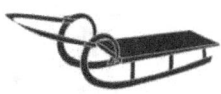

Medical inpatients, including post myocardial infarction	PLR	NLR
o Physical examination		
- Third heart sound (S$_3$)	11	0.88
- Abdominojugular reflux	6.4	0.79
- Jugular venous distention	5.1	0.66
- Chest rales	2.8	0.51
o Chest radiograph		
- Pulmonary venous congestion	12	0.48
- Interstitial edema	12	0.68
- Alveolar edema	6.0	0.95
- Cardiomegaly	3.3	0.33
- Pleural effusion(s)	3.2	0.81
o Electrocardiogram		
- Atrial fibrillation	3.8	0.79
- New T wave changes	3.0	0.83
- Any abnormal finding	2.2	0.64
o Overall clinical impression		
- Initial clinical judgment that the patient is in HF	4.4	0.45

Abbreviations: HF, heart failure; ECG, electrocardiogram; HJ, hepatojugular; JVP, jugular venous pressure; L-CHF, left side congestive heart failure; PLR positive likelihood ratio; NLR, negative likelihood ratio.

Adpated from: Simel DL, et al. *JAMA* 2009, Table 16-12, page 213.

- Give the pathophysiology of systolic (DS) and diastolic dysfunction (DD). Give examples of conditions leading to DD.

Dysfunction	Pathophysiology
o SD	- ↓ contractility
o DD	- ↓ filling, from ↑ stiffness of heart

➢ Causes of DD   o Severe LVH
      – AS (aortic stenosis)
      – HBP (systemic hypertension)
   o Cardiomyopathy
      – Hypertrophic cardiomyopathy
      – Restrictive cardiomyopathy

Abbreviation: LVH, left ventricular hypertrophy

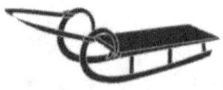

ACC / AHA **Guidelines for Stage of Chronic Heart Failure** in Adults

ACC / AHA Stage	Risk factors*	Structural disease **	Symptoms	Refractory symptoms
A	+			
B		+		
C			+	
D				+

*risk factors
 - Coronary heart disease
 - Hypertension
 - Diabetes
 - Cardiotoxins
 - Familial cardiomyopathy

**structural disease
 - ↓ LV systolic function
 - STEMI
 - Valvular disease

Abbreviations: ACC, American College of Cardiology; AHA, American Heart Association; LV, left ventricle; STEMI, ST-segment elevation myocardial infarction

- Life style
    - ↓ salt / water intake
    - ↓ alcohol
    - ↓ smoking
    - ↓ excess weight
    - Correct hypolipidemia
        - Anemia
        - Hypothyroidism
    - Exercise training

- Pharmacotherapy
    - Vasodilators
        - po
            - Angiotensin-converting enzyme (ACE) inhibitors
            - Angiotensin II receptor blocker
            - Hydrazaline plus isosorbide dinitrate
            - Nitrates

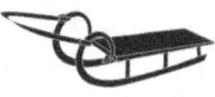

- IV
  - Nitroglycerin
  - Sodium nitroprusside
  - Recombinant BNP (B-type natriuretic peptide)
  - Enalaprilat

- B-blocker
  - Bisoprolol
  - Metoprolol succinate
  - Carvedilol

  o Note:
    - Only 3 B-blockers have been shown to ↓ mortality in HF.
    - This may be a drug effect rather than a drug class effect, so it is suggested that the choice of B-blocker be limited to this list of only 3 beta-blockers

- Diuretics
  - Aldosterone antagonists
    - Spironolactone
    - Eplerenone
  - Thiazides

- Digitalis

- Inotropic sympathomimetics
  - Dopamine
  - Phosphodiesterase
  - Dobutamine
  - Milrinone

- Non-pharmacological non-surgical invasive procedures
  o Coronary revasculization
  o Cardiac resynchronization therapy, biventricular pacing
  o Implantable cardiac defibrillators (ICDs)
  o Intra-aortic balloon pump (IABP)
  o Percutaneous left ventricular assist device (LVDD)
  o Ventricular assist device
  o Cardiac transplantation

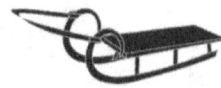

B-blockers (BB)

- o Benefits of BB in HF
    - ↑ survival
    - ↑ functional status
    - ↓ progression
    - ↓ arrhythmia
    - ↓ SCD (sudden cardiac death)

- o BBs with proven benefits in HF
    - Bisoprolol 1.25 mg → 10 mg / day
    - Caredilol 3.125 mg q 12 h → 25-50 mg q 12 g
    - Metoprolol 12.5 – 25 mg → 200 mg/day

- o Note:
    - There may be a slow (2-3 mon) onset of maximum benefit
    - Titrate dose to maximum tolerable in terms SBP / HR (systolic blood pressure and heart rate)

Vasodilators

- A little pathophysiology

- o HF is associated with
    - Abnormalities in
        - Contraction
            - Systolic dysfunction
        - Relaxating and filling
            - Diastolic dysfunction
    - Vasoconstriction
        - Arterial
            - Afterload
        - Venous
            - Preload

- o Venodilators
    - ↓ preload → ↓ ventricular filling pressure

- o Arterial vasodilators
    - ↓ SVR (systemic vascular resistance) → ↓ afterload → ↓ ventricular filling pressure →☐↑ cardiac output

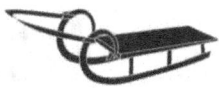

CLINICAL CAUTION

- o Vasodilators are used to ↓ arterial afterload, and are of benefit
  - Systolic dysfunction, but
  - Not of benefit in diasystolic dysfunction

- o When the cardiac output cannot increase, as in aortic stenosis (AS) or hypertrophic cardiomyopathy (HCM), then it is not advantageous to use a vasodilator

Angiotensin-Converting Enzyme (ACE) inhibitors

➤ Pathophysiology

- o HF → ↑ activity of renin-angiotensin system → ↓ Na^+, ↓ K^+, fluid retention
- o ACE inhibitors lessen this enhanced activity, and lessen the hyponatremia, hypokalemia, and fluid retention.

CLINICAL CAUTION

- o Do not use in pregnancy
- o Use cautiously in renal impairment
- o Use cautiously with K^+ supplements or K+ sparing diuretics

ADVERSE ALERT

- Give the reason why the cautions physician may choose to use an ACE inhibitor other than captopril, especially when serum creatinine > 1.5 mg/dL, or if the patient has collagen vascular disease.

  - o The risk is less for the adverse events of angioedema or agranulocytosis in ACE inhibitor other than captopril

  - o This effect of non-captopril ACE inhibitors causing less angioedema and agranulocytosis is even more pronounced when serum creatinine > 1.5 mg/dL or in the patient with collagen vascular disease.

- o Clinical benefit in LV dysfunction
  - ↓ symptoms of HF
  - ↓ progression of asymptomatic to systematic LV dysfunction
  - ↓ mortality

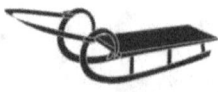

Angiotensin II Receptor Blockers (ARBs)

- ○ ↓ symptoms and ↓ mortality in persons with HF and not on ACE inhibitors

---

SO WHAT

- The ACE inhibitors ↑ bradykinin concentration, but the ARBs do not. Give why this is clinically important.

  - ○ ACE inhibitors cause ↑ bradykinin, which leads to the adverse effects of cough

  - ○ ARBs do not ↑ bradykinin, do not cause cough, so are useful to substitute for ACE inhibitors in the person with intolerable drug-associated cough

---

Hydralazine plus Isosorbide dinitrate

- ○ In HF, this combination therapy is added to B-blockers and ACE inhibitors, and reduce mortality.

- Speculate why you have probability not seen hydralazine +/- isosorbide dinitrate used very often in the patient with HF.

  - ○ HF has many causes, but > 50% of cases are due to coronary artery disease (CAD).

  - ○ When hydralazine is given to patient with HF plus CAD, there is reflex ↑ HR → ↑ myocardial consumption of O_2 → demand ischemia.

Nitrates

- Give the mechanisms by which the nitrates are useful for the patient with HF and symptoms of pulmonary congestion and venous congestion, yet at the same time may cause hypotension.

  - ○ Nitrates
    - – Venodilatory
      - ▪ ↓ pulmonary / venous congestion
    - – ↓ ventricular filling pressures
      - ▪ ↓ myocardial ischemia → ↓ chest pain
    - – Dilate coronary arteries

  - ○ Words of praise: "….nitroglycerin is the preferred vasodilator for treatment of HF in the setting of acute MI or unstable angina."

Larue SJ, et a. The Washington Manual of Medicine Therapeutics 34th Edition. Page 178, 2014, Wolters Kluwer

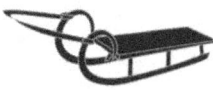

Sodium Nitroprusside

- Give the reason why nitrates are recommended in HF in the setting of acute MI or unstable angina, but **sodium nitroprusside** is not, and why is sodium nitroprusside the ideal parenteral vasodilator in the patient with HF and hypertension, or who have severe aortic or mitral valvular regurgitation.

Drug	Venous or arterial action	Effect on load	Optimal dysfunction benefit	↑ cardiac output
○ Nitroglycerin	Venodilator	↓ preload	Diastolic	No
○ Sodium nitroprusside	Arterial vasodilator	↓ afterload	Systolic	Yes

---

CLINICAL CHALLENGE

The patient with HF, hypotension and renal impairment is treated with IV sodium nitroprusside, initially 0.25 mcg/kg per min, increasing to 10 mcg/kg per min when the hypertension corrects. The serum creatinine concentration slowly rises to 3 mg/dL, but the patient becomes confused, while complaining of nausea, abdominal pain and paresthesias.

- Give the most likely explanation for these new symptoms.

  - ○ Not likely hypertension, which has corrected

  - ○ Not likely the renal failure per se, because it is only moderately impaired

  - ○ A large dose of mitroprusside is being given, its half-life is short, it is metabolized to cyanide, but the hepatic metabolite of the cyanide, thiocyanate, will be only slowly excreted from the kidney because of its impaired excretory function, which is reflected by the rising serum creatinine.

  - ○ This patient's symptoms are due to this cyanate toxicity, which caould be proven by measurement of serum thiocyanate > 10 mg/dL.

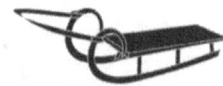

Recombinant BNP (Nisiritide)

➢ Mechanism

    o Arterial and venous vasodilation
        - ↓ RA / ↓ LV end-diastolic pressures (LVEDPs)
        - ↓ SVR
        - ↑ CO

➢ Dose

    o 2 mcg/kg IV bolus, then IV infusion 0.01 mcg/kg per min

➢ Indications

    o Symptoms of acute exacerbation of HF

➢ Outcomes

    o ↓ symptoms of acute HF

    o No Δ hospitalization or survival rate

➢ Contraindications

    o SBP 90 mmHg, including cardiogenic shock

Abbreviations: CO, cardiac output; HF, heart failure; LV, left ventricle; RA, right atrium; SBP, systolic blood pressure; SVR, systemic vascular resistance;

Enalaprilat

➢ Mechanism

    o ACE inhibitor (metabolite of enalapril)

➢ Dose

    o 1.25 mg IV q 6 h → 5 mg IV q 6 h

    o Initial dose is 0.625 mg IV q 6 h for
        - Serum creatinine > 3 mg/dL
        - Creatine clearance < 30 mL/min

➢ Caution

    o Rapid onset of action that is variable and unpredictable

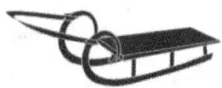

Aldosterone Antagonists

- Spironolactone

➢ Benefit
  - ↓ hospitalization ⎤
  - ↓ deaths   ⎦   NYHA III / IV patients (low EF)

➢ Cautionary use if
  - Serum
    - Creatinine > 2.5 mg/dL
    - Potassium > 5.0 mEq/L
  - Concomitant drugs which may also cause hyperkalemia
    ACE inhibitors
    - NSAIDs
  - The 10% to 20% risk of gynecomastia in men, and this risk is less with eplerenone

- Eplerenone
  - Useful in post MI HF, without the ↑ risk of gynecomastia (as with aldosterone)

Abbreviations: ACE, angiotensin-converting enzyme; HF, heart failure; NSAIDs, non-steroidal anti-inflammatory drug; NYHA, New York Heart Association

Digitalis

➢ Mechanism of action
  - Cardiac glycoside
    - ↑ cardiac contractility
    - "May attenuate the neurohormonal activation associated with HF" (Washington Manual of Medical Therapeutics, Chapter 5, page 179. Wolters Kluwer / Lippincott William & Wilkins, 2014)
  - Dose
    - 0.125 mg to 0.25 mg po per day, with dose adjusted to serum digoxin levels of 0.8 to 2.0 ng/mL
  - Benefits
    - ↓ hospitalizations for HF
    - No Δ in mortality in men

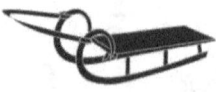

CLINICAL CAUTION

- Give major clinical cautions or concerns about the use of digitalis.

  o Pharmacology
    - Narrow therapeutic index
    - Toxicity may occur even when serum digitalis is in the "therapeutic" range (0.8 ng/mL to 2.0 ng/mL)
    - Clinical improvement does not always correlate with serum concentrations

  o ↑ mortality
    - Women
    - Men and women with serum digitalis concentration 1.2 to 2.0 ng/mL (still in the "therapeutic" range

  o Drug interactions ↑ serum digitalis concentration)
    - Amiodarone
    - Erythromycin
    - Flecainide
    - Quinidine
    - Tetracycline
    - Verapamil

  o Toxicity (↑ risk of ventricular arrhythmias)
    - Drug interactions
    - Hypokalemia
    - Hypoxemia
    - Hypothyroidism
    - ↓ renal function
    - ↓ volume (volume depletion)

Diuretics

  o Thiazides
    - Use cautiously if serum creatinine > 2.5 mg/dL

  o Metolazone
    - A thiazide which ↓ Na+ reabsorption in both proximal and distal renal tubule
    - If ↑ serum creatinine / ↓ creatinine clearance, may be used with loop diuretic

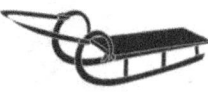

- Loop diuretics
  - May be used alone or with metolazone if there is ↓↓ renal function
  - Furosimide is effective when given IV, both because it is a potent diuretic, as well as because it acts on veins to cause venodilation → ↓ preload
- Aldosterone antagonists
  - Their weak diuretic action means they are best used with an other class of diuretic.
  - Their major advantage is to retain K+, thereby ↓ risk of development of hypokalemia with other classes of diuretic

---

SO YOU WANT TO BE A CARDIOLOGIST!

- A patient with HF and poor renal function also has sulfa-allergy. Give the name of a loop diuretic other than furosemide or butetanide that is safe to give.
  - Ethacrinic acid may be given to the person with sulfa-allergy

---

Inotropic drugs

- Dopamine / dobutamine
  - Use
    - Receptor effect, and mechanism of action depends upon dose
    - Stabilization of hypertension
  - Use for
    - Severe / refractory HF
    - As a bridge to mechanical due to systolic dysfunction
      - Ventricular support or
      - Cardiac transplantation
    - Palliative / end-of-life therapy
  - Adverse effects
    - ↑ risk of myocardial ischemia
    - ↑ mortality from continuous IV dobutamine
    - ↑ severe / life threatening arrhythmia
    - ↑ risk in dwelling of catheter infections

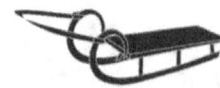

Quick Quiz

- Give the cause of HF in which the sympathomimetic agents are not used.
    - The sympathomimetic agents are not used for heart failure (HF) due to diastolic dysfunction or the high-output failure.

- Phosphodiesterase inhibitors
    - Mechanism
        - ↑ intracellular cAMP (cyclic adenosine monophosphate)
        - ↑ vasodilation
        - ↑ cardiac contractility
- Milrinone
    - Benefit
        - ↑ cAMP → improves hemodynamics when used with sympathomimetic drugs (dopamine, dobutamine) in persons with severe / refractory HF
    - Caution: hypotension is common adverse effect, especially if patient have
        - Intravascular volume contraction
        - Or on concomitant vasodilator
    - Limitations
        - No benefit on hospitalizations for HF, or mortality rate
        - ↓ SVR (systemic vascular resistance
        - Atrial and ventricular tachyarrhythmia

Non-pharmacologic Therapy for Heart Failure (HF)

- Give non-pharmacologic therapy for HF.

    - ↓ intake of salt / (and sometimes water)
    - Treat underlying / precipitating conditions (e.g. anemia, hypertension, stoop apnea, valvular disease, drug toxicity)
    - Avoid
        - NSAIDs
        - Negative inotropics
            - Diltiazem
            - Verapamil
            - OTC B-stimulants

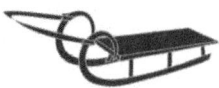

- o Supplemental O2 if patient dyspnic with hypoxemia
- o Dialysis ultrafiltration, therapeutic tap of associated ascites
- o End of life decisions
  - Hospital / palliative care
  - DNR decisions
  - Preparing will
  - Last rights (i.e. decisions based on religious benefits)
- o Coronary revascularization
  - ↓ ischemia ⎤
  - ↑ systolic function ⎦ in CAD
- o Cardiac resynchronization therapy / biventricular pacting
  - ↑ quality of life
  - ↑ survival
  - When
    - EF ≤ 35%
    - NYHA III / IV HF
    - LBBB / AV delay
- o Implantable cardiac defibrillator (ICD)
  - ↓ SCD (sudden cardiac death) by 1% -1.5% per year
  - Used when EF ≤ 35% after optimal medical therapy for 3 mon, or 40 days after acute MI / revasculization
  - Contraindications
    - Inadequate trial of optimal medical therapy
    - Advance age
    - Severe life-shortening comorbidities
    - End-stage HF in non-transplantation eligible patient

- Give the rational for recommending that patients with heart failure avoid use of NSAIDs.

  - o ↑ SBP (systolic blood pressure)
  - o ↓ renal function
  - o Benefit of
    - Diuretics
    - ACE inhibitors
  - o Intra-aortic balloon pump (IABP)
    - Indications
      - Failure of optimal medical therapy for HF
      - Transient myocardial dysfunction

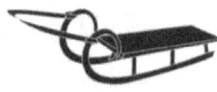

- A bridge to
  - LVAD, or
  - Cardiac transplantation
- Contraindications
  - Severe aortoiliac atherosclerosis
  - Aortic insufficiency (AI), moderate /severe

o Percutaneous LVAD (left-ventricular assist device)
  - Indicated for cardiac genic shock
  - Shorten benefits of LVAD > IBBP, but ↑ survival > 30 days not improved

Surgery for HF

o Ventricular assist devices (VADs)
  - Indications
    - Acute MI complicated by cardiogenic shock
    - Severe HF after cardiac surgery
    - Bridge to heart transplantation
    - Refractory, end-stage HF, non-candidate for transplantation but
  - 1 yr mortality rate > 50% despite optimal medical Rx

o Cardiac transplantation
  - ↑ functional capacity and quality of life in persons who have failed optimal medical therapy, other options exhausted, < 65 yr, no "irreversible extracardiac organ dysfunction, no active infection or malignancy and adequate social / family support

---

Patient Counseling

- Give the major complications, which occur after cardiac transplantation.

  o Heart
    - Acute / chronic rejection
    - Vasculopathy
      - Coronary artery disease (CAD)
      - Chronic rejection

  o Survival rates
    - 1, 5 and 10 yr ~ 90%, 70% and 50%

  o Infection

  o Drug toxicity

  o Malignancy
    - Including post-transplantation lymphoproliferative disorders (related to EBV infection)

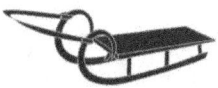

➤ Diagnosis

Performance characteristics of Chest radiograph and electrocardiogram in emergency department patents in HF.

	PLR	NLR
o Chest radiograph		
- Pulmonary venous congestion	12	0.48
- Interstitial edema	12	0.68
- Alveolar edema	6.0	0.95
- Cardiomegaly	3.3	0.33
- Pleural effusion(s)	3.2	0.81
- Any edema	3.1	0.38
o ECG		
- Atrial fibrillation	3.8	0.79
- New T wave changes	3.0	0.83
- Any abnormal findings	2.2	0.64

Abbreviations: CHF, congestive heart failure; ECG, electrocardiogram; PLR, positive likelihood ratio; NLR, negative likelihood ratio.

Note that the presence of pneumonia and hyperinflation on chest x-ray , as well as ECG evidence of either ST elevation or depression have PLRs >2, and are not included here.

Adapted from: Simel DL, et al. *JAMA* 2009, Table 16-7, page 201.

- o Symptoms of HF are neither sensitive nor specific
    - May be vague
    - May relate to systems other than heart and lungs
    - CNS   ▪ Fatigue
    - GI   ▪ Lymphedema (TS)
                   ▪ Nausea / vomiting
                   ▪ Chest / abdominal pain / discomfort
                   ▪ Early satiety

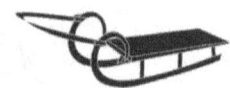

- Take a directed history and perform a focused physcal examination for HF.

  - o Symptoms
    - Paroxysmal nocturnal dyspnea (PND)
    - Orthopnea (SOB, ie shortness of breath)
    - Dyspnea on exertion (SOBOE, shortness of breath on exertion)
    - Chest pain (previous MI, CHF)

  - o Physical examination
    - Jugular venous pressure (JVP) assess
    - Peripheral and sacral edema
    - S3 (ventricular filling gallop)
    - Rales and wheezes
    - Cardiac murmur

  - o Chest radiograph
    - Pulmonary venous congestion
    - Interstitial edema
    - Cardiomegaly
    - Pleural effusion(s)

  - o Electrocardiogram findings
    - Any abnormal result
    - Atrial fibrillation

  - o Brain natriuretic peptide
    - Most useful when < 100 pg/ml for decreasing the likelihood of CHF

Abbreviations: HF, heart failure; LVH, left ventricular hypertrophy; LV, left ventricle; MI, myocardial infarction; PE, pulmonary embolus

Source: Simel DL, et al. *JAMA* 2009, Box 16-1, page 204; and Davey P. *Wiley-Blackwell*, 2006, pages156, 158,160 and 162.

	Approximate Sens, %
o Top 5 signs for sensitivity (sens)	
- Pulmonary crackles	60
- Peripheral edema	39
- ↑ JVP	39
- HJR	24
- S3 gallop	13
o Top 4 signs for specificity (spec)	
- S3 gallop	99
- Ascites	97
- HJR	96
- ↑ JVP	92
- Pulmonary crackles (edema)	78

(sens of ascites, only 1%)

Abbreviations: JVP, jugular venous pressure; HJR, hepatojugular reflex

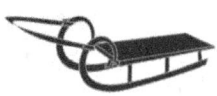

- Give the performance characteristics of findings on history and physical examination in emergency department patients.

Finding	PLR	NLR
o Initial clinical judgment	4.4	0.45
o Past History		
– Heart failure	5.8	0.45
– Myocardial infarction	3.1	0.69
o Symptoms		
– Paroxysmal nocturnal dyspnea	2.6	0.70
– Orthopnea	2.2	0.65
– Edema	2.1	0.64
o Physical examination		
– Third heart sound (ventricular filling gallop)	11	0.88
– Abdominojugular reflux	6.4	0.79
– Jugular venous distention (JVP)	5.1	0.66
– Rales	2.8	0.51
– Any murmur	2.6	0.81
– Lower extremity edema	2.3	0.64
– Valsalva maneuver	2.1	0.41
– Systolic blood pressure < 100 mm Hg	2.0	0.97

Abbreviations: JVP, jugular venous pressure; PLR, positive likelihood ratio; NLR, negative likelihood ratio

- o Note
  - – Many historical points, symptoms and signs on physical examination have a PLR > 2 (and are not included here)

➢ Remember the probability (%)

PLR	Increase	NLR	Decrease
2	15%	0.5	-15%
5	30%	0.2	-30%
10	45%	0.1	-45%

Abbreviations: PLR, positive likelihood ratio; NLR, negative likelihood ratio

Adapted from: Simel DL, et al. *JAMA* 2009, Table 16-6.

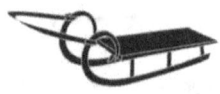

Probability

Decrease | Increase

-45%	-30%	-15%		+15%	+30%	+45%
0.1	0.2	0.5	1	2	5	10

LRs

- Perform a focused physical examination for the causes of right-sided heart failure (R-HF).

    o Any cause of L-HF

    o Cor pulmonale

    o Mitral stenosis, tricuspid incompetence

    o Some forms of congenital heart disease

    o Shunts
    - Heart
    - Peripheral

    o Deformity of chest wall

Diastolic Heart Failure (normal ejection fraction [EF])

➢ Definition

    o Heart failure (HF) in the presence of LV > 40 (preserved LV function; ala HF with preserved ejection fraction (HFpEF)

➢ Demography

    o ~ half of patients hospitalized for HF have HFpEF

    o Most prevalent in older women

➢ Causes / associations

    o Hypertension → LV hypertrophy

    o Diabetes

    o Constriction pericarditis

    o Cardiomyopathy
    - RCM (restrictive cardiomyopathy)
    - HCM (hypertrophic cardiomyopathy)
    - Infiltrative cardiomyopathy

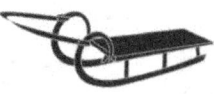

> Diagnosis
  - o Echocardiography
    - LV function normal
    - ↓ diastolic relaxation
    - ↑ filling pressure

D-HF (diastolic heart failure) is aka HFPEF (heart failure with preserved ejection fraction [EV > 50%])

- Give the risk factors and causes of HFPEF (heart failure with preserved ejection fraction).

- Risk factors
  - o Older females
  - o Comorbidities
    - Heart
      - CAD (coronary heart disease)
      - Hypertension

    - Endocrine
      - Diabetes
      - Obesity

    - Renal
      - Chronic renal disease

  - o Lung
    - Lung disease
    - Pulmonary hypertension

  - o Nutrition
    - Obesity
    - Deconditioning
    - Anemia

  - o Extracardiac shunt

- Causes
  - o Heart
    - Heart
      - Lymphedema (TS)
      - Coronary artery disease

    - Wall
      - Intracardiac shunt
      - Cardiomyopathy

    - Valve
      - Valvular disease

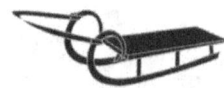

- o Lung
    - Lung disease
    - Pulmonary hypertension
- o Nutrition
    - Obesity
    - Deconditioning
    - Anemia
- o Extracardiac shunt

> Treatment
  - o Treat associated conditions
  - o Empiric therapy for symptoms

- In the context of the use of diuretics in the patient with HF (heart failure), give the conditions to be met to use spironolactone.
    - o NYHA class III or IV

- Give the conditions to be met to use a combination of hydralazine plus isosorbide dinitrate.
    - o When ACE-inhibitor or ARB contraindicated
        - Chronic renal disease
        - Hyperkalemia
    - o NYHA III, IV symptoms in patients with African-inheritance

- Give the conditions to be met in order to use eplerenone.
    - o NYHA class II symptoms, EF ≤ 35%
    - o Persons on spironolactone who develop painful gynecomastia

Note: CCBs (calcium channel blockers) are **not** of benefit in treating 5-HF (↓ EF)

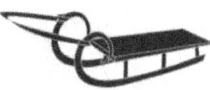

Medical Devices Used to Treat Heart failure

- o ICD (implantable cardioverter-defibrillator)
  - Prevent SCD (sudden cardiac death)
- o CRT (cardiac resynchronization therapy)
  - Restore myocardial –electromechanical coupling
  - ↑ ventricular contraction

- Give the indications for ICD (Implantable Cardioverter-Defribrillator) and for cardiac resynchronization therapy (CRT).

  - o ICD
    - Ischemic cardiomyopathy
      ≥ 40 d post MI, or
      EF ≤ 30% plus NYHA class I-III symptoms
    - Non-ischemic cardiomyopathy
      EF ≤ 35%, or
    - History of cardiac arrest, or
    - Hemodynamically severe ventricular arrhythmia

  - o CRT
    - All of above, plus
    - NYHA class II or IV symptoms, despite optimal medical care
    - EF ≤ 35%
    - QRS > 120 msec

Note: these criteria are limited, since even when following these criteria to use medical devices, the mortality rates (MR) are still high.

Device	MR
ICD	70% (all cause ↓ MR, 30%)
CRT	50% (↓ 50% MR from progressive HF)

- Give the follow-up of outpatients with chronic heart failure (HF).

  - o Clinical
    - Hypotension

  - o Laboratory
    - BNP or proBNP, for patients < 75 yr
    - Hyponatremia

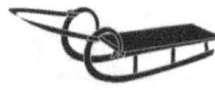

- o Survival scores
  - Heart Failure Survival Score
  - Seattle Heart Failure Model (SHFM; please see www.seattleheartfailuremodel.org)
  - The SHFM is based on numerous factors, such as
    - Patient
      - Age
      - Gender
      - NYHA class
      - Weight

    - Heart
      - EF
      - SBP
      - Etiology (i.e., ischemia)
  - PFT (pulmonary function testing)
    - Labs
    - Medications
    - VO_2 (peak O_2 uptake) with exercise
    - Devices

Acute Decompensation of Heart Failure

- o S-HF (↓ EF)
  - Hypotension of end-organs
  - Hypoperfusion

- o HFPEL (D-HF), normal EF)
  - Common precipitant
  - Poorly controlled hypertension

- Give criteria for admission to hospital for acute decompensated HF.

  - o CNS
    - Δ LOC (altered level of consciousness)
    - CVA /TIA (cerebrovascular accident [stroke], transient ischemic attack)

  - o Heart
    - Decompensation
      - Hypotension
      - ↑ Cr (creatinine; worse renal failure)
      - Altered mentation
    - ACS (acute coronary syndrome)
    - Repeated ICD firing
    - Rapid atrial fibrillation (or other arrhythmias causing hemodynamic instability)

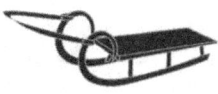

- o Lung
  - Dyspnea at rest
  - Pneumonia
  - PE (pulmonary embolism)

- o Renal
  - Renal failure
  - Electrolyte to disturbance (major)

Evidence based

Yes

- o In the setting of patients with worsening HF and volume overload, modest salt restriction and loop diuretics are used.
- o If the response is inadequate, the po diuretic may be switched to continuous IV infusion, or the loop diuretic may be supplemented with a thiazide diuretic.
- o Also in the setting of volume overload, if hypotension / hypoperfusion develop, add an inotropic agent.

No

- o Limited benefit is achieved by adding
  - Renal ultrafiltration
  - Vasopressin (V) antagonists
    - IV conivaptan (non-selective V 1a / V 2 receptor blocker)
    - po tolvaptan (selective V2 blocker)

Clinical Caution

- o Note: In the setting of worsening HF, do **not** suddenly discontinue a patient's use of ACE inhibitor, unless there are major contraindications, such as
  - Severe hypotension
  - AKI (acute kidney injury)

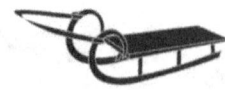

Cardiogenic Pulmonary Edema (CPE)

- Give the mechanism of development of cardiogenic pulmonary edema.
    - Acute LV failure
    - ↓ flow across mitral valve → PCP (PCV > SOP + P IHP) → ↑ fluid in alveoli pulmonary interstitium → ↓ gas exchange
        - Mitral stenosis (MS)
        - Atrial myxoma
    - Pulmonary veno-occlusive disease

Abbreviations: LV, left capillary pressure; PCP, pulmonary capillary pressure; PINP, pulmonary interstitial hydrostatic pressure; SOP, serum osmotic pressure

➢ Treatment
    - Correct precipitating factor
        - Hypertension
        - Myocardial infarction (MI)
        - Myocardial ischemia, acute regurgitation, especially MR (mitral regurgitation, such as with MI)
        - New tachy- / bradyarrhythmias
        - LV dysfunction plus fluid volume overload
    - Improve ventilation / oxygenation
        - Supplemental O2 → ↑ arterial O2 tension > 60 mmHg
        - Mechanical ventilation
        - Sitting upright
        - Bed rest
        - Control pain and anxiety
    - Hemodialysis / ultrafiltration
    - Pharmacotherapy

- Morphine
    - 2 mg to 5 mg IV, repeat q 10-25 min, as needed
    - Mechanism of benefit
        - ↓ pain
        - ↓ anxiety
        - Venodilation
            ▪ Pulmonary veins
            ▪ Systemic veins

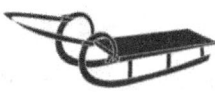

- Furosemide
  - 20 mg to 80 mg IV, repeated as needed to maximum of additional 200 mg
  - Mechanism
    - Immediate
      - Direct effect on venodilation
    - Alter
      - Diuretic
  - May be given with nitroglycerine

- Nitroglycerine
  - Venodilation, which may ↑ early venodilation effect of furosemide

- Nitroprusside
  - Arterial catheterization (used to determine dose of nitroprusside)
    - Systemic
    - Pulmonary
  - Especially useful for acute CPE due to
    - Hypertension
    - Acute regurgitation, such as mitral regurgitation (MR)

- Inotropic agents used to supplement initial therapy if hypotension / shock are present
  - Dobutamine, or
  - Milrinone

- Nesiritide (recombinant BNP)
  - IV bolus → IV infusion
  - Vasodilation → ↓ filling pressures → ↑ CO (cardiac output)
  - Often used with furosemide

CLINICAL GUIDANCE

- In the patient with acute heart failure (HF), give the reason why it is useful to place a Swan-Ganz (right heart) catheter.
  - Differentiate cardiogenic versus non-cardiogenic HF versus non-cardiogenic pulmonary edema
  - Guide therapy

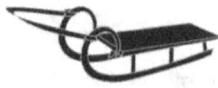

JUGULAR (CENTRAL) VENOUS PRESSURE (JVP)

➢ Definition: The pressure of the internal jugular system and is a direct assessment of the pressure in the right atrium of the heart.

Useful background: The three positive waves of the jugular venous pulse (A, C, V), and the three negative wave forms (X, X_1, Y).

- Perform a focused physical examination for the causes of elevated jugular venous pressure (JVP).

  - o Heart   - HF
    - - Valvular defects
      - ▪ TR (tricuspid regurgitation)
      - ▪ TS (tricuspid stenosis)
      - ▪ PS (pulmonary stenosis)
    - - Conduction defects – complete heart block

  - o Lung   - PHT (pulmonary hypertension; aka cor pulmonale)

  - o SVC (superior vena cava obstruction)
    - - Neck
      - ▪ ↑ JVP prominent veins (neck, chest)
      - ▪ ↑ JVP with pulsations
    - - Face
      - ▪ Pink
      - ▪ Dyspneic
    - - Eyes Horner syndrome
    - - Look for signs of cause
      - ▪ Lung – bronchogenic cancer
      - ▪ Chest – lymphoma
      - ▪ Neck – goiter
      - ▪ Heart – aortic aneurysm, constrictive pericarditis

Mangione Pearl:

"The more severe and acute the condition, the more difficult and inaccurate the bedside determination of jugular venous pulse and pressue"

Source: Mangione S. *Hanley & Belfus* 2000, page 190.

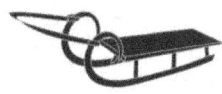

- Give circumstances, other than lack of adequate clinical skill, which make it difficult to access central venous pressure (CVP, from the right atrium).

    o ↓ CVP
    o Short, thick neck
    o Mechanical ventilation
    o Acute attack of asthma (wide respiratory swings in CVP)
    o Critically ill patients
    o Inspection of the external rather than the internal jugular vein

- Give how to distinguish EJV (external jugular vein) from IJV (internal jugular vein).

    o EJV is
    - Above SM (sternomastoids) muscle
    - Lateral to IJV
    - No bulb (bulb at junction of subclavian vein and IJV, between two heads of SM muscle

    o Lateral to IJV
    o Above SM

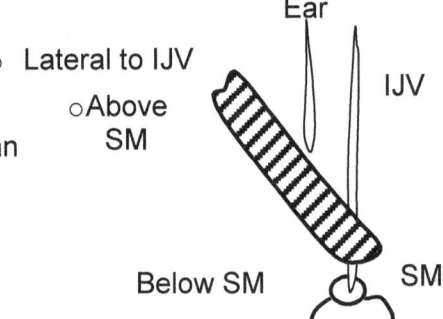

Below SM

Bulb

Evaluation of jugular venous pressure (JVP) and Central Venous Pressure (CVP)

3 cm (from sterna notch)
+ 5 cm (from right ventricle to sternal notch)
8 cm H$_2$O jugular venous pressure

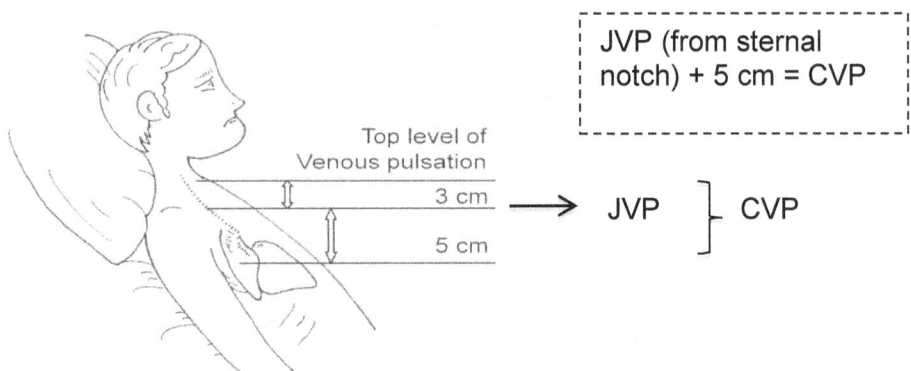

JVP (from sternal notch) + 5 cm = CVP

Top level of Venous pulsation

3 cm → JVP ⎫ CVP
5 cm

Abbreviations: ECG, electrocardiogram; TR, tricuspid regurgitation

Adapted from: Ghosh AK. *Mayo Clinic Scientific Press* 2008, Figure 3-1, page 38.

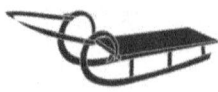

- Give causes of elevation of jugular venous pulse (JVP)

    - SVC   - SVC obstruction

    - RA   - RA thrombus, tumour, Bernheim effect
                                   - ↑ RA filling pressure

    - TR   - Tricuspid stenosis
                                   - Giant 'a' waves, cannon waves, tricuspid incompetence

    - Lung   - Coughing, valsalva maneuver
                                   - Pleural or pericardial effusion
    - RV   - ↓ RV filling
                                     - RV failure
                                     - RV infarction
                                     - Constrictive pericarditis
                                     - Cardiac tamponade
                                   - ↓ RV compliance

    - Circulation   - Increased blood volume
                                   - Bradycardia
                                   - Hyperdynamic circulation

Abbreviations: RA, right atrium; RV, right ventricle; SVC, superior vena cava

Adapted from: Burton JL. *Churchill Livingstone* 1971, page 10.

- Give the physiology of JVP ascents and descents.
    - A wave
        - From right atrium (RA) contraction
        - S_1 and carotid upstroke
        - Coincides with S_4
        - Follows p wave on ECG
        - More permanent than V wave
    - C wave
        - Poorly visible
        - from both bulging of tricuspid cusps into right atrium, as well as from transmitted carotid pulsation
        - Coincide with ventricular contraction
        - Interval between a and c wave of JVP coincides with P-R interval or RV coinciding with RV contraction
        - Occurs between S_1 and S_2
        - More prominent than Y descent

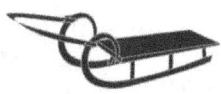

- o V wave
  - - At end of ventricular systole and at the early phase of ventricular diastole
  - - Less prominent than A wave
- o Y descent
  - - At beginning of ventricular diastole
  - - Caused by opening of the tricuspid valve and emptying of R. Atrium
  - - Corresponds to S_3
  - - Less prominent than X descent

Adapted from: Mangione S. *Hanley & Belfus* 2000, pages 193 and 194.

Jugular venous pressure, wave forms, and their relationship to the normal heart sounds

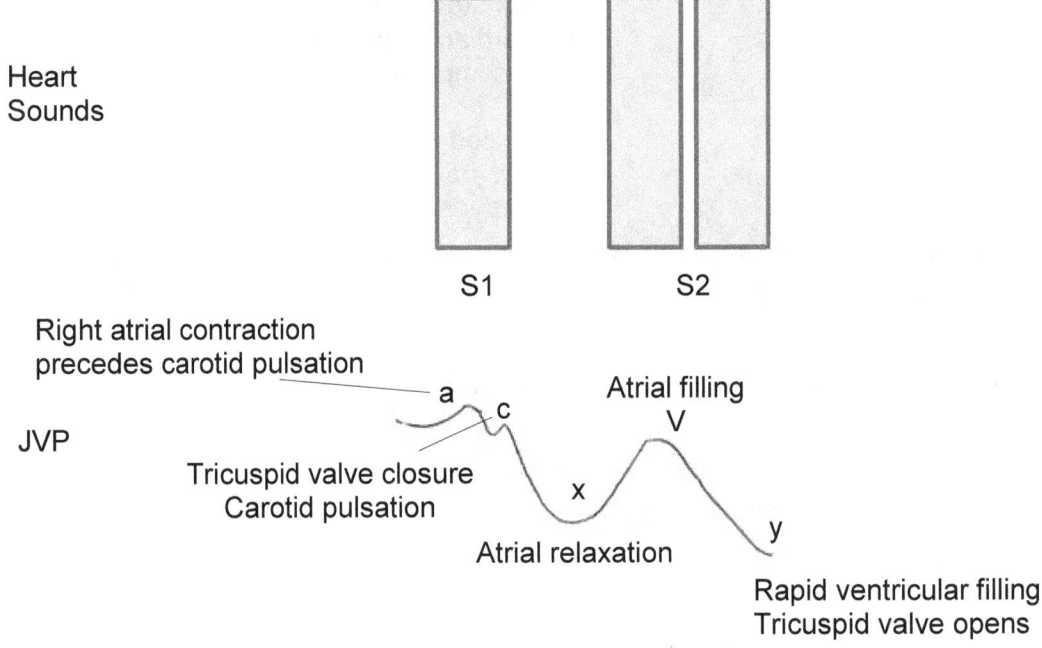

Abbreviations: CCF, congestive cardiac failure; CVP, central venous pressure; HJR, hepatojugular reflex; JVP, jugular venous pressure

Source: Talley NJ, et al *Maclennan & Petty Pty Limited* 2003, page 47.

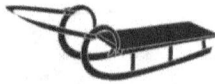

Clinical Gems and Pearls

- Give the normal range for JVP.
  - Normal range is 4-5 cm above the sternal angle, with the patient at a 45° angle, sitting.

- Give when the abdominojugular reflux (AJR; aka hepatojugular reflux) is abnormal.
  - Abnormality is indicated when there is a sustained rise in JVP > 4cm
  - After applying abdominal pressure for a minimum of 15-30 seconds.
  - R-HF (not in L-HF)
  - Tricuspid regurgitation or stenosis
  - Contructive pericarditis or pericardial tamponade
  - IVC obstruction
  - Hypervolemia

AJR has 66% sensitivity and 100% specificity distinguishing Tricuspid (TR) from mitral regurgitation (MR) (Note: AJR⁺ in TR, AJR⁻ in MR).

Adapted from: McGee SR. *Saunders/Elsevier* 2007, page 381, 382; and Mangione S. *Hanley & Belfus* 2000, page 199.

- Give how to estimate JVP pulsations when there is markedly increased JVP pressure and pulsations are not visible.
  - Use a higher elevation of the head (>30°) until pulsations are seen.

- Give the normal effect of inspiration on JVP pressure.
  - Normal inspiration - ↓JVP

- Give the meaning and significance of the Kussmaul sign - ↑ JVP on inspiration (opposite to normal, ie abnormal inspiratory increase in JVP).
  - Paradoxical increase in JVP with inspiration
  - Kussmaul sign occurs because the heart is unable to accommodate the increase in the venous return that accompanies the inspiratory fall in intrathoracic pressure.
  - R-HF
  - SVC obstruction
  - Tricuspid stenosis (TS)
  - Restrictive cardiomyopathy
    - Hemochromatosis
    - Sarcoidosis
    - Amyloidosis
  - RV infarction

Abbreviations: JVP, jugular venous pressure; R-HF, right sided heart failure; RV, right ventricle; SVC, superior vena cava; TS, tricuspid stenosis

Adapted from: Filate W, et al. *The Medical Society, Faculty of Medicine, University of Toronto* 2005, page 57.

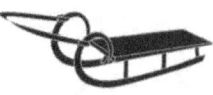

Abnormalities of the venous waveforms

Waveform		Cardiac Condition
• A waves	○ Absent	- Atrial fibrillation, sinus tachycardia
	○ Flutter	- Atrial flutter
	○ Prominent	- First degree AV block
	○ Large	- TS
		- Right atrial myxoma
		- PHT
		- PS
	○ Cannon wave	- AV dissociation
		- Ventricular tachycardia
• X descent	○ Absent	- TR
	○ Prominent	- Conditions causing enlarged a waves
	○ Large *cv* waves	- TR
		- Constrictive pericarditis
• Y descent	○ Slow	- TS
		- Right atrial myxoma
	○ Rapid	- Constrictive pericarditis
		- Severe R-HF
		- TR
		- ASD
	○ Absent	- Cardiac tamponade

Abbreviations: ASD, atrial septal defect; AV, atrioventricular; PHT, pulmonary hypertension; PS, pulmonic stenosis; R-HF, right sided congestive heart failure; TR, tricuspid regurgitation, TS, tricuspid stenosis

Adapted from: Simel DL, et al. *JAMA* 2009, Table 11-1, page 126, and Mangione S. *Hanley & Belfus* 2000, pages 194 and 195.

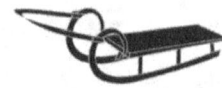

- Give the performance characteristics of inspection of the neck veins.

Finding	PLR
o Elevated venous pressure at the bedside	
– Detecting measured CVP > 8 cm H_2O	9.0
– Detecting measured CVP > 12 cm H_2O	10.4
– Detecting elevated left heart diastolic pressures	3.9
– Detecting low left ventricular ejection fraction	7.9
– Predicting postoperative pulmonary edema	11.3
– Predicting post-operative myocardial infarction or cardiac death	9.4
o Positive abdominojugular test	
– Detecting elevated left heart diastolic pressures	8.0

Abbreviation: CVP, central venous pressure; PLR, positive likelihood ratio; NLR, negative likelihood ratio; NS, not significant

Adapted from: McGee SR. *Saunders/Elsevier*, 2007, Box 32-1, page 378.

- Perform a focused physical examination to determine if a patient's elevated JVP is due to SVC (superior vena caval) obstruction?

  o Face
  - Edema
  - Cyanosis
  - Collateral vessels

  o Eyes
  - Exophthalmosis
  - Papilledema

  o Signs in face and eyes become worse when the patient leans forward.

Germs and Pearls

Under which circumstance does the patient's pulse rate reduce the specificity of the finding of an elevated JVP to suggest CHF?

  o In the presence of bradycardia

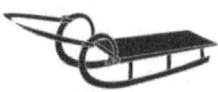

Mastering the Boards: Cardiology A.B.R. Thomson

- Perform a focused physical examination to determine if a patient's elevated JVP is **not** due to heart failure.

  - Heart
    - HF (heart failure)
    - TR (tricuspid regurgitation)
    - ↑ blood volume
    - Bradycardia

  - VC (vena cava)
    - SVC obstruction
    - ↑ intra-abdominal pressure on IVC

  - Neck
    - Compression of neck veins

  - Lung
    - Pleural effusions
    - ↑ intrathoracic pressure

Trick Questions

- Give how to tell if, the vessel in the neck is the jugular vein (JV) or the carotid artery (CA).

	JV	CA
o Inwards x,y waves	✓	No
o Upper level	✓	No
o Upper level falls with inspiration	✓	No
o Seen, better than felt	✓	No
o Felt, better than seen	No	✓

Jugular Venous Pressure (JVP)

'a'
  - o Atrial contraction
    - absent in AF
    - prominent in
      - PHT
      - PS
      - TS

'x'
  - o Atrial relaxation
'y'
  - o Tricuspid valve opens
'c'
  - o Tricuspid valve closes
'v'
  - o Venous blood returns to RA
  - o Not due to contraction of ventricle
  - o Often prominent in TR

Movement

Outwards   Inwards

a, v ←   → x, y

Abbreviation: PHT, pulmonary hypertension; PS, pulmonary stenosis; TS,

---

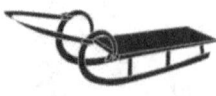

Mastering the Boards: Cardiology   A.B.R. Thomson

Trick Questions

- What are the performance characteristics of a "carotid shudder"?

A palpable thrill on the slow stroke (pulsus tardis)
- Definition of carotid shudder
- Carotid shudder arises from the transmission of the murmurs of AS, AR, or AS plus AR to the artery.
- "... relatively specific but insensitive sign of aortic valvular disease"

Source: Mangione S. *Hanley & Belfus* 2000, page 186.

- Give in which side of the neck the carotid bruit is best auscultated in the person with an iatrogenic forearm AV fistula prepared for hemodialysis.

    - Louder carotid bruit on the same side as the AV fistula.

- Atherosclerotic disease is common in persons with chronic renal failure (CRF). In the CRF patient with an AV fistula for hemodialysis, what sigh if present favors the cause of the carotid bruit to be due to the fistula rather than being due to a carotid stenosis?

    - An Associated subclavian bruit.

- Give what is the clinical significance of auscultating a carotid bruit.

o Asymptomatic	- Age 50, male - preoperative	▪ 3 x ↑ annual risk of CVA, TIA, death from coronary heart disease ▪ ↑ risk of postoperative dysfunction and behavior problems (but <u>not</u> predictive of ↑ post-op risk of CVA)
o Symptomatic		▪ ↑ risk of 70% to 99% stenosis ("high-grade" stenosis)

- Give how you can assess central venous pressure (CVP) from the left internal jugular vein (IJV).

    - The right IJV more directly reflects right atrial pressure, and CVP measured on left side is higher than on the right side.

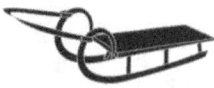

- Perform a direct physical examination to distinguish between the JVP and carotid waveforms.

Characteristic	Venous Pulse	Carotid Pulse
o Location	Low in neck and lateral	Deep in neck and medial
o Contour	Double-peaked and diffuse	Single-peaked and sharp
o Character	Undulant, not palpable	Force, brisk, easily felt
o Waveform	Diffuse biphasic	Single sharp
o Positional change	Varies with position	No variation
o Respiratory variation	Height falls on inspiration	No variation
o Effect of palpation	Wave nonpalpable, pressure obliterates pulse, vein fills	Pulse palpable, not compressible
o Abdominal pressure	Displaces pulse upward	Pulse unchanged

Abbreviation: JVP, jugular venous pressure

Adapted form: Simel DL, et al. *JAMA* 2009 Table 11-2, 127; and Mangione S. *Hanley & Belfus* 2000, page 192.

Cardiac Apex Beat

Clinical Tricks

- Give how would you modify the physical examination of the precordium to determine if there is systolic retraction of the apex beat (PMI).
  - o Have patient sit upright, and inhale

- Give what conditions are associated with systolic retraction of the apex beat.
  - o Pericardial adhesions
  - o Right ventricular hypertrophy

- Give what conditions give a weak apex beat.
  - o Obesity
  - o Emphysema
  - o Pleural effusions
  - o Dextro cardia
  - o CHF (congestive heart failure)

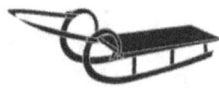

Peripheral Edema

➢ Causes

- Unilateral
    - ○ Vein
        - Deep vein thrombosis
        - Varicose veins
        - Postphlebitic limb
        - Venous valve incompetence
        - Compression of large veins by tumour or lymph nodes
    - ○ Artery
        - Arterial occlusion
    - ○ Lymphatic obstruction
    - ○ Tissue
        - Cellulitis
        - Trauma
        - Arthritis
        - Cellulitis
        - Ruptured Baker cyst
        - Localized immobility (e.g. hemiparesis)
        - Filariasis
    - ○ Congenitial

Adapted from: Baliga RR. *Saunders/Elsevier* 2007, page 560.

- Pitting bilateral lower limb edema
    - ○ Cardiac
        - Heart failure
        - Constrictive pericarditis
        - Beri beri
    - ○ Gastrointestinal tract
        - Malabsorption
        - Starvation
        - Protein losing enteropathy
    - ○ Endocrine
        - Hypothyroidism
    - ○ Hepatic
        - Cirrhosis

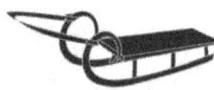

- o Renal
    - Renal failure
    - Nephrotic syndrome

- o Cyclical edema

- o Drugs
    - NSAIDs
    - Calcium channel blockers

- o Lymphatic obstruction
    - Tumor
    - Allergy
    - Infection
    - Idiopathic (Milroy disease)

- Deep vein obstruction

Abbreviation: GI, gastrointestinal; R-CCF, right-sided congestive cardiac failure

Adapted from: Talley NJ, et al. *Maclennan & Petty Pty Limited* 2003, Table 3.11, page 64; Davey P. *Wiley-Blackwell* 2006, page 1.

- ➢ Non-pitting lower limb edema
    - o Hypothyroidism
    - o Lymphedema
        - Infectious (e.g. filariasis)
        - Malignant (tumour invasion of lymphatics)
        - Congenital (lymphatic development arrest)
        - Allergy

    - o Ideopathic
        - Milroy disease (unexplained lymphedema which appears at puberty and is more common in females)

Abbreviations: DVT, deep vein thrombosis; NSAIDs, nonsteroidal anti-inflammatory drugs.

Adapted from: Talley NJ, et al. *Maclennan & Petty Pty Limited* 2003, Table 3.11, page 54; Davey P. *Wiley-Blackwell* 2006, Table 5.1, page 15.

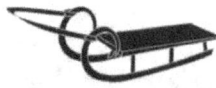

- Perform a focused physical examination to differentiate between venous edema versus lymphedema.

Feature	Venous	Lymphedema
o Bilateral	+/-	+/-
o Foot involved	+	+
o Toes involved	0	+
o Thickened skin	0	+
o Stasis	+	0

Source: Ghosh AK. *Mayo Clinic Scientific Press* 2008, Table 25-7; page 1049.

- Perform a focused physical examination for causes of bilateral leg swelling:

o Heart	– Cardiac failure
o Kidney	– Renal failure
o Skin	– Cellulitis
	– Trauma
	– Burn
o Vessels	– Deep vein thrombosis
	– Arterial occlusion
	– Venous causes

- Varicose veins
- Post-phlebitic limb

o Joints	– Arthritis
o Lymphatics	– Milroy disease
	– Filariasis (in the tropics)
o GI	– Hypoproteinemia
o Ideopathic congenital	– Congenital

Adapted from: Baliga RR. *Saunders/Elsevier* 2007, page 560.

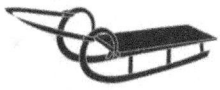

- Perform a focused physical examination to differentiate between the types of regional edema.

	Feature	Venous	Lymphedema	Lipedema
o	Bilateral	Occasional	+/-	Always
o	Foot involved	+	+	0
o	Toes involved	0	+	0
o	Thicken skin	0	+	0
o	Stasis changes	+	0	0

Source: Ghosh AK. *Mayo Clinic Scientific Press* 2008, Table 25-7, page 1049.

➢ Laboratory

- Give the chest X-ray changes seen in pulmonary edema.
    - o Costophrenic angles
        - Kerley "B" lines (septal lines)
            - Small, horizontal, parallel lines from dilated lymphotics in the inter lobar septa
        - Pleural effusions
            - Also seen in the transverse or oblique fissures
    - o Hilum
        - Fuzzy, homogeneous opacities radiating outwards from hilum
        - Hazy hilar vessels
    - o Lung fields
        - Fuzzy lower zone, or all of lung
        - Upper lobe, dilated veins

- Pulmonary edema (PE) is often associated with cardiomegaly. Give conditions in which PE is not associated with cardiomegaly.
    - o CNS
        - Head injury
        - CVA
    - o Lung
        - Viral pneumonia
        - Chemical pneumonitis
        - Pneumoconiosis, silicosis
    - o Heart
        - Mitral stenosis
        - Constrictive pericarditis
        - Constrictive cardiomyopathy

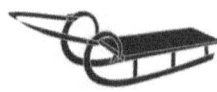

- Give 3 causes of a carotid bruit.

    - Carotid stenosis
    - High-output states
    - AV fistula of the forearm
    - Normal finding in children (~20% of children < 15 years)

- HF (heart failure) is suspected from a clinical syndrome comprised of symptoms and signs, plus clinical evidence of the causes and complications of HF. Give 4 laboratory or diagnostic imaging tests used to make the diagnosis of HF.

    - BNP (brain naturetic peptide, or terminal pro BNP levels in blood performance characteristics depend upon clinical presentation.

o BNP	- ER, dyspnea	▪ < 100 pg/mL excludes compensated HF
	- Outpatient established HF	▪ May be up to 500 pg/mL look changes above patient's previous baseline valves

B-type Naturetic Peptide (BNP)

- B-type naturetic peptide (BNP) is released from cardiac cardiac myocytes when there is
    - ↑ preload
    - ↑ afterload
    - ↑ stress in cardiac wall
- BNP is increased in the serum of patients with acute heart failure.

- Give one non-cardiac condition that will lower BNP levels, and which will increase BNP.

o Increase	- Age
	- Gender
	▪ Women
	- Kidney
	▪ CKD
o Decrease	- ↑ BMI (obesity)

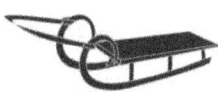

- o Chest X-ray   - Assess for
  - Heart > ½ transverse measurement
  - Enlarged chambers
  - May still be ↑ intravascular and ↑ filling pressures
  - Pulmonary edema
  - May be falsely negative

- o Cadiopulmonary exercise testing
  - May be vague
  - Functional capacity
  - Evaluation of exercise limitation
  - Evaluation for heart transplantation
  - Gas exchange

- o CMR (cardiac MR)
  - May be vague
  - Improved diagnosis of cardiomyopathy

- o ECG
  - Q wave
    - Lymphedema (TS)
    - Possible old MI
  - ↑ HR
    - Lymphedema (TS)
    - Possible tachycardia-mediated cardiomyopathy
  - ↑ voltage
    - Lymphedema (TS)
    - Pericardial effusion
    - Cardiomyopathy
  - Obesity (↑ BMI)
  - Emphysema
  - Arrhythmia
  - QRS interval

- o Echocardiogram
  - May be vague
  - Ejection fraction
  - LV hypertrophy or infiltration (cardiomyopathy)
  - Wall movement
  - Pulmonary hypertension
  - Pericardial effusion
  - Assessment of murmurs, shunts
  - Diastolic filling across mitral valve poor prognosis

- o Coronary angiography
  - Assess candidacy for revascularization

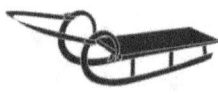

Clinical Gem

o A pleural effusion usually has features of a transudate when caused by heart failure (HF), but if the HF-patient has been on diuretics, the pleural effusion may have borderline exudative chemical characteristics. For example, the modified Light criteria are usually ~ 100% sensitive and 83% specific for an exudate process, except when there is concurrent therapy with diuretics.

o When the

- Albumin gradient between serum to pleural fluid > 1.2 g/dL, or

- Total protein gradient between serum to pleural fluid > 3.1 g/dL (31 g/L)

- The pathophysiological process can be transudative or exudative

- Said another way, finding a pleural effusion in patient with HF on diuretic cannot with certainty be considered to be non-exudative

Superior Vena Cava Obstruction

- Take a directed history and perform a focused physical examination for superior vena cava (SVC) obstruction.

   o History
      - Headache
      - Blackouts
      - Swelling of the face
      - Dysphagia
      - Dyspnea
      - Wheezes

   o Examination
      - General
         • Dyspnea
      - Face
         • Plethora
         • Dyspnea
         • Edema

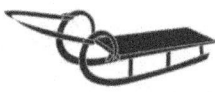

- Eyes
  - Horner syndrome
  - Signs of radiation marks
- Neck
  - Tortuous, visible and dilated veins on the chest wall and neck
  - Neck veins non pulsatile
- Signs of brochogenic carcinoma
  - Clubbing
  - Tar staining (tobacco smoking)
  - Lymph nodes
  - Chest signs

➤ Causes
  - ○ Bronchogenic carcinoma (commonest cause, 70% of cases)
  - ○ Lymphoma – in young adults
  - ○ Other causes:
    - Aortic aneurysm
    - Mediastinal goitre
    - Mediastinal fibrosis (due to methysergide, histoplasmosis or TB)
    - Constrictive pericarditis

Adapted from: Baliga RR. *Saunders/Elsevier* 2007, pages 593 and 594.

➤ Treatment

Systolic Heart Failure (↓ ejection fraction [EF])

Once HF has been diagnosed, it is important to access the patient's functional therapy, so as to better advise optimal therapy.

- Give the New York Hear Association (NYHA) functional class of HF.

New York Heart Association (**NYHA**) functional classification of congestive heart failure

Class	Activity evoking angina	Limits to physical activity
I	None	None
II	Ordinary physical activity	Slight
III	Walking < 2 blocks or < 1 flight of stairs	Marked
IV	Minimal or at rest	Severe

Abbreviation: NYHA, New York heart association

Source: Filate W, et al. *The Medical Society, Faculty of Medicine, University of Toronto* 2005, Table 3, page 55.

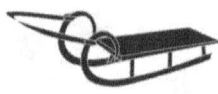

➢ NYHA I, II
  ○ ACE inhibitor, plus
    - ↓ afterload
    - ↓ activation of renin0angiotensinaldosterone system
      ▪ LV dysfunction
      ▪ ↓ development after MI
      ▪ LV dysfunction
    - ↓ hospitalization
    - ↓ mortality
    - Do **not** combine ACEI with ARB (angiotensin-receptor blocker)
    - Do **not** use with Hypovolemia
  ○ β-blocker
    - ↓ myocyte function → ↓ LV remodeling
    - Vasodilation (in β-blockers with α1-receptor blocking properties)
    - ↓ mortality
    - LV dysfunction
      ▪ ↓ progression
    - Caution: do not use with decompensated HF

➢ NYHA III, IV
  ○ ACE inhibitor, plus β-blocker, plus or eplerenone
  ○ Spirolactone or eplerenone, plus hydrazalazine-isosorbide dinitrate (especially in African-Canadian)
    - Guideline for use of spironolactone
      ▪ NYHA III-IV symptoms
      ▪ K^+ < 5 mmol/L (5 mEq/L)
      ▪ Creatinine < 221 mmol/L (2.5 mg/dL)
      ▪ ↓ mortality, ↓ hospitalization, ↓ NYHA symptom class
    - Eplereone may also have role in NYHA class II HF after MI when EF ≤ 35%

Clinical Caution

• Give the β-blockers which are **not** to be used in HF (heart failure).

  ○ Acebutolol and pindolol must not be used in persons with HF because of their sympathomimetic activity.

  ○ Digoxin
    - ↓ symptoms in S-HF (systolic HF, i.e. HF with ↓ EF)
    - Control of heart rate in AF (Atrial fibrillation); follow K^+_s to avoid ↑ risk of dig' toxicity

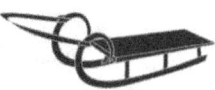

Peripartum Vascular Disorders

- Give cardiovascular changes which occur in the peripartum period.

    - o Blood
        - ↑↑ plasma volume
        - ↑ RBC mass
        - ↑ total blood volume
        - Dilutional anemia
        - Mild peripheral edema

    - o Heart
        - ↑ HR (heart rate, 20-30%)
        - ↓ systemic vascular resistance
        - ↓ BP (blood pressure (~ 10 mm Hg)
        - ↑ CO (cardiac output)
        - 1/6 -2/6 systolic murmur (80%)

    - o S3 gallop
        - APB (atrial premature beats)
        - VPB (ventricular premature beats)

- Give 7 factors important for prenatal risk stratification for Maternal Cardiovascular Complication during pregnancy.

    - o Previous
        - HF (heart failure)
        - TIA (transient ischemic attack)
        - CVA (cerebrovascular accident)
        - Arrhythmia

    - o Cyanosis
    - o NYHA class III or IV for baseline symptoms
    - o Left-side obstruction
        - MVA (mitral valve area) < 2 cm^2
        - AVA (aortic valve area) < 1.5 cm^2
        - RPLVOTG (resting peak left ventricle outflow tract gradient) > 30 mm Hg

    - o Ventricular systolic function
        - ↓ EF < 40%

    - o Pulmonary hypertension (PAP ≥ 2/3 SBP, Maternal mortality ~ 50%)

Abbreviations: PAP, pulmonary artery pressure; SBP, systolic blood pressure

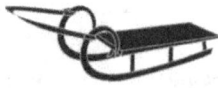

SYNCOPE

- Take a directed history and perform a focused physical examination for syncope.
  - Vasovagal
    - Emotional, heat, standing still
    - Postural hypotension
      - Prolonged recumbency
      - Vasodilator drugs
      - Autonomic neuropathy: familial, diabetes, etc.
      - Micturition syncope
      - Swallowing syncope
      - Carotid sinus hypersensitivity
      - Cough syncope
  - Cardiac
    - Tachycardia
    - Strokes-Adams
    - Aortic stenosis, HOCM
    - Atrial myxoma, ball-valve thrombus
    - Constrictive pericarditis
    - Cyanotic congenital heart disease
  - Cerebral
    - Anoxia
      - High altitude
      - CO poisoning
      - Anemia
      - Atheroma, embolus
      - Cervical spondylosis, strangulation
      - Subclavian steal syndrome
    - Hypoglycemia
    - Hypocapnai
  - Hysterical

Adapted from: Burton JL. *Churchill Livingstone* 1971, page 17.

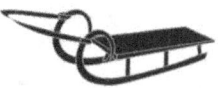

- ➢ Pathophysiological types
  - o Neurocardiogenic
    - – Vasovagal
      - Cardioinhibition ($\downarrow\downarrow$ AR, asystole)
      - Vasodepression (peripheral vasodilation)
    - – Carotid sinus hypersensitivity
    - – Situational
      - Pass urine stool
      - Coughing
      - Swallowing
  - o Orthostatic hypotension
    - – Hypovolemia
    - – Autonomic dysfunction
    - – Drugs
  - o Cardiovascular
    - – Arrhythmia
      - Dysfunction of
        - Sinus node
          - Conduction system
          - AV block
        - Pacemaker
      - %VT
      - VT
      - WPW syndrome
        - Long QT syndrome
    - – Mechanical
      - Heart stenosis
        - Aortic stenosis
        - Hypertrophic cardiomyopathy
        - Atrial myxoma
      - Aorta
        - Dissection
      - Lung
        - Pulmonary hypertension
      - Subclavian artery
        - Subclavian "steal" syndrome
  - o Pseudo-syncope
    - – Psychogenic
    - – Lung
      - Hypoxia
    - – CNS
      - Seizure
      - CVA / TIA
      - Severe atherosclerotic
      - Obstruction of 4 cerebral vessels
    - – Endocrine
      - Hypoglycemia

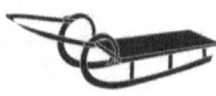

Postural (Orthostatic) Hypotension And Hypovolemia

➢ Definition

   o With a change in body position
- ↓ systolic BP >15 mmHg
- ↓ diastolic BP >0-10 mmHg
- And/or ↑ heart rate >20 bpm

   o Seen in conditions of autonomic dysfunction or volume depletion.

Abbreviation: BP, blood pressure

To examine a patient for orthostatic hypotension measure BP in supine patient, then have the patient sit up with the legs down or have patient stand for 2 minutes before reassessing BP.

Source: Jugovic PJ, et al. *Saunders/ Elsevier*, 2004, page 187.

- Take a directed history for the causes of postural hypotension.

   o Hypovolemia
- Bleeding, dehydration

   o Drugs
- Vasodilators
- Diuretics
- Anticholinergics (including TCAs)

   o Endocrine
- Diabetes
- Addison disease
- Hypopituitarism

   o Autonomic neuropathy
- Diabetes
- Amyloidosis
- Shy-Drager syndrome

   o Idiopathic

Abbreviation: TCAs, tricyclic antidepressants.

Adapted from: Talley NJ, et al. *Maclennan & Petty Pty Limited* 2003, page 44.

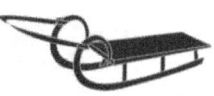

- Give the use of postural tachycardia to predict the severity of blood loss causing hypovolemia.

Supine to standing, PR ↑ 30 bpm	Sensitivity (%)	Specificity (%)
○ Moderate blood loss < 630 mL	22	98
○ Severe blood loss > 630 mL	97	-

Abbreviation: bpm, beats per minute

Source: Simel DL, et al. *JAMA* 2009, Table 24-9, page 327.

➤ Causes of hypovolemic shock

- ○ Abnormal distribution
  - CNS
    - Neurogenic
  - GI
    - Hepatic failure
    - Pancreatitis
  - CVS
    - Thiamine deficiency
    - Anaphylactic
  - Infection
    - Sepsis
  - Adrenal crisis

- ○ ↑ loses
  - GI
    - Bleeding
    - Vomiting
    - Diarrhea
  - Skin
    - Burns
    - Exudative skin lesions
  - Lung
    - Bronchorrhea
    - Allergic alveolitis
  - Kidney
    - Diuretics
    - Diabetes mellitus
    - Diabetes insipidus
    - Lack of access to water (e.g bedbond)

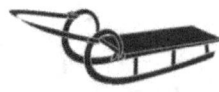

- Trauma
  - Pancreatitis
  - Crush injuries
- Malnutrition/ dehydration

Adapted from: Ghosh AK. *Mayo Clinic Scientific Press* 2008, Table 3.29, page 107, Table 4-18 and Table 4-19, page 161.

- Perform a directed physical examination for hypovolemia (volume depletion).

  - Tilt test: (supine or standing) – postular ↑ HR by 30 bpm (sensitivity of 97%, specificity of 96% for blood loss >630 ml)
  - Supine SBP <95 mmHg, HR > 100 bpm
  - Poor skin turgor, seen as "tenting" of skin when pinched
  - Slow capillary refill time (2 sec for children and adult males, 3 sec for adult women, 4 sec for elderly) (sensitivity for hypovolumia only 11%, but specificity of 89%)
  - Drug mucous membranes and axillae
  - Sunken eyes
  - Longitudinal tongue furrows

Adapted from: Mangione S. *Hanley & Belfus* 2000, pages 3 to 4.

- Give the performance characteristics of hypotension and its predicting mortality.

Finding	PLR
o Systolic blood pressure <90 mm Hg	
- In intensive care unit	4.0
- In patients with bacteremia	4.9
- In patients with pneumonia	10.0
o Systolic blood pressure ≤ 80 mm Hg	
- Predicting mortality in patients with acute myocardial infarction	15.5

Source: McGee SR. *Saunders/Elsevier* 2007, Box 15.1 page 161.
THERAPEUTICS

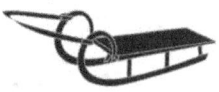

Mastering the Boards: Cardiology   A.B.R. Thomson

B-blockers

- o Avoid B-blockers with ISA (intrinsic sympathetics mimetic activity) e.g.
  - Acebutolol
  - Carteolol
  - Pendolol
  - Pindolol

- o Use cautiously in present if
  - Reactive airway disease
  - Bradyarhythmias
  - HF (heart failure)
  - Vasospastic / Prinzmetal variant angina

- o May be coadministered with CCBs (calcium channel blockers)

Calcium Channel Blockers (CCB)

- o Use alone, or with B-blockers
- o Avoid short-activity dihydropyridine nifedipine
- o In presence of systolic dysfunction ($\downarrow$ LV EF) avoid long-activity non-dihydropyridines
  Diltiazem
  Verapamil

Nitrates

- o Useful for $\downarrow$ symptoms, but do not $\downarrow$ risk of death
- o Do not use with phosphodiesterase-5 inhibitors (stop for 48 hr if using sildewafil or vardenafil, and 48 hr if using tadalafil)

Angiotensin Converting Enzyme Inhibitors (ACEI) / Angiotensin receptor blockers (ARB)

- o Indications of ACEIs: All persons with
  - Stable angina
  - LV EF < 40%
  - Hypertension
  - Diabetes
  - Chronic renal disease

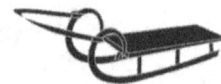

- o Indications of ARBs: same as for ACEIs, plus
  - Intolerance to ACEIs
    - Angioedema
    - Cough
    - ↑ creatinine
  - Bilateral renal stenosis
  - With NSAIDs
  - Dehydration
  - Severe retention of Na^+

LDL-Cholesterol Lowering Agents

- Give which of the several classes of drugs which are used for secondary prevention to ↓ LDL-C / ↓ TG (triglycerides), (such as resins, statins, fibrates, nicotinic acid derivatives) have been shown to ↓ mortality.

  - o Easy, simple
    - The statins

Coronary Revascularization Surgery (CABG, coronary artery bypass grafting)

- o Failed medical therapy failure when 3 classes of anti-anginal drugs use
- o Stable angina patient with no high risk factors or ↓ LV-EF = PCI CV outcomes
- o Note
  - Medical therapy of angina does not ↓ risk of
    - MI
    - Death
- o CABG > Rx therapy for survival
- o CABG rather than PCI
  Left disease with artery
  Low comorbidities
- o Calculate STS (Society of Thoracic Surgeons) risk score used to help decide between CABG vs PCI
  http://riskcalc.sts.org/STSWebCalc2731

- o Calculate Syntax score to determine suitability of anatomy for PCI
  http://www.syntaxscore.com/

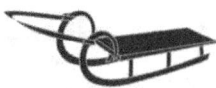

- o CABG > PCI when
  - LV EF < 35%
  - Non-invasive stress testing shows-reversible ischemia, or
  - 3-vessel disease, or
  - Proximal left-anterior descending (LAD) viable myocardium artery plus a second artery
  - 2-vessel disease causing severe ischemia on stress imaging (e.g. > 20% myocardial ischemia)
  - Multi-vessel disease in diabetes, placing left interval mammary artery (LIMA)

- o CABG = PCI
  - Acute coronary syndrome (ACS)
  - Survival from SCD (sudden cardiac death) due to ischemic ventricular tachycardia
  - Multi-vessel disease in diabetics and a syntax score < 22 (less post-PCI CVA than post-CABG)

- o CABG and PCI have not been evaluated and compared for ↓ LV EF

- o CABG = PCI for rates of
  - Myocardial infarction (MI)
  - Stroke
  - Death

- o PCI > CABG for recurrent angina after CABG

Outcomes	CABG	Elective PCI
o Operative mortality	1-3%	< 1%
o Perioperative MI	5-10%	2-5%
o Perioperative CVA		Likely lower than with CABG
o Need for emergent CABG for failure of PCI		< 1%
o Graft patency		
- Saphenous vein graft	40-50% (10 yr)	
- Internal mammary artery graft	90% (10 yr)	
- Radial artery graft	80% (5 yr)	

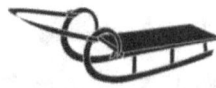

- Late (> 10 yr) recurrent
  Angina / other adverse cardiac events, 50%
- Need for repeat procedure PCI > post-CABG
- Follow-up
  - Secondary prevention measures (similar to primary prevention)
  - Cardiac rehabilitation program, with exercise
  - Minor angina post-CABG / post-PCI
    - Antianginal drugs
  - Significant angina
    - Stress testing with imaging, or
    - Cardiac angiography

CLINICAL CAUTION

Post-PCI patients require both ASA plus P2Y12 antagonist for months, depending on type of PCI stent used

- **Do not** perform PCI if patient is unlikely to be adherent to taking ASA plus P2Y12 (↑↑ risk of restenosis)

Non-ST-Segment Elevation Myocardial Infarction (NSTEMI)

➢ Definition
- No ST-segment elevation
- ↑ CK-MB (creatitine kinase MB) or troponin

➢ Clinical

- Give the presentations of unstable angina.

  - Rest — Occurs at rest and lasts > 20 min

  - New onset

  - Progressive — More frequent
    - Lasts longer
    - Precipitated by less excretion

  - Acute coronary — Severe
    syndrome: angina — Long
    — At rest

  - Angina equivalents

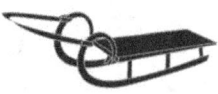

- Give characteristics of the chest pain, which may represent angina equivalents.

    o Pain radiating to
      - Jaw
      - Arm
      - Epigastrium
      - Neck
      - Back

CLINICAL ALERT

In patient with CHD, give the most common symptom which occur in the absence of pain.

   o Dyspnea is the most common presentation in "silent MIs"

SO YOU WANT TO BE A CARDIOLOGIST!

- Give the cardiac and the intracranial lesions associated with:

    - T-wave inversion > 5 mm
    - QT prolongation in V2 to V1

  o Cardiac
    - Critical stenosis in LAD distribution

  o Intracranial
    - Bleeding

- Give the clinical significance of non-specific / non-diagnostic

    - ST-segment changes
    - T-wave inversion

  o Non-diagnostic / non-specific ST-segment changes and T-wave inversion
    - Do **not** suggest current acute ischemia, but
    - Do suggest ↑ risk of future cardiac ischemic events

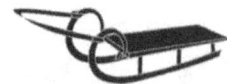

CLINICAL TIPS TO REMEMBER

- o A transient ST-segment elevation does not equal STEEMI
- o 50% of NSTEMI patients have ECG changes
  - ST-segment
    - Elevations, transient
    - Depressions, in a2 contiguous leads
  - T-wave inversion > 5 mm
- o There are many causes of ST-segment elevation other than CAD
- o Q waves are normal if seen only in lead III ("isolated Q wave")

- o The diagnosis of NSEMI requires no persistent ST-segment elevation, possible other ECG changes such as ST-depression or T-wave inversion, and importantly a demonstrated ↑ in troponin, CK-MB and possibly myoglobin.

- o Because of the diagnostic importance of these biomarkers, it is important to appreciate the time when they become detectable (time of onset of detectability, peak concentration, and time of offset of detectability (return to normal).

- o For onset, peak and offset, the relative order in the kinetics of these biomarkers is M-C-T (myoglobin, CK-MB, troponin I, T):

	Onset, h	Peak, hr	Offset, hr
o Myoglobin	1-2	6-8	12-24
o CK MB	2-6	12-18	24-48
o Troponin I, T	3-6	24-36	120 (5R) to 336 (14 d)

- Suggestion
  - Draw blood for measurement of biomarkers within 6 hr of onset of chest pain, then repeat assessment in 8-12 hr
- o Myoglobin
  - Very early after onset of chest pain (within 1-2 hr)
  - Disadvantage
    - Non-specific
- o Troponin
  - Sensitivity and specificity
  - Usually absent in blood, so presence of troponin I or T is clinically important
  - Direct relationship between ↑ troponin and ↑ risk of MI size and prognosis

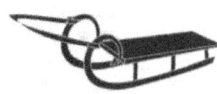

Mastering the Boards: Cardiology   A.B.R. Thomson

- o CK-MB
  - CK MB / total CK fraction > 2.5% → suggests myocardial injury
  - Useful to diagnose
    - Re-infarction (post-infarction ischemia)
    - Post-PCI infarction
  - Lack the higher specificity of ↑ troponin

- o Approach to ACS (acute coronary syndrome) base on presentation
  - UA
  - NSTEMI
  - STEMI

- o Risk characteristics

- o Diagnosis (stress testing, ejection fraction [EF]

- o Wall motion abnormality [WMA]

- o Treatment strategy
  - Early invasive
  - Early conservative

- ➢ Assessment of risk

- • Give the high-risk characteristics of ACS.

  - o Angina
    - Despite medical treatment
    - Recurrent
    - Accelerating

  - o Complications
    - HF (heart failure)
    - PE (pulmonary edema)
    - Shock
    - MR (mitral regurgitation)
      - New
      - Worsening

  - o ECG / monitoring
    - LBBB (new left bundle branch block)
    - VT (ventricular tachycardia)

- • Give the scoring systems to access risk of ACS.

  - o Risk of MI, cardiac death or revascularization
    - Grace (Global Registry of Acute Coronary events)
    - TIMI (Thrombolysis in myocardial infarction)
      - Score from 0 to 7 predicts 14 day rate of non-fatal MI, death, or revascularization, ranging from 5% to 40%

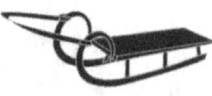

SO YOU WANT TO BE A CARDIOLOGIST!

The TIMI risk score may be used in the patient with ACS (acute coronary syndrome) to predict then 14-day risk of MI, death or need for revascularization. One part is scored for each of seven points, and the TIMI score guides subsequent investigation and management

- Give the components, which are used to calculate the TIMI risk score for NSTEMI.

  - Age > 65 yr
  - ≥ 2 pain episodes in 24 hr
  - Known CAD stenosis ≥ 50%
  - ASA used with in last 7 days
  - ↑ troponin / CK-MB
  - ECG changes in ST-segment or T-waves
  - ≥ 3 of the following risk factors for CAD
    - Diabetes
    - Hypertension
    - Hyperlipidemia
    - Smoking
    - Family history of CAD

➢ Types of initial approaches

- Medical treatment approaches, then testing

  - Low TIMI score (0-1), some selected intermediate TIMI score patients
    - Non-invasive cardiac stress test

  - Intermediate / high TIMI score
    - 72 yr after peak value of ↑ troponin, Ck-MB
    - No pain in past 12 yr
    - Submaximal exercise test, or pharmacologic test

  - Invasive approach preferable
    - For high-risk ACS
    - Coronary angiography early, before
    - Revascularization within 12-48 hr

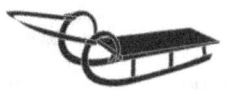

- Give the indications for coronary angiography is done for

  o High-risk ACS when revascularization planned within 12-48 hr, or
  o Intermediate-risk ACS patient who has
    - Angina at low level of exercise during stress test
    - High-risk stress test
    - LV EF < 40%

- Give the characteristics of the patient, which make the initial strategy preferably the invasive approach.

  o Low- / intermediate risk ACS patient treated medically but who experience repeated ACS
  o High-risk ACS patient
    - ↑ TIMI / GRACE risk score
    - Diabetes
    - Renal failure
    - LV EF < 40%
    - CABG, or PCI with last 6 mon
    - ↑ troponin / CK-MB
    - New ↓ ST-segment

Important Exception

  o The presence of renal insufficiency is a factor which in the high risk ACS patient makes the initial invasive strategy preferable.
  o However, severe renal insufficient (creatinine clearance test < 30 ml/min) or these are dialysis may do better on a conservative medical approach

---

Medications

  o Anti-platelet
  o Anti-coagulant
  o Anti-angina
    - Note: use O_2 supplementation only for
      - Hypoxemic < 90%
      - Dyspnea (SOB, shortness of breath)
      - Otherwise
        - Do **not** give unnecessary O_2 supplmentation

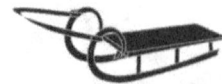

Antiplatelet Therapy

- o Types
  - - Aspirin (ASA)
  - - Thienopyridine PY12 receptor antagonist
    - • Clpidogrel
    - • Ticlopidine
    - • Prasugrel
  - - Reversible non-thienopyridine P2Y12 receptor antagonists
    - • Ticagrelor
  - - Glycoprotein (GP) IIb / IIIa antagonists
    - • Abciximab
    - • Eptifibatide
    - • Tirofiban

Aspirin

- o 1° / 2° prevention for CVA, CHD
- o ↓ risk of MI, SCD, repeat need for CABG 33%
- o Dose
  - - ASA 75-162 mg/d
  - - Clopidogrel 75 mg/d for ASA-sensitivity
- o Rapidly block platelet aggregation for days after even just one dose
- o Dosing
  - - Initial
  - - Maintenance
    - • 81 mg po od forever   Bare metal ASA 162-325 mg for 1 mon ⎤
    -                                       ⎬ Then 75-162 mg forever
    - • Following a PCI stent   Drug eluting ASA 162-325 mg for 6 mon ⎦

- o If patient is
  - - Allergic to ASA, or
  - - May be allergic to ASA 9asthma, nasal polyps, bronchospasm)
  - - Do not give ASA → bolus clopidogrel 300 – 600 mg

- o If patient on ASA with high risk of upper GI bleeding (UGIB, previous UGIB peptic ulcers H. pylori infection, comorbidities, drugs [NSAIDs, warfarin, corticosteroids), including use of ASA plus clopidogrel → PPI for gastroprotection

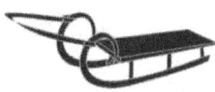

Clopidogrel

- o Prodrug converted to active metabolite by CYP2C19 activity
- o Metabolite inhibits P2Y12 receptor, so slower onset of anti-platelet activity
- o Low risk of bleeding TTP, neutroponin
- o Useful to use for
    - Dual or triple (e.g., ASA, clopidogrel, warfarin)
    - For both early conservative or invasive strategies
    - For NSTEMI or for STEMI
- o Dosing
    - 300-600 mg loading dose, then 75 mg od

- o Used much more now than ticlopidine, because of better safety profile

- Give the pharmacogenetic reason for the wide variation in patient response to clopidorel, and the way in which this resistance may be predicted and treated.

  o The prodrug clopidogrel is converted to the active metabolite (which blocks the P2Y12 receptor) by the gene CYP2C19
  o ↓ activity of CYP2C19 → ↓ active metabolite → ↓ antiplatelet activity
  o ↑ activity of CYP2C19 → ↑ active metabolite → ↑ antiplatelet activity

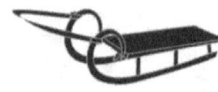

- Low activity of CYP2C19, causing clopidogrel resistance, can be determined by screening for
  - Genotyping for polymorphisms in CYP2C19 activity, or
  - Platelet inhibition
- If clopidogrel resistance is identified
  - ↑ dose of clopidogrel
  - Add glycoprotein IIb / IIIa inhibitors
  - Add prasugrel or ticagrelor

Prasugrel

- Prodrug with faster onset of uniform and greater action than with clopidogrel, but with ↑ risk of bleeding
- **Do not** use
  - 75 yr
  - < 60 kg
- Dosing
  - 60 mg loading dose, then 10 mg od

- Use only after coronary angiogram and when PCI is planned (invasive strategy)

Ticagrelor

- Used in either early conservative and early invasive strategies
- ↑ risk of bleeding, so **do not** use with prior TIA / CVA
- Dosing
- When given with ASA, after the loading dose of ASA is switched to maintenance ASA, the maintenance dose of ASA is < 100 mg when coadministered with ticagrelor

---

CLINICAL TRADE-OFF

- Prasugrel and ticagrelor have
  - Greater benefit than clopidogrel in ↓ risk of
    - MI
    - Stent thrombosis
    - CVA
    - Death
  - < but ↑ risk of bleeding

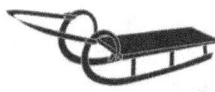

Anti-platelet drug	↓ in MI, CVA, CV death by	Bleeding
o Clopidogrel	18% - 30%	1%
o Prasugrel	10%	2.8%
o Tacagrelor	10%	4.5%

- Give the times prior to CABG revascularization surgery that the antiplatelet drugs are stopped.

Antiplatelet drug	Drug stopped prior to CABG
o Clopidogrel	5 days
o Prasugrel	7 days
o Tacagrelor	3-5 days
o GP IIb / IIIa	4 hr

Glycoprotein (GP) IIb / IIIa antagonist

- o ↓ platelet aggregation by ↓ interaction between platelets and ffibrinogen
- o Indications for use of eptifibatide or tirofiban
  - Add-on therapy to ASA plus heparin in ACS for ↑ ischemia
  - Troponin-positive during PCI
  - Sometimes for troponin-negative during PPI
  - Add-on therapy for troponin-positive
    - TIMI > 3
    - Diabetes
    - ↓ ST-segment (significant depression)
- o Relative contraindications
  - ↑ risk of bleeding
  - Thrombocytopenia
    - Monitor
    - Treat by platelet transfusion as needed
- o Benefits ↓ risk of MI or death
- o Dosing
  - Eptifibatide
    - 180 mcg/kg IV bolus, then 2 mcg/kg per min
  - Tirofiban
    - 0.4 mcg/kg IV bolus, then 0.1 mcg/kg per min
  - Abciximab
    - 0.25 mg/kg IV bolus, then 10 mcg per min

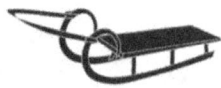

- Give the name of the glycoprotein IIb / IIIa antagonist which is used only for the indication of achieving antiplatelet activity during **PCI**.

  o Abciximab may be started up to 4 hr before or during PCI

Anticoagulation Therapy

  o Types
  - Indirect thrombin inhibitors
    - UFH (unfractionated heparin)
    - LMWH (low molecular weight heparin), enoxaparin
  - Direct thrombin inhibition
    - Bilvalirudin
  - Selective factor Xa inhibitor
    - Fondaparinux

  o Indication
  - All UA (unstable angina) / NSTEMI patients require anti-coagulant plus dual antiplatelet therapy for both conservative and for invasive strategies

Anticoagulant	Route / dose	aPTT monitoring	Risk of HIT	Caution	Strategy
o UFH	IV (target 1.5-2x control) 60 U/kg bolus to max 400 U, then 12-14 U/kg per hr	Yes	High		Both CON and INV
o LMWH (enoxaparin)	1 mg/kg SC bid	No	Low	- Stop on an angiography - ↑ risk of bleeding	CON, INV in CON, preferred t(UFN
o Fondaparinux	2.5 mg SC od	No	No	- In CON, preferred to UFN - In INV with PCI, must add UFN	CON, INV
o Bivalirudin	IV 0.75 mg/kg bolus, then 1.75 mg/kg per hr	Yes	No		

Abbreviations: HIT, immune-mediated heparin-induced thrombocytopenia; CON, conservative strategy; INV, invasive strategy

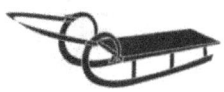

Comparisons

- ○ Lowest risk of HIT
  - Fondaparinux
  - Bilvalirudin

- ○ Highest risk of bleeding
  - LWMH (enoxaparin) plus dual antiplatelet therapy
  - Use of concern with history of TIA / CVA

- ○ Previous or current HIT
  - Bivalrudin

- ○ Conservative strategy
  - Fondaparinux (rather than UFN)

- ○ Superior outcome (compared to enoxaparin [LMWH])
  - Fondaparinux

- ○ No data for use in invasive strategy
  - Bivalirudin

*Superior outcome: lowest risk of
  - MI (myocardial infarction)
  - Refractory ischemia
  - Major bleeding
  - Death

CLINICAL REMINDER

While anti-platelet, anticoagulation and anti-ischemia therapy is indicated in UA / NSTEMI, **do not** use thrombolytic therapy (thrombolytic therapy used for NSTEMI)

Anti-anginal Medication

CLINICAL ALERT

- ○ A successful trial of nitroglycerine (NTG, sublingual, topical, IV) to relieve chest pain is not a specific test for angina
- ○ NTG will ↓ chest pain in ~ half (40%) of persons whose chest pain is not from CAD

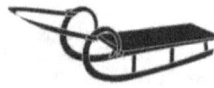

TREATMENT TIP

- o Anti-anginal medications may ↓ chest pain, but only B-blockers also ↓ risk of MI, recurrent ischemia and death

---

- Give the cautionary factors (contraindicated or relatively contraindicated) arising from serious adverse effects (AEs) of nitroglycerine, B-blockers and calcium channel blockers when used for control of angina.

Drug	Serious AEs
o Nitroglycerin	- Right-sided infarction - Preload-dependent ▪ AS (aortic stenosis) ▪ HOCM (hypertrophic obstructive cardiomyopathy) - Recent users of phosphodiesterase-5 inhibitors (PDEs) ▪ Sildenafil within 24 hr ▪ Tadalafil within 48 hr ▪ Vardenafil within time safety unknown – do not use - Use with caution in ▪ Vasospasm ▪ Prinzmetal angina
o B-blocker	- Do not use in ▪ Patients at risk for cardiogenic shock: - > 70 yr ▪ AV block (severe) ▪ Hypotension, bradycardia - SBP < 120 - HR < 60 > 110 bpm ▪ Active bronchospasm
o Calcium channel blockers	- Nifedipine - Verapamil, diltiazem ▪ Do not use if there is - ↓↓ LV EF - ↓ pulmonary edema - AV block

Abbreviations: AV, atrioventricular: LV EF, left ventricular ejection fraction SBP, systolic blood pressure

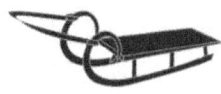

Mastering the Boards: Cardiology   A.B.R. Thomson

SO YOU WANT TO BE A CARDIOLOGIST!

- Give the explanation for why nitroglycerin (NTG) is not recommended in men with ED (erectile dysfunction) treated with a PDEs (phosphodiesterase inhibitors).

  o Both agents cause vasodilation, and the combination may result in severe hypotension.

- Give the reasons why calcium channel blockers are not considered to be first-line agents for the treatment of angina.

  o The calcium channel blockers are vasodilators if the coronary arteries, and as such may ↓ cardiac output (CO)
    - Short-acting nifedipine → ↑ risk of MI and death, so must be used with B-blocker
    - Long-acting diltaizem, verapamil → ↑ risk if used in presence of
      - ↓ LV EF
      - AV block
      - Pulmonary congestion
  o No benefit upon the risk of recurrent MI or death

Angiotensin Converting Enzyme Inhibitor (ACEIs)

  o Use in ACS plus
    - Diabetes
    - LV EF < 40%
    - Hypertension

  o Add aldosterone as long as no
    - Hyperkalemia (K+ > 5 mEq/L)
    - Renal insufficiency (creatinine clearance 30 ml/min)

  o Use ARB (angiotensin receptor blocker) if ACEI is not tolerated

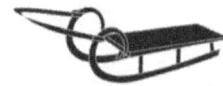

High dose statins

- ○ Use within 24 hr of ACS to rapidly ↓ LDL-C < 70 mg/dL
- ○ Benefits: ↓ risk of
  - MI
  - Peri-PCI MI
  - Recurrent ischemia
  - Death
- ○ Mechanism of benefit in ↓ LDL-C
- ○ Screen for depression, and treat as appropriate
- ○ Assessment and intervention as needed
- ○ Cardiac rehabilitation program

CLINICAL ALERT

- • Give the classes of medications which must not be used for analgesia of musculoskeletal pain in UA / NSTEMI.

  - ○ NSAIDs and COXIBs should not be used in ACS because of ↑ risk of
    - MI
    - Myocardial rupture
    - Death

SO YOU WANT TO BE A CARDIOLOGIST!

The non-cardiac patient with a GI bleed is transfused to a target hemoglobin of 7 mg/dL, and the cirrhotic patient with bleeding varices is transfused to a target of 9 g/dL.
- • Give the target outcome of blood transfusion in the patient with a NSTEMI who suffers from a GI bleed.

  - ○ Anemia is dangerous in the presence of NSTEMI because of
    - ↓ O_2 carrying capacity
    - ↓ myocardial O_2 supply

  - ○ Transfuse packed red blood cells to target values
    - Hemoglobin 10 mg/dL
    - Hematocrit 30%

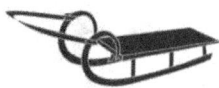

Invasive Strategy

- o Options
  - - PCI (percutaneous coronary intervention)
    - ▪ DES (drug eluting stent)
      - - ↓ ISR
      - - ↑ late stent thrombosis (especially if clopidogrel incorrectly stopped in year 1 after PCI)
    - ▪ BMS (bare metal stent)
  - - CABG (coronary artery bypass grafting)
    - ▪ Internal mammary artery
    - ▪ Long saphenous vein

- o Indications in
  - - Stable angina   Abnormal coronary vessels
  - - Unstable angina   Initial conservative strategy, or PCI
  - - NSTEMI   1-2, or 3 moderate
  - - CABG, PCI   Severe or left main coronary artery

- o CABG best for
  - - 1 vessel
    - ▪ Significant disease in left main coronary artery
  - - 2 vessels
    - ▪ In which there is complicated disease, and significant stenosis of left LAD (left anterior descending artery)
  - - Multi-vessel disease
  - - Diabetes

- • Give the role of FFR (fractional flow reserve ≤ 0.8) in deciding between PCI vs CABG (especially with multi-vessel CAD).

  - o ↓ FFR suggests CABG optimal to PCI for revascularization
  - o Using FFR testing and making an evidence-based decision for CABGs PCI results in ↓ 1 yr risk of
    - - Recurrent MI
    - - Revascularization
    - - Death

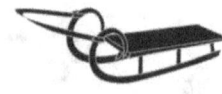

ST-segment Elevation Myocardial Infarction

- ➢ Demography
  - o A medical emergency due to high mortality rate
    30 day mortality rate
    - Half of this mortality rate predicted by TIMI-STEMI risk score > 8-35%
    - Mortality rate ~90% of a mechanical complication develops
      - VSD (ventricular septa defect)
      - PMR (papillary muscle rupture)
      - Free wall rupture

- ➢ Risk stratification

- • Give a comparison of TIMI risk score for STEMI versus NSTEMI.

		TIMI Risk Scores			
	Factors STEMI	Points	Factors	NSTEMI	Points
o Age	65-74	2	Age	> 65 yr	1
	≥ 75	3			
o ≥ 2 pain episodes in 24 hr					1
o Known CAD stenosis ≥ 50%	SBP < 100 mmHg	3			1
	HR > 100 bpm	2			1
o ASA used within last 7 days	Diabetes angina or hypertension	1			1
o ↑ troponin / CK-MB	Time to reperfusion > 4 hr Weight < 67 kg	1			1
o ECG changes in ST-segment or T-waves	ECG: anterior STEMI, or LBBB	1			1
	Killip class II-IV	2			1
o ≥ 3 of the following risk factors for CAD - Diabetes - Hypertension - Hyperlipidemia - Smoking	30-day mortality rate, TIMI STEMI risk score > 8 – 35%				

SO YOU WANT TO BE A CARDIOLOGIST!

- Give the physical findings used to determine the Killip risk score for STEMI and for each class give the approximate 30-day mortality rate.

Physical sign	Killip risk class	Approximate 3-day mortality
o No HF (heart failure)	1	5%
o S3 gallop, or pulmonary rules	2	15%
o Pulmonary edema	3	30-40%
o Cardiogenic shock	4	60-80%

- Give the ST-segment elevation (in two consecutive ECG leads) equivalents to make an ECG diagnosis of STEMI.

  - o New LBBB (left bundle branch block)
    - Suggests large infarct of anterior wall
      - Very bad prognosis
  - o Posterior MI (V7-V9)
    - ↑ ST-segment at J point > 0.5 mm

SO YOU WANT TO BE A CARDIOLOGIST!

- In addition to the individual components being different, give other variations between TIMI-NSTEMI, TIMI-STEMI and Killip class risk stratification.

  - o TIMI-NSTEMI
    - Model developed to predict 14-day mortality rate, MI, or revascularization

  - o TIMI-STEMI
    - Model developed to predict 3-day mortality rate (MR) in STEMI in the presence of PSI or CABG (invasive reperfusion strategy)

  - o Killip class
    - 30 day MR in STEMI in the absence of PSI or CABG

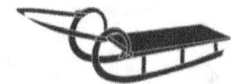

ECG

- ↑ ST-segment in two contiguous leads is suggestive of STEMI, and there is ↑ specificity if there are reciprocal ↓ ST-segment is opposite the area of suspected infarction; or new pathologic Q waves or peaked upright T waves are suggestive of myocardial damage.
- In addition to hyperkalemia and pulmonary embolism, there are many cardiac causes of ↑ ST-interval

- Give the criteria for pathological Q waves

  - V2, V3 ≥ 0.02 sec, or Q5 complex

Note: A Q wave in V1 or III (isolated Q wave) is a **normal** finding

- Give the non-STEMI causes of ↑ ST-segment.

  - Normal variant, arising from early repolarization
  - Myocardium
    - HTC hypertrophic cardiomyopathy
    - Vasospasm
      Prinzmetal angina
      Cocaine
    - Pericarditis
    - Myocarditis

  - Aorta
    - Aortic dissection involving coronary artery
    - LVH / AS with strain
  - Brugada syndrome

Abbreviations: AS, aortic stenosis; LVH, left ventricular hypertrophy

- Diagnostic criteria for STEMI ↑ ST-segment in ≥ 2 anatomically contiguous ECG leads)

  - J point ST elevation, V2 and V3

J point ST elevation, V2 and V3	Men < 40 yr	≥ 2 mm in V2 and V3
	Men > 40 yr	> 1 mm in other leads
	Women	> 1.5 mm in V2 and V3 > 1 mm in other leads

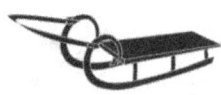

- o J-point ↑ ST, right side leads, V3R and V4R
  - Males < 30   1 mm
  - Males > 30, women   0.5 mm
  - Suspect proximal RCA (right coronary artery) lesion and RV infarction

- o J-point ↑ ST, posterior leads V7 to V9   0.5 mm

  - ↑ ST in II, III, AVF   Suspect posterior wall ischemia from
  - ↓ ST in V1 to V2   obstruction of the circumflex (CX)
  - R waves in V1 or V2   coronary artery

  - ↑↑ T waves in V1 to V2   The ECG may be normal / unchanged in ischemia of CX (circumflex coronary artery)

Because a new onset LBBB (left bundle branch block) suggests

- o Large anterior wall MI with a poor prognosis, it is important to recognize the criteria for ST-segment-elevation equivalent in the patient with previous LBBB, or paced RV (right ventricle)

Criteria			ST-change
o ST-elevation	-	Positive QRS complex	> 1 mm
	-	Negative QRS complex	> 5 mm
o ST-depression in V1-V3			> 1 mm

ST-elevation	Myocardium	Arterial blood supply
V1, V2	Septum	Septal branch and pLAD
V1 to V6	Septum, anterior wall	pLAD and left main
V2 to V4	Anterior wall	LAD
V5-6	Lateral wall	LCX
I, aVL	High lateral wall	pLCX, diagonal
II, III, aVF	Inferior wall	LCX, or RCA

Abbreviations: CX, circumflex; LAD, left anterior descending; LCX, left circumflex; pLAD, proximal left anterior posterior wall; pLCX, proximal left circumflex; RCA, right coronary artery

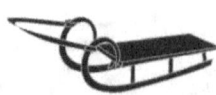

Mastering the Boards: Cardiology   A.B.R. Thomson

- Give the use of measuring blood concentrations of cardiac-specific troponin in STEMI when CR-MB is negative.

    o CK-MB returns to baseline at 24-48 hr, whereas troponin remains increased for 5 to 14 d
    o May be used to estimate the size of the myocardial infarction
    o May be raised to predict risk of SCD (sudden cardiac death)

JUMP To IT – ACT NOW !

    o A STEMI is a medical emergency. The benefit of PCI or CABG reperfusion is inversely related to ischemia time.
    o An ECG is a "must do now" in the patient presenting to the ER with chest pain, with ↓ mortality of 90% with reperfusion within 90 min ("pain-to-balloon time < 90 min), but ~ 0% ↓ mortality after 24 hr

---

CLINICAL ALERT

    o If STEMI is suspected, do not do early non-invasive imaging.
    o If imaging is necessary, perform
        - TTE (transthoracic echocardiogram, or)
            ▪ Detect abnormalities of myocardial wall
        - TEE (transesophageal echocardiogram)
            ▪ Detect dissection of aorta

- Give the clinical significance of normal chest X-ray to exclude aortic dissection.

    o A normal chest x-ray (no mediastinal widening) does not exclude an aortic aneurysm
    o If aortic aneurysm is suspected and chest x-ray does not show mediastinal widening, consider performing TEE (transesophageal echocardiogram)

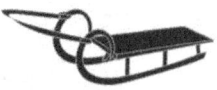

➢ Treatment

- Immediate medical therapy
  - ○ PCI capable facility
  - ○ STEMI protocol
  - ○ Immediate ECG (serial ECGs id ST-segment-elevation not seen initially [may be "evoluting"])
  - ○ 2 IV lines
  - ○ Draw blood for laboratory testing
  - ○ Telemetry
  - ○ Pain relief only if dyspnea or hypoxemia
  - ○ Supplemental O_2
  - ○ Antiplatelet
    - AA, plus
    - P2Y12 inhibitor / GP IIb / IIIa inhibitor, plus
    - Anticoagulation
  - ○ Anti-angina
    - Symptom onset to time ECG shows STEMI
      - ▪ < 30 min, thrombolysis
      - ▪ < 90 min, PCI (percutaneous coronary intervention)
  - ○ Dosing
    - Aspirin (chewable)
      - Naïve 325 mg
      - On ASA 162 mg

		Clopidogrel	
		Loading	Maintenance
- P2Y12 inhibitors	- < 75 yr	300 mg	75 mg
	▪ < 24 hr after fibrinolytic therapy (FT)	600 mg	75 mg
	▪ > 75 yr- No loading dose		
	- > 75 yr No loading dose		

- GP IIb / IIIa inhibitor
  - ▪ During PCI, already on clopidogrel + UHF or bivaliridin
  - ▪ In place of P2Y12 inhibitor in STEMI needing urgent surgery (CABG)
  - ▪ Mitral regurgitation (ischemia)
  - ▪ Ruptured papillary muscle
  - ▪ Ventricular septal defect (VSD)
- Anticoagulation
  - ▪ Give to all for up to 8 days
  - ▪ STEMI patients, along with ASA and P2Y12 inhibitor
  - ▪ Regardless of PCI or thrombolytic therapy

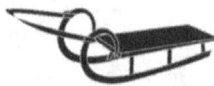

- Therapy before PCI
  - ASA (continue indefinitely), P2Y12 inhibitor (continue for up to 1 yr), bolus of UFA or LMWH
  - Anti-ischemic therapy
    - Nitroglycerine
    - Morphine
      - 2-4 mg IV for pain refractory to nitroglycerine
    - Po B-blocker
      - IV only for arrhythmias
        - Acute accelerated hypertension

CAUTION

- Within first 24 h, as long as **no**
  - > 70 yr
  - SBP < 120 mmHg
  - PR < 60 - > 110 bpm
  - Advanced heart block
  - New heart failure
  - Cardiogenic shock

Note: Do **not** give NSAIDs while STEMI patient is in hospital

- ACEIs
  - Within first 24 hr to
    - ↓ mortality
    - ↓ heart failure
    - ↓ recurrent MI
      - Especially useful for
        - EF < 40%
        - Large anterior MI
        - Previous MI

- Statin
  - ↓ LDL > 50%, or < 70 mg/dL

- Aldosterone receptor antagonist
  - EF < 40%
  - Diabetes
- Reperfusion
  - Thrombolysis
  - Primary PCI
  - Emergency CABG

- Cardiac rehabilitation

- Primary PCI

  - Indications
    - Within

  - Benefits (vs fibrinolysis)
    - ↑ perfusion
    - ↑ survival
    - ↓ bleeding (intracranial)
    - ↓ reinfarction

  - Choice of PCI over fibrinolysis
    - Heart failure, severe
    - Cardiogenic shock (Killip class III/IV or TIMI risk score ≥ 5)
    - Recent PCI or Previous CABG
    - Contraindication to fibrinolysis

  - Technical considerations
    - Experienced operative: restoration of normal coronary blood flow in > 95%
    - Step-wise revascularization, starting with IRA (infarct –related artery)
    - Coronary stenting better than just balloon angiography
    - Before PCI, do not ↓ GP IIb / IIIa inhibitors and / or fibrinolytic agent → ↑ bleeding

Fibrinolytic Therapy

  - Fails to provide patency of coronary artery and restoration of normal flow in 30%
  - Use when PCI is not available within
    - 2-3 hr and in STEMI with   ↑ ST segment
    - Contraindications to fibrinolysis   New LBBB
  - < 5 risk factors for intracerebral bleeding (risk < 4%)

- Give the risk factors for intracerebral hemorrhage in patient undergoing for STEMI.
  - Age ≥ 75 yr
  - Female
  - African origin
  - Weight
    - Men ≤ 80 yr
    - Women ≤ 65 yr
  - Prior smoking
  - SBP ≥ 160 mmHg
  - INA > 4 (PT > 24)
  - Use of alteplase (rt-PH)

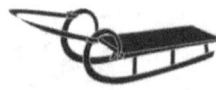

- o Choice of agents
  - Fibrin-selective
  - Non-selective
  - Note:
    - ▪ Fibrin-selective agents are used with ASA, clopidorel plus anticoagulation
    - ▪ Do not use with GP IIb/ IIIa inhibition

The patient given fibrinolysis for STEMI develops sudden neurological symptoms and signs. There were only < 4%, CT scan configured this diagnosis.
- • Give the non-consultative management of intracerebral hemorrhage of the patient with STEMI given fibrinolytic therapy.

  - o Stop   - Anticoagulation and fibrinolysis

  - o Give   - FFP (fresh frozen plasma)
    - Cryoprecipitate ↑ fibrinogen and ↑ factor VIII)
    - Platelet transfusion   }   For ↑ BT (bleeding
    - Protamine zinc sulfate   time)
    - Blood transfusion, as needed

  - o Pharmaco-invasive strategy
    - - Failed fibrinolysis
      - ▪ Ischemic symptoms
      - ▪ New symptoms of heart failure
      - ▪ The elevated ST segments fall < 50% within 90 men of fibrinolysis
      - ▪ Instability
        - - Hemodynamic (SBP, HR)
        - - Electrical (ECG)
    - - Benefit
      - ▪ While fibrinolysis helps in 70% of STEMI patients, it fails in 30%
      - ▪ Of these 30% who fail fibrinolysis, rescue PCI provides benefit in ~ 50%
      - ▪ ↓ death
      - ▪ ↓ heart failure
      - ▪ ↑ reinfarction

- • Give indications for emergency CABG post STEMI.

  - o Mitral regurgitation (ischemic)
  - o Rupture papillary muscle
  - o VSD (ventricular septal defect)
  - o Ventricular aneurysm plus intractable ventricular arrhythmias

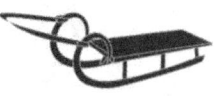

- ➤ Causes of RBBB
    - o Normal (variant)
    - o RV strain (especially pulmonary embolism)
    - o ASD
    - o Myocardial ischemia
    - o Myocarditis

- ➤ Effects of digitalis
    - o Bradycardia
    - o PR prolongation
    - o QT shortening
    - o ST depression
    - o T inversion
    - o Any arrhythmia

- ➤ Hyper-/ hypokalemia

	↑ K⁺	↓ K⁺
o P	Absent	-
o PR	-	Long
o QRS	Wide	-
o T	Tall	absent
o ST	-	Depressed
o U	-	Tall

- ➤ Hyper-/ hypocalcemia

	↑ Ca²⁺	↓ Ca²⁺
QT	Short	Long

Adapted from: Burton JL. *Churchill Livingstone* 1971, page 21.

"A Child's mind is a fire to be kindled, not a vessel to be filled."

Anonymous

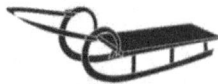

Mastering the Boards: Cardiology   A.B.R. Thomson

Clinical Gem

> Severe hypothermia (< 28 °C, 82.4 °F): there may be
>   o CNS   - Coma
>   - Areflexia
>
>   o Lung   - Pulmonary edema
>
>   o Heart   - Ventricular arrhythmias
>   - Cardioversion
>   - Bradycardia
>   - Tachycardia
>   - Sinus
>   - AF (atrial fibrillation)
>   - Myocardial ischemia
>   - Cardiac arrest
>
>   o MSK   - Loss of shivering

- In the context of hypothermia, and hyperkalemia, give the meaning of Osborne waves on ECG.

   o "Hump" between QRS and ST segments
   o Do **not** mistake for
      - Acute myocardial ischemia
      - ICD (intraventricular conduction defect)

> Diagnosis
>   o 12-lead ECG
>   o Rhythm strip focus on right atrium
>   Leads II, III, AVF, V1
>   o Identify the anatomical position of the conduction defect
>   o Correlate symptoms with onset of bradycardia (symptom association)

- Sinus node dysfunction (aka sick sinus syndrome)
   o Chronotropic incompetence
   o Heart rate does not increase normally after demand such as exercise, metabolic need
   o Sinus bradycardia
      – Rhythm   regular
      – Rate< 60 bpm
      – Upright sinus P waves in I, III and AVP

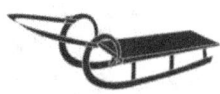

- o Sinus arrest / sinus pause
  - – Periods of < 3 sec with on P waves (representing atrial asystole)
  - – May be accompanied by
    - ▪ Ventricular asystole
    - ▪ Ventricular escapes beats

- o Sinus exit block
  - – Short periods where the R-R interval is a multiple of the R-R which preceeded the bradycardia
  - – Wave of normal depolarization from the sinus node does not pass beyond the perinodal tissue

- o "Tachy-brady syndrome"
  - – Tachyarrhythmia alternating with bradycardia
  - – Often associated with atrial fibrillation
  - – The rapid atrial rate → ↓ sinus node (SN) output → SN dysfunction → bradycardia
    - • AV conduction disturbances

- ➢ Treatment
  - o Overview
    - – For acute symptoms, ↓ perfusion, ↓ hemodynamic stability
      - • Atropine 0.4 mg – 2.0 mg IV
    - – Consider short-term pacing
      - • Transvenous
      - • Transcutaneous
    - – Treat any underlying disorder / precipitating condition, including drugs e.g.
      - • B-blocker
      - • CCBs
      - • Digoxin and electrolyte disturbance
    - – Assess for class I or IIa indications for permanent pacemaker
  - o Treatment of sick sinus syndrome and proximal dysfunction of conduction system are safely and efficiently treated with atropine
  - o Distal dysfunction of conduction system (Mobitz type II) ↑ severity with atropine
  - o Situational or prodromic
    - – Suggests neurocardiogenic Consider tilt table testing
    - – Treatment
      - ▪ Position
      - ▪ Hydration
      - ▪ Isometric exercise
      - ▪ Midodrine 5-15 mg po tid

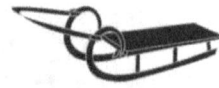

- Permanent dual-chamber pacing for selected patients with a prominent cardioinhibitory component
- Cardiac pacing for carotid sinus hypersensitivity

- Postural (orthostatic) changes
  - Suggests orthostatic hypotension
  - Treatment
    - Position
    - Hydration
    - Salt tablets
    - Compression stockings
    - Midodrine plus fludrocortisone
- Abnormal neurological examination suggests cardiovascular disease or abnormal ECG
  - Abnormal cardiac echocardiogram
  - Abnormal electrophysiological study
  - Non-pharmacological
    - ICD (intracardiac defibrillator (VT and EF < 35%, use with syncope even without arrhythmia)
    - Pacing
    - Radiofrequency ablation
- Abnormal neurological examination suggests neurological disease

➢ Indications for permanent pacemaker

Please refer to the ACC / AHA / HRS guideline for using cardiac pacemakers

The topic is beyond the knowledge requirement for Cardiology for Internist. Only a brief outline is provided here, further details may be obtained from UpToDate or a current textbook of cardiology or cardioelectrophysiology, or the reader's choice.

➢ Most common pacing system
  - AAIR
    - Sinus node dysfunction, without
    - AV conduction abnormalities
    - Meaning
      - **A** the atrium is paced
      - **A** the atrium is sensed
      - **I** inhibition
      - **R** rate adaptive (modulated) pacing

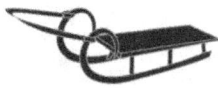

- o DDDR
    - – AV nodal disease
    - – HIS-Purkinje disease
    - – Meaning
        - **D** dual (A+V) is paced
        - **D** dual (A+V) is sensed
        - **D** dual inhibition and triggering: response to pacemaker
        - **R** Rate adaptive pacing

- o VVIR
    - – Chronic AF
    - – Meaning
        - **V** ventricle is paced
        - **V** ventricle is sensed
        - **I** response to pacemaker inhibition
        - **R** rate-adaptive pacing

- Give 3 categories of pacemaker malfunction.

    - o Failure to pace (output failure)
    - o Failure to capture
    - o Failure to sense (undersense)
    - o Pacemaker-mediated dysrhythmia

CLINICAL CHALLENGE

The patient with a rate-adaptive (modulated) pacemaker developed wide-complex tachycardia.

- Give the way to make the diagnosis of pacemaker-mediated tachycardia (PMT).

    - o Rate of arrhythmia
        - – ≤ programmed URL – PMT
        - – > URL – not pacemaker-mediated tachycardia

- Give the indications for a permanent pacemaker.

    - o Any type of heart block with symptoms

    - o Second-degree block
        - – Transient, with RBBB / LBBB
        - – Persistent, Mobitz type 2 constant PR interval R-R (contains dropped [non-conducted] beat) as long as P-P intervals

    - o Third-degree block

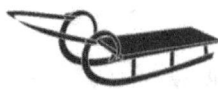

➢ Treatment

- Give the treatment for sustained VT (ventricular tachycardia) or VF (ventricular fibrillation).

  - Stable
    - BB (beta blocker)
  - Unstable
    - Electrical cardioconversion

Sudden Cardiac Death (SCD)

➢ Causes

- Give causes of SCD (Sudden Cardiac Death).

  - Prolonged QT syndrome
  - WPW syndrome
  - Brugada syndrome
    - Incomplete RBBB
    - Inherited
    - ↑ ST in V_1, V_2 ("coved" ST-segments)
  - Dysrhythmias
  - Structural heart disease

The **long QT syndrome** may be inherited.

- Give acquired associations with the long QT syndrome.

  - Female
  - Structural heart disease
  - Electrolyte disturbances
    - ↓ K^+, ↓ Mg^{2+}
  - Alcohol
  - "street" drugs
  - Drugs e.g. cisapride, antibiotics (macrolide, fluoroquinolone), antihistamine, anti-depressants, antipsychotics

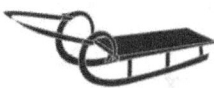

> Treatment

- Give indications for intracardiac defibrillation (ICD) to prevent SCD.

  - Female
  - MI with EF < 30%
  - Cardiomyopathy (ischemic or non-ischemic), EF < 35%
  - HCM, high risk
  - Inherited syndromes
    - Long QT
    - Brugada
  - Syncope plus sustained VT / VF structural heart disease plus sustained VT
  - Cardiac arrest survivors, with no reversible cause of VT / VF
    - > 40 days after MI
    - > 30 month after PCIOR CABG
    - EF < 30%

Atrioventricular (AV) **Block**

> First degree

  - PR interval > 200 msec
  - ↑ risk of
    - AF (atrial fibrillation)
    - Need for pacemaker
    - ↑ mortality rate

> Secondary-degree

  - Mobitz type I (Wenckebach)
    - Disease in AV node
    - Progressive ↑ PR interval, then
    - A dropped QRS complex

xxxxxxxxxxxxxxxxxxxxxxxxxxxxxxxxxxxxxxxxxxxxxxxxxxxxxxxxxxx

SO YOU WANT TO BE AN HCM CARDIOLOGIST ARRHYTHMIOLOGIST!

- Give the circumstance when it is not possible to distinguish between Mobitz type I and type 2 second-degree block.

  - In the presence of 2:1 AV block, it may not be possible to see the progressive ↑ PR interval and to distinguish between Mobitz type 1 and 2 block.

 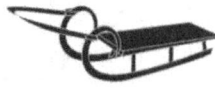

➢ Third-degree (complete heart block)

    o Failure to maintain a relationship between P waves and QRS complex (i.e., a P wave and a QRS complex are not necessarily associated with each other)
- Disease in bundle of HIS or below

Sweet Nothing

- Give the name of the infection which commonly causes complete heart block.

    o Lyme disease

Pacemakers are indicated for symptomatic bradycardia, or asymptomatic complete heart block.

- Give additional indications for a pacemaker use besides symptomatic bradycardia and asymptomatic third-degree (complete) heart block.

    o Atrial fibrillation plus pauses ≥ 5 sec

    o Alternating bundle branch block (BBB)

SO YOU WANT TO BE A CARDIOLOGIST!

- In the context of finding an arrhythmia, give what is the "holiday heart syndrome".

    o Transient supraventicular arrhythmias (usually atrial fibrillation or atrial flutter) following an acute alcoholic binge in chronic alcoholics.

Source: Baliga RR. *Saunders/Elsevier* 2007, pages 32 and 33.

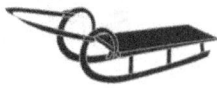

Anti-arrhythmic Medications

- Give a classification of anti-arrhythmic medications.

Vaughan-Williams classification of anti-arrhythmic medications

	Contraindication	Example	Atrial fibrillation	Atrial flutter	SVT	SVT Termination	VA	AA	TA	HF, LVH	Special Comments
Class I Na⁺-channel blockers	■ Ventricular arrhythmias (AE)										
A		Procainamide	+				+				
B	■ Post-MI	Lidocaine	+		+						
C	■ Coronary artery disease	Flecanide	+				+				
Class II β-blocker	■ Decompensated S-HF ■ WPW syndrome	Metoprolol	+	+	+		+				Add an AV nodal blocker

Class III K⁺-channel blockers	■ Ventricular arrhythmias
	■ ↑ QTc
	■ Amiodarone
	  * ↓ BP (thyroid toxicity, liver dysfunction, skin hypersensitivity)
	  - ↑ Cr$_s$ NYHA class II, III, V with recent compensation or class IV
	  - AF (permanent)
		Sotalol
		Amiodarone
			+
			
				+
				
							+
							
										+	

Class IV Calcium channel blockers	■ Decompensated S-HF WPW syndrome	Verapamil Diltiazem			+ 	 	+ 	+ 	+ 		
A1 receptor	■ Agonist of AV node	Adenosine Digoxin				+ 					

*Dronedarone, A class III K⁺ channel blocker, does not have the same AEs as does amiodarone

Abbreviations: AA, atrial arrhythmias (rate control); AE, adverse effects; Cr$_s$, serum creatinine; QTc, corrected AT interval; S-HF, systolic heart failure; SVT, supraventricular tachycardia; TA, triggered arrhythmias; VA, ventricular tachycardia; WPW, Wolff-Parkinson-White syndrome

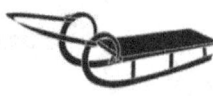

Cardiac Resynchronization Therapy (CVT)

- o Patients with heart failure (HF) have a much worse prognosis if they also have disease of the conduction system
- o About 1/3 of patients with HF have a delay in the interventricular conduction system
- o The septum and the lateral wall of the ventricle do not contract in harmony (dyssynchronous ventricular contraction, DVC)
- o DVC → ↓ LVEF (LV ejection fraction)
- o SVT (biventricular pacing) partially corrects dyssynchronous contraction of septum and lateral wall of the ventricle

- ➢ Indications
  - o LVEF < 35%, QRS > 150 ms, asymptomatic
  - o LVEF 35%, QRS > 120 ms, HF symptoms – NYHA III / IV
  - o LVEF < 35%, HF-symptoms – NYHA I / II

- ➢ CRT pacemaker plus ICU device

Old age makes you redundant

So

It's OK to be redundant – if you're a gene!

 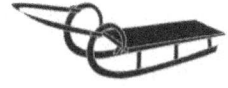

THE PERIPHERAL PULSE

➤ Classification of AV blocks

- o Diverted   - Fascicular
                              - Bundle branch
- o Delayed   - First-degree AV
- o Frequently blocked   - High-degree
- o Complete block   - Third degree
- o Occasional delay   - Second degree
                              - Mobitz type I block (Wenckebach)

- o First-degree AV block
  - – PR > 200 ms
  - – P wave for every QRS (no dropped beats)

- o Second-degree AV block
  - – P wave missing ("dropped") before some QRS complexes
  - – Mobitz type I block (proximal interruption)
    - Progression ↑ PR interval → dropped QRS
    - ↓ PR interval before the dropped beat
    - RR interval of dropped beat < 2x the shortest RR interval
    - Regularly irregular grouping of QRS complexes (group beating)
    - Little progression to complete (third-degree) AV block, since type I second-degree AV block arises within AV node
  - – Mobitz type II block (distal interruption)
    - Abrupt AV conduction block (no progression of ↑ PR as in Mobitz type I) → sudden loss of P wave
    - ↑ risk of progression to third-degree AV conduction block, especially if associated with a BBB (bundle branch block)
  - – AV 2:1 block
    - Distinguish Mobitz type I and II ↑ sinus rate (SR) / ↑ sympathetic input

- o ↑ SR (sinus rate)
  - – Mobitz I → concomitant
    - First-degree block
    - Periodic AV Wenckebach
    - Improved conduction (1:1)
  - – Mobitz II → Concomitant
    - BBB (bundle branch block)
    - Fascicular block
    - Worse conduction (e.eg 3:1)

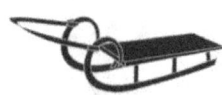

- Advanced (high-degree) AV block
  - Consecutive P waves without QRS, but
  - Some P:QRS conduction (e.g. 3:1, 4:1 block; > 1 consecutive atrial depolarization fails to conduct to ventricle)

- Third-degree (complete) AV block
  - Atrial rate > ventricular rate (from complete dissociation)
  - No P wave associated with QRS complex

SO YOU WANT TO BE A CARDIOLOGIST!

When "A > V" rates, there is complete dissociation between the atrial and ventricular rates, and the diagnosis is third-degree complete AV block.

- Give the ECG diagnosis when "V > A".

  - Dissociation with competition at the AV node causes "V > A" rates

---

- Give the abnormalities in the pulse rate

  - Bradyarrhythmias-
    - Sinus bradycardia
    - Sick sinus syndrome
    - Junctional and ventricular escape rhythmias

  - Conduction delays
    - 1°, 2°, or 3° AV nodal block
    - Fascicular block
    - Bundle branch block (BBB)

  - Irregular Tachyarrhythmias
    - Sinus arrhythmia
    - Atrial fibrillation
    - Multifactorial atrial tachycardia
    - Atrial flutter with variable block
    - Atrial or ventricular premature beats
    - Extrasystoles (ventricular or supra-ventricular)
    - 2° heart block
    - Ventricular fibrillation
    - Irregularity of volume also occurs in pulsus paradoxus and pulsus alternans

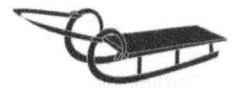

Mastering the Boards: Cardiology   A.B.R. Thomson

o Regular Tachyarrhythmias - **narrow complex**:
  - Supraventricular tachycardia
  - Atrial flutter
  - Wolfe-Parkinson-White syndrome
  - AV node re-entry tract
o Wide complex:
  - Supraventricular tachycardia with aberrance or bundle branch block
  - Ventricular tachycardia, torsades de pointes
  - Unstable arrhythmia
  - Arrhythmia plus hypotension, dyspnea, chest pain, presyncope, or syncope.

Abbreviation: AV, atrioventricular; $1^0/2^0/3^0$ – first, second or third degree heart block

Adapted from: Jugovic PJ, et al. *Saunders/ Elsevier* 2004, page71 and 72; and Burton JL. *Churchill Livingstone* 1971, page 12.

Tachycardia

➢ Definition
  o "cardiac rhythm whose ventricular rate exceeds 100 beats per minute (bpm)" (Sharma S, et al. The Washington Manual of Medical Therapeutics. Godara H, et al. Eds, 34th edition, 2014, Wolters Kluwer, Chapter 7, 220-67).

• Take a directed history for the causes of tachycardia.

  o Sinus tachycardia
    - Exercise or emotion
    - Constitutional
    - Anemia
    - Thyrotoxicosis
    - Fever
    - Congestive heart failure
    - Constrictive pericarditis
    - Drugs (e.g adrenaline, atropine, nitrites)
    - Acute hemorrhage
  o Supraventricular (atrial or nodal) tachycardia
  o Atrial flutter
  o Atrial fibrillaton
  o Ventricular tachycardia
  o Ventricular flutter

Abbreviation: AV, atrio-ventricular

Printed with permission Burton JL. *Churchill Livingstone* 1971, pages 11 and 12.

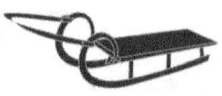

- Give the effect of exercise and vagal stimulation on tachyarrhythmias.

		Vagal stimulation	Exercise
o Atrial	– Flutter	↓	↑
	– Fibrillation	-	↑
	– PAT	↓	
	– APC	-	↓
o Sinus	– Bradycardia	-	↑
	– Arrhythmia	-	↓
	– 2^0 HB	-	↑
	– 3^0 HB	-	-

> Easy to Remember: Exercise ↑ all atrial and sinus tachyarrythmias except
>
> o APC ↓
>
> o 2^0 HB ↓ / 3^0 HB -

Abbreviations: APC, atrial premature contraction; HR, heart rate; PAT, paroxysmal atrial tachycardia; $2^0/3^0$ HB second/third degree heart block

Adapted from: Talley NJ, et al. *Maclennan & Petty Pty Limited* 2003, page 41.

Subventricular Tachycardia

➤ Prevalence

- o AF >> AFL (9:1)

- o Paroxysmal STV
  - < 40 AVRT + WPW (Wolff-Parkinson-White) syndrome
  - > 40 AVNRT

Classification of tachyarrhythmia	QRS, MS	Name	Origin	Activation of ventricles
o Narrow-complex tachycardia (NCT)	< 120	Supraventricular (SVT)	Atrium or AV node	His-Purkinje system AV node maintains this arrhythmia Holding breath / Valsalva maneuver improves symptoms

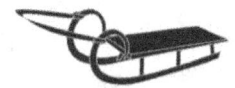

Classification of tachyarrhythmia	QRS, MS	Name	Origin	Activation of ventricles
o Wide-complex tachycardia (WCT)	> 120	Ventricular Supraventricular tachycardia	Outside AV node	Slowly

➢ Mechanism

- o Impulse conduction

- o A region of the myocardium that was initially refractory to antegrade conduction of an electrical wave front becomes activated by retrograde recently of the electrical wavefront

- o Impulse formation
  - ↑ automaticity
    - ↑ junctional and ↑ ideoventricular rhythm

➢ Clinical

- History

  - o Tachyarrhythmia

  - o Supraventricular tachyarrhythmia (SVT)
    - Improvement with Valsalva maneuver / holding breath

Arrhythmias

- o Atrial
  - Sinus bradycardia
    - Dysfunction of
      - Sinus node
      - AV node
      - His-Purkinje system
  - AV (atrioventricular) block
  - Atrial fibrillation and flutter

- o Supraventricular
  - AV nodal re-entrant tachycardia
  - AV reciprocating tachycardia
  - Premature atrial contractions and atrial tachycardia

- o Ventricular
  - Ventricular tachycardia with structural heart disease
  - Idiopathic ventricular tachycardia

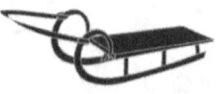

Sinus Bradycardia (< 60 bpm)

➢ Causes

- o Physiological
  - Athlete
  - Aging

- o Pathological
  - ↑ Vagal tone
  - Drugs
  - Infarction
  - Surgery

Bradycardia

➢ Definition

- o Bradyarrhythmia is a heart rate < 60 beats per minute (bpm)

SO YOU WANT TO BE A CARDIOLOGIST!

Ischemia due to coronary artery disease may result in different bradyarrhythmias depending upon the blood supply to the components of the cardiac conduction system,

- Give the arterial blood supply to parts of the cardiac conduction system (**cardioanatomy**).

  - o Sinus
    - Sinus nodal artery
      - Right coronary artery (RCA) (65%)
      - Circumflex artery (CA) (25%)
      - Both RCA and CA (10%)

  - o AV node
    - AV nodal artery
      - Posterior descending artery (PDA, proximal portion) (80%)
      - Circumflex artery (CA) (10%)
      - Both PDA and CA (10%)

  - o Bundle of His and right bundle
    - AV nodal artery
    - Left anterior descending (LAD), septal perforations

  - o Left bundle (LB)
    - Anterior fascicle
    - Posterior fascicle
      - Septal perforations
      - PDA
      - LAD, septal perforations

 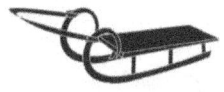

- ➢ Pathophysiology
  - ○ Sinus node (SN) in right atrium (RA) 50-90 bpm
    ↓
  - ○ AV node in RA interatrial septum (40-50 bpm)
    55 to 110 ms delay in wave of depolarization
    ↓
  - ○ Bundle of His in membranous septum
    ↓   ↓
    LBB   RBB
    - Posterior / anterior fascicle

- ➢ Classification
  - ○ Sinoatrial block
  - ○ AV block:
    - 1°, P.R>0.2 sec
    - 2° Mobitz (fixed PR)
    - Wenkebach (varying PR)
    - High grade (2:1, 3:1, etc)
    - 3° complete
  - ○ Bundle branch block
  - ○ Short PR with long QRS (Wolff-Parkinson-White)

- ➢ Causes
- • Take a directed history for the causes of sinus bradycadia.

  - ○ Sinus bradycardia
    - Physiological (conditioning)
    - Hypothyroidism
    - Jaundice
    - Increased intracerebral pressure
    - Mumps
    - Amebic abscess
    - Drugs
    - Familial
    - Congenital
  - ○ Causes of slow regular pulse
    - Sinus bradycardia
    - Complete heart block
    - 2:1 AV block
    - Atrial flutter with 4:1 AV block
    - dionodal rhythm
    - Idioventricular rhythm

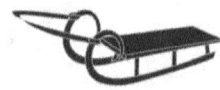

- o Causes of a 'dropped beat'
  - Sinoatrial block
  - Blocked atrial extrasystole
  - 2nd degree heart block

Printed with permission Burton JL. *Churchill Livingstone* 1971, pages 11-12.

- o Heart
  - Athletes
  - Sleep
  - Apparent (pulse deficit [PR<HR] in AF, ventricular bigeminy)
  - Block (3° AV block, or type I or II 2° AV block)
  - Myocardial infarction (MI; ischemic heart disease)
  - Vasovagal episode
  - Cardiomyopathy
  - Sinus arrhythmia (↓PR with expiration)
  - Heart failure (HF)
    - Constrictive pericarditis
    - Myocardial infarction (MI)
    - Myocarditis
    - Aortic stenosis
    - Hypertension
  - Rhythm
    - Supraventricular tachycardia
    - Ventricular tachycardia – hyperthyroidism, acute hypoxia or hypercapnea, sick sinus syndrome
    - Atria flutter with 2:1 AV block, or with variable block
    - Multifocal atrial tachycardia
  - Hyperdynamic circulation
    - Exercise
    - Emotion
    - Fever
    - Hypolemia
    - Anemia
    - Hyperthyroidism
    - Pregnancy
    - AV fistula (Paget's disease)
    - Beriberi
- o Head
  - Increased intracranial pressure
  - Trauma
- o Hypothermia
- o Hypothyroidism

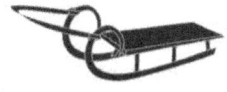

- o Hepatic
  - – Severe jaundice
- o MSK
  - – Collagen vascular disease
- o Drugs
  - – B-blockers, digoxin, amiodarone
  - – Anticholinergics
  - – Sympathomimetics
- o Tachycardia

Abbreviations: AF, arterial fibrillation; AV, atrioventricular; CCF, congestive cardiac failure; HR, heart rate; MI, myocardial infarction; MSK, musculoskeletal system; PR, pulse rate;

Adapted from: Talley NJ, et al. *Maclennan & Petty Pty Limited* 2003, Table 3.5, page 41; Burton JL. *Churchill Livingstone* 1971, pages 12 and 13; and Baliga RR. *Saunders/Elsevier* 2007, page 37.

- Give the types of tachyarrhythmia associated with MVP (mitral valve prolapse).
  - o Supraventricular
  - o Ventricular

- Give the commonest causes of atrial fibrillation (AF), and atrial flutter (ALF).

  - o Heart   - Atrial enlargement
               - Post-cardiac surgery

  - o Lung   - Pulmonary disease

  - o Thyroid   - Thyrotoxicosis

CLINICAL TIP

Atrial fibrillation (AF) is described as being irregularly irregular. Sinus tachycardia (ST) with frequent premature atrial complexes (PACs), as well as ectopic atrial tachycardia (EAT) and multifocal atrial tachycardia (MAT). Atrial flutter (AFL) is usually regular, but sometimes becomes irregularly irregular.
- Give the electrophysiological explanation for AFL being sometimes irregularly irregular.

  - o AFL will be irregularly irregular when the AV block is variable (e.g. 2:1 → 4:1 → 3:1 → 2:1)

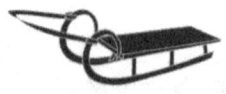

EXPLAINING "CANNON" A WAVES IN JVP

- o "Cannon" A wave seen on inspection of the are caused by contraction of the right atrium against a closed tricuspid valve.

- o When "cannon" A waves of the JVP occur in a 1:1 ratio with the peripheral pulse, the causative tachycardia (AVRT, AVNRT, JT) causes retrograde activation of the right atrium at the same time as contraction of the right ventricle.

Abbreviations: AVNRT, atrioventricular nodal reentrant tachycardia; AVRT, atrioventricular reentrant tachycardia; JT, junctional tachycardia; JVP, jugular venous pressure;

SO YOU WANT TO BE A CARDIOLOGIST!

- • Perform a focused examination of the pulse and the JVP (jugular venous pressure), and suggest the type of tachyarrhythmia.

- • Pulse
  - o Atrial
    - - Irregular, no pattern ("irregularly irregular"), regular rhythm
      - ▪ AF (atrial fibrillation)
      - ▪ MAT (multifocal atrial tachycardia) SVT
    - - ~ 150 bpm
      - ▪ AFL (atrial flutter) with 2:1 block (atrial rate / ventricular rate, 2:1)
      - ▪ "saw tooth" ECG in II, III, av5
      - ▪ "SVT with regular ventricular rate if 150 bpm should raise suspicion for AFL"
    - - > 150 bpm
      - ▪ AVNT (atrioventricular nodal tachycardia)
      - ▪ AVNRT (atrioventricular nodal reentrant tachycardia)

  - o Second-degree heart block
    - - "group beating" (irregular pulse, with a discernible pattern)

- • Jugular venous pressure (JVP)
  - o ↑ JVP plus S3 gallop
    - - Malignant ventricular arrhythmia

  - o With "Cannon" A wave
    - - Irregular
      - ▪ AV dissociation
    - - Regular 1:1 ratio with peripheral pulse
      - ▪ AVRT
      - ▪ AVNRT
      - ▪ Junctional tachycardia (JT)

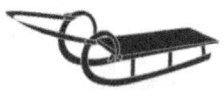

➢ Diagnostic testing

- ○ ECG, exercise ECG, continuous rhythm stop, continuous ambulatory ECG monitoring

- ○ Telemetry with
    - Implantable loop recorder
    - Insertable loop recorder

- ○ Electrophysiology
    - Catheter-based study
    - Best used to study reentrant mechanisms
    - Used with catheter ablation

Narrow Complex Tachycardia

- ○ Irregular rhythm
    - Atrial flutter
    - Multifocal atrial tachycardia (MAF)

- ○ Regular rhythm
    - Sinus tachycardia
    - AV nodal re-entrant tachycardia (AVNRT)
    - AV reciprocating tachycardia (AVRT)
    - Atrial tachycardia
    - Supraventricular tachycardia (SVT)
    - Ventricular tachycardia (VT)
    - WPW syndrome
    - Heart block

Atrial Flutter

- ○ Usually associated from atrial scar from "trauma'

- ○ Conduction through AV node

- ○ Treated similarly to atrial fibrillation, except recommended ablation
    - ↑ success
    - ↓ complications

- ○ A re-entrant arrhythmia

- ○ Atrial rates 250 to 340 / min, with 2:1 conduction giving ventricular rate ~ 150 / min

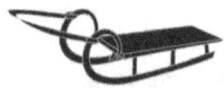

- Give conditions commonly associated with atrial flutter.

  - Heart
    - Intermittently occurring with AF (atrial fibrillation)
    - After treatment of AF
    - Pericardial
    - Open heart surgery
  - Lung
    - Worsening of pulmonary disease, e.g. COPD

- Give the treatment of atrial flutter.

  - Anti-coagulation, as for AF
  - RCA (radiofrequency catheter ablation) recommended rather than BB, CCB or digitalis

Abbreviation: BB, beta-blocker; CCB, calcium channel blocker

Multifocal Atrial Tachycardia (MAT)

  - Irregularly irregular
  - 3 distinct P-wave morphologies in ECG leads II, III and V
  - Associations
    - Heart
      - HF (heart failure)

    - Lung
      - COPD (chronic obstructive pulmonary disease)

    - Metabolic
      - Hypokalemia
      - Hypomagnesemia
      - Glucose intolerance
      - Chronic renal failure
      - Drugs (e.g. theophylline)

- Give the treatment of MAT (multifocal atrial tachycardia).
  - Indications
  - BB or CCB
  - In patient with bronchospasm, se
    - BB – Metoprolol
    - CCB – verapamil
  - Treat underlying disease / disorder
    - Heart disease
    - Lung disease
    - Electrolyte disturbance
      - $\downarrow K^+$
      - $\downarrow Mg^{2+}$

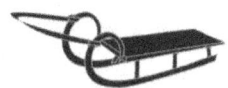

Mastering the Boards: Cardiology A.B.R. Thomson

Sinus Tachycardia

- o Irregularly irregular when ST occurs with PACs (premature atrial complexes)
- o Long RP tachycardia
- o Associations
  - Hyperadrenergic states

  - Drugs
    - Cocaine
    - Amphetamine
    - Methamphetamine

  - Rx drugs
    - Atropine
    - Theophylline
    - B-adrenergic agonist

Ectopic Atrial Tachycardia (EAT)

- o Irregularly irregular → P wave morphology outside sinus node → long RP tachycardia
- o Digoxin toxicity → EAT with variable block → irregularly irregular

- Give the distinction between AFL plus VB and EAT plus VB.

  - o Both AFL (atrial flutter) with variable AV block and EAT (ectopic atrial block) with variable block (VB), may be irregularly irregular, but EAT + VT has an atrial rate of 150-200 bpm, whereas the atrial rate in AFL + VT is 250-350 bpm.

Atrial fibrillation (AF)

- ➢ Definition
  - o Absence of content P waves on 12-lead ECG

- ➢ Demography
  - o Age > 75 yr, AF in > 10%

- ➢ Types
  - o First
    - Symptoms, or no symptoms
    - Spontaneous remmission rate > 50%
  - o Paroxysmal
    - Recurrent episodes of < 7 days

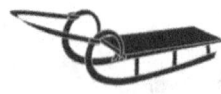

- o Persistent
  - Recurrent episodes of > 7 days, or
  - Termination by electrical conversion
- o Digoxin toxicity → EAT with variable block → irregularly
  - Permanent
  - Failed therapy, or
  - Accepted because of few symptoms
  - Risks of cardioconversion

➢ Terms

- o Paroxysmal AF - AF which stops on its own (50%)
- o Persistent AF - AF for > 7 d
- o Permanent AF - AF which continues despite cardioversion
- o Lone AF - When patient < 60 yr and AF occurs by itself (lone), not associated with another condition

---

ECG TIP

- o The absence of P waves on all ECG leads makes the diagnosis of AF (atrial fibrillation) difficult.

- o Look carefully to ensure that an absence of P waves is not form AF, but rather simply that the P waves are obscured by
  - Deformed T waves
  - ST segments

➢ Differential
- Give conditions which on ECG may be easily confused with AF, and which the clinician must distinguish from AF.

- o Atrial tachycardia
  - With block (digitalis toxicity)
  - Multifocal, in chronic pulmonary disease
- o Sinus tachycardia, with premature atrial beats
- o Second degree
  - AV block, Mobitz type I (Wenckebach)
- o Atrial tachycardia
  - With block (digitalis toxicity)
  - Multifocal, in chronic pulmonary disease
- o RBBB (right bundle branch block)
- o Tachycardia, with accessory pathway

Abbreviation: COPD, chronic obstructive pulmonary disease

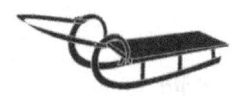

➢ Risk factors

- o Age
- o Males
- o Obesity
- o Cardiac   - Hypertension
  - Valvular disease
  - Previous MI (myocardial infarction)
  - HF (heart failure – cardiothoracic surgery (common 20-50%)
- o Lung
  - OSA (obstructive sleep apnea)

- o Endocrine   - Diabetes
  - Hyperthyroidism

➢ Pathogenesis

- o Inflammatory, fibrous and remodeling → rapid electrical firing ectopic focus in pulmonary veins → rapid conduction to atria → multiple variable reentrant circuits → rapid atrial and ventricular ratio with variably variable conduction block

➢ Clinical

- Perform a focused physical examination for atrial fibrillation (AF.

- o Pulse   – Irregularily irregular pulse
  - Differentiate from other causes of irregularily irregular pulse
    - AF (atrila fibrillation)
    - MVE (multiple ventricular ectopics (unlike AF, MVE become less frequent with exercise)
    - Atrial flutter plus varying block
    - Complete heat block (pulse rate is slow, but irregularily irregular)
  - Deficit
    - HR > PR (heart rate [HR] is greater than pulse rate [PR])
    - Pulse deficit increases when HR increases
  - Exercise
    - ↑ pulse deficit
    - No effect on frequency of AF

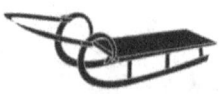

- o JVP   – ↓'a' waves

- o Heart sounds   – S_1 varies in intensity
                            – S_2 split

- o Sign of causes   – Heart
  of AF
    - Mitral valve disease
    - Ischemic heart disease
    - Hypertension
    - Constrictive pericarditis
  - – Thyroid - hyperthyroidism
  - – Lung – chronic pulmonary disease
  - – Congenital
    - ASD (atrial septal defect)
    - Ebstein anomaly
  - – "lone" atrial fibrillation

- Perform a focused physical examination to determine the cause of atrial fibrillation.

  - o Heart
    - – Mitral valve disease
    - – IHD
    - – HBP
    - – Constrictive pericarditis
    - – Cardiomyopathy
    - – ASD
    - – Ebstein anormaly

  - o Lung   – Chronic pulmonary disease

  - o Thyroid   – Thyrotoxicosis

  - o Ideopathic   – 'Lone fibrillation'

Abbreviation: IHD, ischemic heart disease; HBP, hypertension (systemic); ASD, atrial septal defect

Adapted from: Baliga RR. *Saunders/Elsevier* 2007, pages 32 and 33.

- Give the major complication of AF (atrial fibrillation), for which anti-coagulation prophylaxis is required.

  - o Clot in LA (left atrium) → embolization to brain → embolic CVA (cerebrovascular disease)

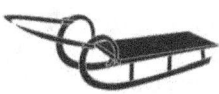

➢ Causes / associations

• Give the conditions which are commonly associated with AF (atrial fibrillation).

- o Heart
  - HF (heart failure)
  - Hypertension
  - WPW (Wolff-Parkinson-White)
  - Myocardial infarction
  - Myocarditis
  - Rheumatic MS (mitral stenosis)
  - Cardiac surgery

- o Lung
  - Acute pulmonary disease

- o Endocrine
  - Hyperthyroidism

➢ Prevention
  - o Statins
  - o ACE-1 /ARBs
  - o B-blockers
  - o Omega-3 fatty acids
  - o Magnesium

➢ ECG diagnosis
  - o Absence of consistent P waves in 12-lead ECG
  - o P waves vary in size, shape, timing
  - o Ventricular response in regular, with tachycardia > 100 bpm
  - o Differentiate from other tachyarrhythmias which are irregularity irregular
    - AFI with variable AV block
    - MAF (multifocal atrial tachycardia)
    - ST with PACs (sinus tachycardia with premature atrial complexes)
    - EAT (ectopic atrial tachycardia)

CLINICAL ALERTS

Prolonged tachycardia from atrial fibrillation → cardiomyopathy (tachycardia-induced)

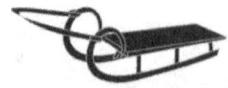

American Heart Association (AHA) / American College of Cardiology (ACG) / European Society of Cardiology (ESC) Guidelines for Chronic Anti-thrombotic Therapy in AF

> ➤ Treatment
>   o Anticoagulation
>   - Warfarin or ASA, depending upon the risk assessed by CHADS2 score
>
>   o Atrial fibrillation and flutter are supraventricular tachyarrhythmias in which there is an increased risk of thromboembolism stroke.
>   o The CHADS$_2$ score is a useful tool
>   - To stratify the risk of stroke in persons with non valvular atrial fibrillation or flutter, and
>   - To determine who should be treated with ASA, clopidogrel or warfarin.

- Take a directed history and perform a focused physical examination to calculate the CHADS$_2$ score.

	CHADS$_2$ risk criteria	Assigned score
C	Congestive heart failure	1
H	Hypertension	1
A	Age > 75 years	1
D	Diabetes mellitus	1
S	Prior stroke or transient ischemic attack	2

Quoted from: Birnie D and Nery P. Chapter 42. In: Therapeutic Choices. Grey J, Ed. 6th Edition, *Canadian Pharmacists Association* 2012, page 578.

CHADS score	Treatment
0	None, or ASA =/- clopidogrel
1	ASA, or warfarin (INR 2.0 – 3.0) or dabigatran*
≥ 2	Warfarin or dabigatrin

Clinical Caution

   o CHADS2 score
      - Is **not** used for patients with significant valve disease
      - Does **not** include all the risk factors for thromboembolism in persons with AF (atrial fibrillation).

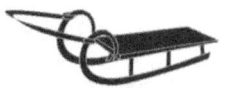

- Give the risk factors for AF which are **not included** in the calculation of the CHADS2 score.
  - MS (mitral stenosis)
  - Mechanical heart valve
  - Systolic dysfunction
  - Previous thromboembolism

Sweet Nothing

In patients with appropriate CHADS2 score, or rheumatic mitral stenosis, the target INR is 2.0 – 3.0.

- Give the target INR for patients with a mechanical valve.
  - INR > 2.5

---

* Rivaroxaban (oral inhibitor factor Xa) may also be used in patients with AF to ↓ risk of systemic embolization and embolic CVA.

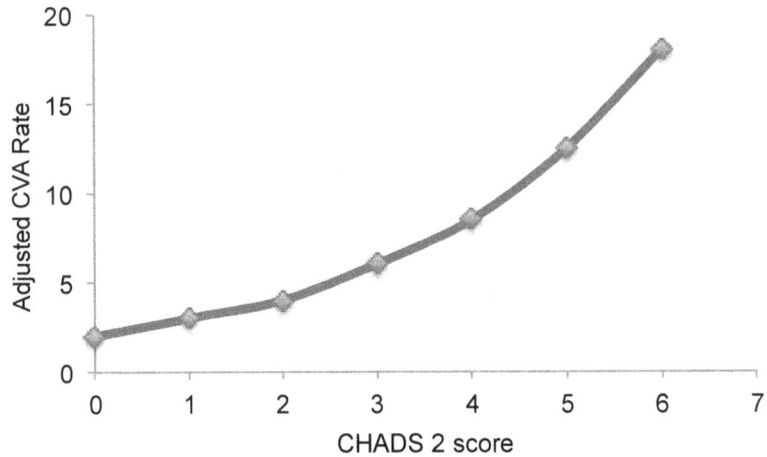

CLINICAL TIP

- Non-pharmacological methods of rhythm control (cardioversion) are superior.

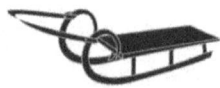

Mastering the Boards: Cardiology

A.B.R. Thomson

- Pharmacological
  - Control rate
    - CCBs (non-dihydropyridine)
    - B-blockers
    - Digoxin
      - Rate control at rest (not with exercise)
      - Useful in LV dysfunction plus HF in AF
      - Combination with CCBs or B-blockers (caution: verapamil and diltiazem → ↑ [digoxin] → ↑ toxicity

- Give the commonest arrhythmias associated with digitalis (digoxin) toxicity, and their management.

  - Stop digitalis; correct K+, renal failure
  - AV block – temporary pacemaker
  - Bidirectional VT

- Non-pharmacological

  - AV nodal ablation, with PPM (permanent pacemaker) implantation

  - Control rhythm

- Pharmaceutical induction of rhythm control
  - Ibutidine
    - For AF < 7 days duration
    - Conversion rate
    - 1 mg (0.01 mg/kg if < 60 kg)
    - IV area 10 min (slow to prevent TdP)
    - ~4% - 8% risk of Torsade de pointes (TdP), especially within first 4 hr
  - Shorter duration AF
    - Dofetilide
    - Sotalol
    - Flecainide
    - Propafenone
    - Amiodarone of limited use for achieving rhythm control, but is used for maintenance

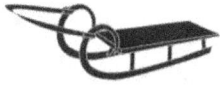

- Pharmaceutical Maintenance of Rhythm Control Therapy for Rhythm Control in Atrial Fibrillation (AF).

Vaughan Williams Classification	Mechanism of Action	
I c	Block fast Na+ channel Normal heart structure	Flecainide Propafenone
II	B-adrenergic blockers	
III	Block K+ channel blockers	D-sotalol Dofetilide Ibutilide
IV	Calcium channel blockers	Dronedarone Amiodarone

Class 10	↑ QRS	Negative inotrope (↑ HF)	Use with AV node blocker	Paradoxical ↑ HR	↑ HF risk
○ Flecainide	+	+	+	+	+
○ Properfenone	+	+	-	-	+

Abbreviations: HF, heart failure; HR, heart rate; VWO, Vaughan Williams classification

- In the context of the use of VW class Ic anti-arrhythmic drugs used for maintenance of sinus rhythm after conversion of AF to sinus rhythm, give the meaning of "use dependence " of flecainide, and explain why flecainide must be used with an AV nodal blocker.

  - ○ ↑ QT with tachycardia: as the heart rate increases, as with exercise, flecainide preferentially blocks active Na+ channels
    - ↑ risk of drug toxicity ("use dependence")
    - ↑ risk of conversion of AF → AFL, and
    - ↑ risk of prodoxical ↑ ventricular rate (VR)

  - ○ Because of these paradoxical ↑ VR, flucainide must be used with an AV nodal blocker when used to maintain conversion of AF to sinus rhythm
  - ○ As HR increases, toxicity increases
  - ○ Perform exercise ECG to establish possible toxicity at ↑ HR

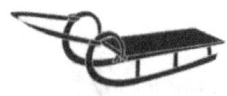

Class III	↑ QT interval	TdP	↑ HF risk	Sinus bradycardia	AV conduction abnormalities
o Desotalol	+ Contraindicated use: - QTc > 440 ms - BBB, Qtc > 500 ms	+	-	+	+
o Dofetilide	+ Contraindicated use: - QTc > 500 ms	+	-	-	-

- Give the drugs which ↓ renal secretion and ↑ toxicity of dofetilide.

    o Verapamil
    o Cimetidine
    o Prochlorperazine
    o Trimethroprim
    o Megestrol
    o Ketoconazole

Classes I to IV

    o Dronedarone
        - Maintains sinus rhythm after successful cardioversion
        - Less effective maintenance than amiodarone, but with fewer adverse effects
        - Contraindicated in
            ▪ HF (heart failure)
            ▪ Severe hepatic dysfunction
        - Safe to use in renal insufficiency

    o Amiodarone
        - 5-yr rates of adverse events
            ▪ High dose 75%
            ▪ Low dose 25%-50%

        - Eye
            ▪ Corneal microdeposits incidental finding by slit-lamp in all patients
            ▪ Optic neuritis

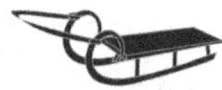

- Skin
  - Blue-grey photosensitivity in sun-exposed areas
  - May persist after amiodarone stopped

- Heart
  - ↑ PR interval
  - Bradycardia
  - High-grade AV block (with pre-existing conduction abnormalities)
  - ↑ QT intervals (but TdP is rare)

- Lung
  - Interstitial pulmonary fibrosis ~5% (especially at doses < 300 mg per day)
  - Reversible only if diagnosed early and amiodarone stopped

- Thyroid
  - Hypo- / hyperthyroidism
  - ~2% - 5% per yr
  - Monitoring TSH q 6 mon
  - If hypothyroidism develops
    - Levothyroxime and continue amiodarone

- Liver
  - ↑ ALT, ↑ AST monitor q 6 mon
  - Stop amiodarone if ↑ transaminases
    - 3x ULN
    - 2x if initial reading of ALT / AST ↑

- Drug interaction
  - ↑ effect of warfarin
  - ↑ digoxin

Useful background: Summary of major adverse events with drugs used for rate control in atrial fibrillation

Drug	↓ BP	↓ HR	HB	HF	Bronchospasm
No accessary pathway					
○ Esmolol					
○ Metoprolol	+	+	+	+	+
○ Propanolol					
○ Diltazem	+	-	+	+	-
○ Verapamil					
○ Digoxin	-	+	+	-	-
Accessary pathway					
○ Amiodarone	+	+	+	-	-

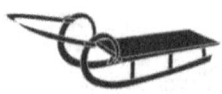

Abbreviations: BP, blood pressure; HB, heart block; HF, heart failure; HR, heart rate

Source: Washington Manual of Medical Therapeutics, 2014Chapter 7, page 220-267. Wolters Kluwer / Lippincott William & Wilkins)

For doses of commonly used anti-arrhythmic drugs used in atrial fibrillation, please see Washington Manual of Medical Therapeutics, 2014, Table 7-6, page 238-239. Wolters Kluwer / Lippincott William & Wilkins)

- Non-pharmacological Therapy for Rhythm control in Atrial fibrillation

- DC cardioversion (DCCV; external cardioverter-defibrillator)

Anti-coagulation

- o 3 wk prior anticoagulation with warfarin with warfarin is essential if AF present for > 48 hr, but not always possible when urgent cardioversion is necessary (AF plus rapid ventricular response) in association with
  - MI (myocardial infarction)
  - Hypertension
  - Respiratory distress
- o Alternatively to anti-coagulation, perform TEE and if no left atrial appendage thrombus, perform cardioconversion without warfarin anti-coagulation
- o Continue warfarin
  - For > 4 wk (INR, 2-3), and lifelong in persons at ↑ risk for CVA
- o Sedation
  - Synchronization of cardioversion with patient's QRS
    - Place the two DCCV patches > 6 cm
    - From PPM, or
    - From defibrillation generators
  - Atropic available at bedside for rapid retreatment of any developing bradyarrhythmia
- o Catheter ablation
  - Purpose
    - Electrical isolation of pulmonary veins sometimes requires targeted ablation of positions of atrial to ↓ reentrant triggers
  - Indication
    - Young patients, structurally normal heart, paroxysmal tachycardia after ≥ 1 failure of antiarrhythmic
  - Success rate
    - 80% to 90%, often require ≥ attempted catheter ablation

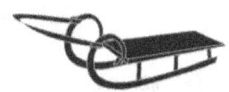

Mastering the Boards: Cardiology   A.B.R. Thomson

- o Cox Maze procedure
  - Indication
    - Failed catheter ablation
    - Other cardiac surgery planned
  - Success rate ~ 90%

- ➢ Treatment

- • Give the treatment of AF (Atrial fibrillation).

- • Pharmacological

- ➢ Acute
  - o Anticoagulation
    - CHADS2 score = 0; ASA (aspirin)
    - CHADS2 score ≥ 2; warfarin, dose adjusted for INR of 2.0-3.0
    - Procedures bridging anticoagulation not required
  - o No complications
    - Warfarin for 3 wk → cardioversion plus warfarin for 4 wk
    - Warfarin (INR 2.0 – 3.0)
    - TEE → (no clot) cardioversion plus warfarin for 4 wk

Note: this treatment plan also applies for **atrial flutter**

  - o Rate control
    - Hemodynamically stable → rate control: IV
      - β-blocker
        - Metoprolol
        - Esmolol
      - CCB
        - Verapamil
        - Diltiazem
      - Digoxin
    - Target rate
      - Young, with symptoms – target < 80 bpm (resting ventricular rate)
      - Old, no symptoms; target < 110 bpm
    - Indications
      - Chronic HF
      - AF of unknown duration (with **no** WPW syndrome)
    - No symptoms from AF

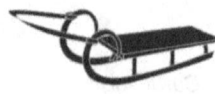

- Across adequacy with
  - Exercise test, or
  - Ambulatory monitoring
- Continue anti-coagulation based on CHADS2
- Medications (with **no** WPW syndrome)
  - BB (atenolol, metoprolol), or
  - CCB (diltiazem, verapamil)
  - If rate not controlled by BB or CCB, add digoxin (do **not** use digoxin on its own)

THERAPEUTIC ALERTS

  o In the presence of AF plus WPW syndrome, do **not** give BB, CCB or digoxin (↑ risk of AF → VT or VF)

---

o Rhythm control
  - Goal to relieve symptoms after rate central score
  - Episode AF may still occur despite cardioconversion / anti-arrhythmic agent
  - Continue anti-coagulation based on CHADS2 score

o Cardioconversion (rhythm control)
  - Unusual AF
    - Urgent procedure
    - Angina
    - Low BP
    - HF
  - Elective (stable AF)
    - Young, persistent symptoms
    - TEE to rule out clot
    - If no TEE, anticoagulate (AC) for 3 weeks before cardioconversion
  - Medications, synchronized cardioversion, ablation therapy, cardiac surgery
    - After cardioconversion, AC for 4 weeks
    - If high risk, A/C long-term after cardiocersion

➢ Chronic

  o Anti-coagulation for non-valvular atrial fibrillation based on CHAD2 score

Abbreviation: AF, atrial fibrillation; BB, beta-blocker; bpm, beats per minute; CCB, calcium channel blocker; VF, ventricular fibrillation; VT, ventricular tachycardia

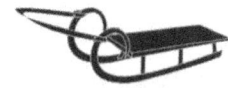

- Give the recommendations for when to use bridging anti-coagulation in AF (atrial fibrillation).

	Clinical situation	Planned duration of stopping anti-coagulation	Need for bridging anti-coagulation
o CHADS2	0-2	< 7 d	No
o CHADS2	5-6 Or Recent CVA Rheumatic or Mechanical MV	> 7 d	Yes
o Cardioconversion		4 wk	Yes

Abbreviation: MV, mitral valve

- Non-pharmacological
  - o Atrial fibrillation ablation
    - - Indication
      - ▪ Symptoms despite ≥ 1 anti-arrhythmic agent
    - - Principle
      - ▪ Exercise test, or
      - ▪ Isolate pulmonary vein so premature atrial contractions do not cause AF
    - - Anti-coagulation
      - ▪ For 2-3 mon after ablation, then
      - ▪ Continue based on CHADS2 score
    - - Outcomes
      - ▪ Success, 84%
      - ▪ Complications ~ 4%
  - o AV node ablation
    - - Indication
      - ▪ Exercise test, or
      - ▪ Not a candidate for atrial fibrillation ablation (and thus also have symptoms despite ≥ anti-arrhythmic agent)
    - - Principle
      - ▪ Prevent AF by destroying aV node
      - ▪ Must insert pacemaker to control
        - - Rate of ventricle
        - - Treat possible complication of polymorphic VT
  - o Maze surgery
    - - Open heart
    - - Multiple incisions made in RA and LA to interrupt any re-entrant pathways

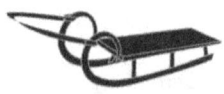

Supraventricular Tachycardias (SVTs)

- o SVT
  - Initiated or maintained by atrial tissue or AV node
  - QRS complex usually narrow

- Give the types short- and long- RP SVT (supraventricular tachycardia)

  - o Short-PR
    - AVNRT (AV nodal re-entrant tachycardia)
    - AVRT (AV reciprocating tachycardia)
    - JT (junctional tachycardia)

  - o Long-PR
    - AT (atrial tachycardia)
    - ST
    - Atypical AVNRT
      - Fast-slow
      - Slow-slow

  - o The distance from P wave to the preceding QRS complex determines whether the SVT is short- or long- RP tachycardia.

  - o Patients with SVT (supraventricular tachycardia) and aberrant conduction usually convert with IV adenosine, whereas VT (ventricular tachycardia will not convert with adenosine.

  - o Therefore, "do not treat irregular wide-complex tachycardia or polymorphic tachycardia with adenosine" (Source: Board Basics 3, 2012, page 39.)

  - o AV-Nodal re-entrant tachycardia
    - Treat with
      - IV adenosine, BB or CCB
      - Valsalva maneuver, or unilateral carotid sinus massage

Atrial Nodal Reentrant Tachycardia (AVNRT)

- ➢ Demography
  - o Usually middle aged females
  - o Most common SVT when > 40 yr
  - o Often occurs with Wolff-Parkinson-White (WPW) syndrome

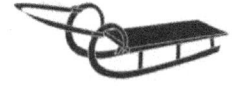

> Types
  o Typical
    - Conduction   ↗ Antegrade to ventricle Slow
                                              pathway   Short RP
                    ↖ Retrograde to atrium   tachycardia
                                              Fast
                                              pathway
    - ECG   P wave in QRS
                    To find retrograde P wave
                    Compare QRS and ST segment in tachycardia and sinus
                    rhythm

  o Atypical
    - Conduction   ↗ Antegrade to ventricle   Fast pathway
                                                            Long RP
                    ↗ Retrograde to atrium   Slow pathway tachycardia
    - ECG
      ▪ To find retrograde P wave
      ▪ After QRS complex, second half of PR interval

> Causes / associations (commonest)
  o Commonest cause of SVT

  o AV node pathway   - Slow
                         ▪ Slow down conduction pathway
                       - Fast
                         ▪ Return conduction up fast pathway

  o Atypical AVNRT   - Fast
                       - Slow

  o Treatment   - Vagal maneuvers
                         ▪ Massage of carotid sinus
                         ▪ Adenosine
                         ▪ β-blockers
                         ▪ CCB (not dihydropyridine)
                         ▪ Anti-arrhythmic agents
                         ▪ Cardioconversion
                         ▪ Catheter ablation

Atrioventricular Reentrant Tachycardia (AVRT)

➢ Types

  o Typical (in 95%): orthodromic AVRT (o-AVRT) form of SVT

	Antegrade to ventricle	AV node	
- Conduction			Short RP
	Retrograde to atrium	Accessory "by pass" tract	tachycardia

  - ECG
    ▪ To find retrograde P waves
    ▪ > 70 ms after QRS complex

  o Uncommon (5%): antidromic AVRT (A-AVRT) form of SVT

	Antegrade to ventricle	Accessory bypass tract	Long RP
- Conduction			tachycardia
	Retrograde to atrium	AV node / second bypass tract	

  - ECG
    ▪ Look for preexcitation on baseline QRS for WPW syndrome (short PR, delta wave on upstroke of QRS

Atrioventricular Reciprocating Tachycardia (AVRT)

  o Direction of electrical signal
    - Down AV node → up the bypass pathway (Kent bundles, between atrium and ventricle), or
    - Down bypass pathway → up the AV node → "preexcitation pattern"

  o Preexcitation pattern plus symptomatic tachycardia = WPW (Wolff-Parkinson-White) syndrome
    - 1/3 of patients with WPW syndrome develop AF, which may cause VF (ventricular fibrillation)
    - Do **not** treat with BB, CCB

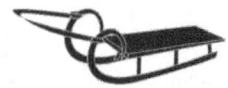

Mastering the Boards: Cardiology   A.B.R. Thomson

- Give risk factors for AF (atrial fibrillation) turning into VF (ventricular fibrillation) in persons with WPW syndrome.

    o AVRT (AV reciprocal tachycardia)

    o Rapid conduction down bypass pathway

    o Multiple bypass pathways

    o Ebstein abnormality

➢ Treatment

    o No reexcitation
      - Catheter ablation
      - β-blockers
      - Anti-arrhythmic agents

    o Preexcitation (WPW syndrome)
      - Catheter ablation
      - Avoid nodal blockers → will ↑ VR (ventricular rate)

Junctional Tachycardia

AV junction   ↑ automatically   electrical impulse   Atrium / Ventricle

Sinoatrial Nodal Reentrant Tachycardia

    o Sudden atrial complexes

    o Premature atrial complexes (PACs)

    o Retrograde conduction in sinoatrial (SA) node

    o ECG P-wave in SVT similar to native P-wave morphology / axis during sinus rhythm

- Give the electrophysiological reason why atrial fibrillation (AF) and atrial flutter (AFL) supraventricular tachycardias (SVTs) fail to respond to slowing of the ventricular rate by the use of AV blocking maneuvers (carotid sinus massage, Valsalva to ↑ vagal activity) or drugs (adenosine).

    o AF / AFL have partial AV nodal blockade, so unlike some other SVTs, they do not respond to carotid sinus message on the Valsalva maneuver to stimulate vagal activity, or drugs like adenosine

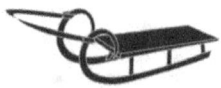

- ➢ Treatment
  - ○ General treatment of SVTs
    - – If not AF, AFL
      - ▪ ↑ vagal tone
        - - Carotid sinus massage
        - - Valsalva maneuver
      - ▪ Drugs
        - - Adenosine
    - – Correct associated electrolyte abnormalities and any other pathophysiologic processes
  - ○ Radiofrequency ablation (RFA)
    - – ~ 90% cure rate
      - ▪ Focal AF
      - ▪ AFL
      - ▪ AVNRT
      - ▪ AVRT

Arrhythmia	Anticoagulation	Medications	RFA	Cardioversion
○ AF				
○ AFL				
○ MAT		B-blockers CCBs		
○ EAT - Acute		B-blockers, CCBs		
- Chronic		B-blockers, CCBs Amiodarone Propafenone Flecainide		
○ AVNRT		B-blockers, CCBs Digoxin Amiodarone, Propafenone, flecainide		
○ AVRT - Acute		VMM, adenosine CCB, B-blockers, procainamide		
- Chronic		Flecainide, procainamide		

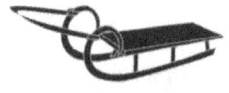

Mastering the Boards: Cardiology   A.B.R. Thomson

Arrhythmia	Anticoagulation	Medications	RFA	Cardioversion

o A-VRT
   - Acute   Ibutilide, procainamide, flecainide

   - Chronic   Flecainide, propafenone

Note: Do not use adenosine for AV node blockade in acute A-AVRT

Abbreviations: A-AVRT, antidromic AV reentrant tachycardia; AF, atrial fibrillation; AFL, atrial flutter; AVNRT, AV nodal reentrant tachycardia; EAT, ectopic atrial tachycardia; MAT, multi-focal atrial tachycardia; O-AVRT, orthodromic AV reentrant tachycardia; VMM, vagal massage maneuvers

Wolf-Parkinson-White (WPW) Syndrome

➢ Pathogenesis

   o   Accessory bypass conduction tract causes pre-excitation

   o   Typical mechanism of supraventricular tachycardia in patients with Wolff-Parkinson-White syndrome (WPS syndrome)

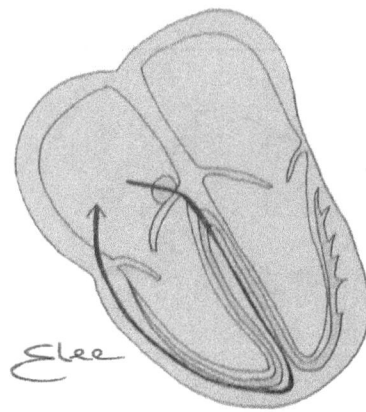

          – WPS syndrome arises from orthodromic atrioventricular re entry.
          – The resulting WPS syndrome is a narrow QRS complex because ventricular activation is over the normal conduction system.

Adapted from: Ghosh AK. *Mayo Clinic Scientific Press* 2008, Figure 3-33, page 88.

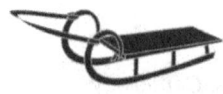

o   Mechanism of supraventricular tachycardia in patients with WPW syndrome

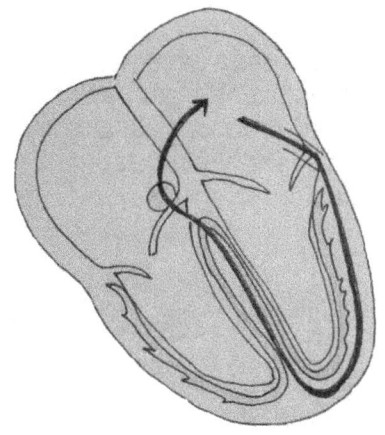

- The result is a wide QRS complex because ventricular activation is over an accessory pathway.
- This arrhythmia is difficult to distinguish from ventricular tachycardia.

Adapted from: Ghosh AK. *Mayo Clinic Scientific Press* 2008, Figure 3-34, page 88.

o   Conduction of sinus impulses in Wolff-Parkinson-White syndrome

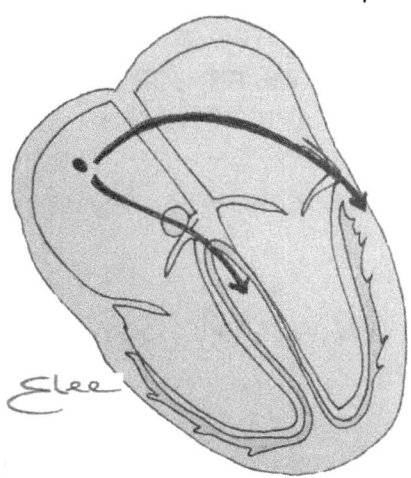

- The ventricles are activated over the normal atrioventricular node – His-Purkinje system and accessory pathway
- The result is a fusion complex (QRS and delta wave).

Adapted from: Ghosh AK. *Mayo Clinic Scientific Press* 2008, Figure 3-35, page 88.

 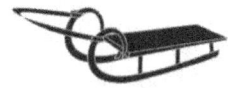

o Pacemaker syndrome

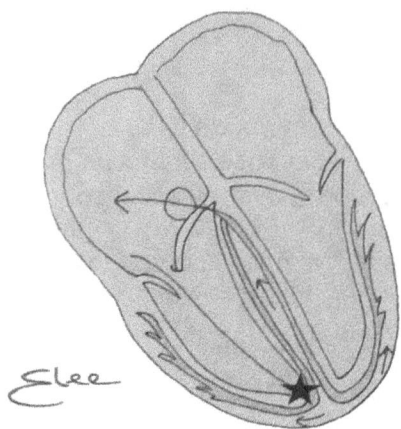

– Retrograde atrial activation during ventricular pacing (star) produces simultaneous atrial and ventricular contractions.

Adapted from: Ghosh AK. *Mayo Clinic Scientific Press* 2008, Figure 3-19, page 75.

The importance of the WPW Syndrome relates to the **Clinical Cautions**

o WPW is a risk factor for SCD (sudden cardiac death)

o If patient with AF (atrial fibrillation) has missed WPW syndrome and the AF is incorrectly treated with BB, CCB or digitalis, the AF may convert to VT (ventricular tachycardia) or VF (ventricular fibrillation).

➢ ECG

• Give the ECG findings and treatment of WPW (Wolf-Parkinson-White) syndrome.

o ECD
  - Short PR interval
  - QRS – long or normal
  - Slurred onset (delta wave)

o Treatment
  - Unstable
    ▪ Cardioversion
  - Stable
    ▪ Procainamide
    ▪ If drug resistant → ablation (of accessory byoass conduction tract)

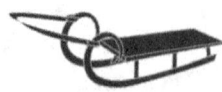

Premature Atrial Contractions (PAC) and Atrial Tachycardia (AT)

- o Treatment
  - β-blockers
  - CCB
  - Digoxin
  - Catheter ablation
- o Multifocal AT
  - Treat associated lung disease
  - Maintain normal electrolytes
  - β-blockers
  - CCB

Ventricular Arrhythmias

- o PVC (premature ventricular contractions)
- o VT (ventricular tachycardia) plus structural heart disease
- o Idiopathic VT

Premature Ventricular Contractions (PVCs)

PVCs are common, and patients with symptoms may be worried that they have underlying heart disease such as CAD (coronary artery disease), hypertension or LVH (left ventricular hypertrophy). These factors can readily be excluded in the patient. However, the symptomatic patient with PVCs may still vary.

- Give the risk factors for the patient with PVCs (premature ventricular contractions) about which they can be reassured.

  - o No
    - Syncope
    - Structural heart disease
    - Family history of SCD (sudden cardiac death)

Ventricular Tachycardia

➢ Definitions
  - o Ventricular tachycardias (VT): "......≥ 3 consecutive ventricular complexes at a rate > 100 BPM on an ECG recording".
  - o Ventricular fifibrillation (VF): "....a rapid, disorganized rhythm without recognizable QRS complexes on the ECG".

Dorian P, et al. Chapter 43. In: Therapeutic Choices. Grey J, Ed. 6th Edition, *Canadian Pharmacists Association* 2012, page 587.

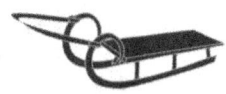

> Useful background
  - Premature ventricular complexes are usually benign
  - There are three types of wide QRS ventricular tachyarrhythmias (QRS > 0.12 sec plus AV dissociation): VT, Tde P (torsades de pointes), and VF (ventricular fibrillation)
    - VT (ventricular tachycardia)
      - Monomorphic QRS complexes have varying contour
      - Polymorphic QRS complexes have varying contours
      - Torsades de pointes a form of polymorphic QRS complexes
      - Associated with long QT syndrome
      - May progress to VF / SCD

(Washington Manual of Medical Therapeutics, 2014, Chapter 7, Wolters Kluwer / Lippincott William & Wilkins)

> Types
  - Usually wide-complex tachyarrhythmias, WCT

  - Non-sustained ventricular tachycardia (VT)
    - "three or more consecutive ventricular complexes (> 100 bpm) that terminates spontaneously within 30 sec without significant hemodynamic consequences or need for intervention"

  - Sustained monomorphic VT
    - "....a tachycardia composed of ventricular complexes of a single QRS morphology that lasts longer than 30 sec or requires cardioconversion due to hemodynamic compromise".

  - Polymorphic VT
    - Ever-changing QRS morphology
    - TdP (Torsade de pointe) is a type of polymorphic VT that is proceeded by a long QT interval during sinus rhythm

  - Ventricular fibrillation (VF)
    - "... irregular and rapid oscillations (250 to 400 bpm / g highly variable amplitude without uniquely identifiable QRS complexes or T waves..... associated with disorganized mechanical contraction, hemodynamic collapse, and sudden [cardiac] death " (SCD).

CLINICAL ALERTS

  - Sudden cardiac death (SCD) is associated with
    - Ventricular arrhythmias
    - Previous myocardial infarction
    - Non-ischemic cardiomyopathy

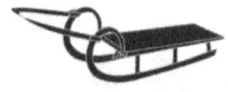

- ➤ Etiology
- No associated structural heart disease
  - ○ Brugada structural heart disease ⎤ - Inherited ion channelopathies
  - ○ Long QT syndrome ⎦ - Polymorphic VT
  - ○ Familial exercise-induced VT ⠀⠀⠀ - Catecholaminonergic polymorphic VT (CPVT)
  - ⠀⠀⠀⠀⠀⠀⠀⠀⠀⠀⠀⠀⠀⠀⠀⠀⠀⠀⠀⠀⠀⠀ - Abnormal processing of Ca^{2+}
- Structural heart disease
  - ○ Arrhythmogenic substrate
    - Ischemic scar / post-infarction area → reentry of sustained mono- / polymorphic VT
    - RV dysplasia fibrofatty replacement of RV / LV → LBBB morphology VT → SCD
    - Non-ischemic / infiltrative cardiomyopathies
    - BBRVT (bundle branch reentry VT)
    - Congenital heart disease
  - ○ Ideopathic
    - Diagnosis of exclusion
    - Types
      - ▪ RVOT-VT (right ventricular outflow tract VT)
      - ▪ LVOT-VT (left ventricular outflow tract VT)
      - ▪ Fascular VT LBBB, anterior and posterior divisions

- ➤ ECG diagnosis of wide complex tachyarrhythmias (WCT)
  - ○ Ventricular tachycardia (consider all WCTs to be ventricular [and not supreaventricular (SVT)] until proven otherwise)
    - WCT is usually (80%) VT
    - In those with previous MI, 98% of WCT are VT
    - In those with pacemaker or ICD (implanatable cardiac defribrillator)
    - In those with prior LBBB, RBBB, IVCD (intraventricular cardiac defribrillator) causing conduction
      - ▪ QRS morphology similar to baseline → SVR
      - ▪ QRS morphology different from bedside → VT
      - ▪ Narrow QRS at baseline → WCT (due to SVT with aberrancy)
    - In those on medications
      - ▪ Class I and III antiarrhythmics
      - ▪ Selected antibiotics
      - ▪ Antipsychotics
      - ▪ Digoxin
      - ▪ Diuretics
      - ▪ ACEI / ARBs

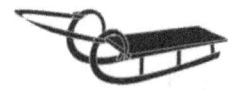

For assessment of possible drug adverse effects causing WCT, please see
http://www.qtddrugs.org

- - Telemetry artifact / tremor may mimic VT / VF
- o Antidromic AVRT
- o Arrhythmia causes by hyperkalemia

- ➢ Differentiated diagnosis of VT [clinical alert]
  - o Use Brugada criteria to distinguish SVT with aberancy from VT
    - - Absent RS complex in precordia leads → VT
    - - RS complex in precardial leads but RS interval > 100 msec in any precardial lead → VT
    - - RS complex in precardial leads, RS > 100 msec, but AV dissociation → VT
    - - RS complex in precordial leads (V1-V6), RS > 100 msec, no AV dissociation, but morphology criteria for VT in V1-2 and V6 → VT

  - o SVT with aberrant conduction
    - - RS complex
    - - No
      - ▪ AV dissociation
      - ▪ QRS characteristic
      - ▪ Morphology criteria in V1-2, V6

- • Give the treatment of acute ventricular tachyarrhythmias.

SVT	VT	Pulseless VT / VF
o B-blocker	o Autoarrhymic drugs	o DCCV
o Adenosine	o Intracerdiac defibrillator	
o Calcium channel blockers - Caution - Hemodynamic instability	- IV amiodarone - B-blockers - ACE inhibitors - Sotalol - IV lidocaine - po mexiletine - IV phenytoin	
o RFA (radiofrequency catheter ablation)		

Abbreviations: DCCV, DC cardioversion; SVT, supraventricular tachycardia; VT, ventricular tachycardia

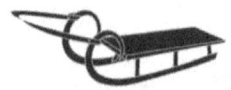

SO YOU WANT TO BE A CARDIOLOGIST!

- Give the ECG characteristics of the following types of VTs.
  - Arrythmogenic RV dysplasia: baseline
    - Epsilon wave after QRS
    - ± wide QRS
    - ± T-wave inversion in V1, V2
  - Brugada pattern: baseline
    - Pseudo-RBBB
    - ST-segment elevation ⎫ V1, V2
    - T-wave inversion ⎭
  - Bundle branch reentrant VT
    - IVCD (intraventricular conduction delay)
    - VT: LBBB morphology
      "down: the right bundle
      "up" the left bundle
  - Fascicular VT
    - VT: superior axis
    - RBBB morphology
  - Long QT
    - Baseline
      QT > 50% of RR-interval when HR 60-100 bpm
      QTc ≥ 400 ms
    - VT;TdP → VF

Abbreviations: LBBB, left bundle branch block; RBBB, right bundle branch block; TdP, Torsade de Pointes; VF, ventricular fibrillation; VT, ventricular tachycardia

---

CLINICAL CAUTION

- Give a major reason for a "falsely positive" ECG for VT (ventricular tachycardia) / VF (ventricular fibrillation) (i.e., condition or circumstances which mimics VT / VF on ECG.
  - Telemetry of a shaking patient (e.g. tremor) during telemetry may give an artifact which mimics VT / VF.

VT diagnostic criteria
  - QRS characteristic morphology criteria
  - AV dissociation
  - No RS in precordial leads (V1-V6) LBBB plus RAD

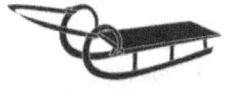

```
TREATMENT ALERT

Be      Careful
           Critical
               For this
                   Crucial distinction of
                       SVT plus aberrancy from VT
```

Non-pharmacologic Therapies of VT: ICD and RFA

- ➤ Intracardiac defibrillator (ICD)

  - o Primary prevention of sudden cardiac death (SCD)
    - - High risk factors for SCD
      - ▪ Arrhythmogenic cardiomyotomy
      - ▪ Brugada syndrome
      - ▪ Hypertrophic cardiomyotomy
      - ▪ Syncope
      - ▪ Family history of SCD
      - ▪ Prior to cardiac transplantation (especially if hemodynamically unstable and requiring inotropes)

  - o Secondary prevention of SCD
    - - Indications
      - ▪ Persons surviving resuscitation from ventricular arrhythmias (often having LV-EF < 35% despite 3 mon of optimal medical therapy)
    - - Contraindications
      - ▪ Myocardial infarction within last 40 days
      - ▪ Incessant VT
      - ▪ Major psychiatric illness
      - ▪ Morbidities limiting life expectancy to < 12-24 mon

- ➤ Radiofrequency catheter ablation (ATA)

  - o Indications
    - - Patients with "…. Hemodynamically stable forms of idiopathic VT that is anot associated with structural heart disease" (Sharma S et al. Washington Manual of Medical Therapeutics, 2014, Chapter 7, page 220-267. Wolters Kluwer / Lippincott William & Wilkins)
    - - VT refractory to pharmacological

  - o Ildeopathic VT (structurally normal heart)
    - - RVOT-VT (RV outflow tract VT)
    - - LVOT-VT (LV outflow tract VT)
    - - RFA (but not ICU) useful

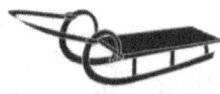

Mastering the Boards: Cardiology   A.B.R. Thomson

- o BBRVT
  - Reentrant through His-Purkinje system
  - RFA (radiofrequency catheter ablation)
  - ICD (intracardiac defribrillator)

- o Ischemia-associated VT
  - Use RFA for VT that is refractory to optimal medical therapy
  - RFA may be used in patients with an ICD and refractory ischemia-associated VT
- o Non-ischemic cardiomyopathy-associated VT
  RFA is center specialized to perform intra- / epicardial ablation

Pharmacological Therapies of VT/VF

- Acute
  - o Resistant external DCCV (DC cardioversion)
    - Add
      - ▪ IV amiodarone
      - ▪ IV lidocaine
    - Continue IV antiarrhythmic agents until reversible causes have been corrected
- Chronic
  - o Recurrent and symptomatic VT / VF
    - ICD ± drug therapy

CLINICAL TIP

When idiopathic VF occurs within 3 days after AMI, it is unlikely to become chronic and does not require treatment with longterm use of antiarrhythmic drugs.

- o Diphyalkylamine CCB such as verapamil or benzodiazepine CCB such as diltiazem have negative cardiac inotropic and negative chromotropic effects so may ↑ HF (heart failure) in a patient who has ↓ LV function and a cardiac conduction abnormality.

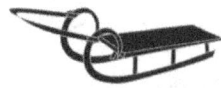

- **Amiodarone**
  - 1 wk to see any benefit
  - 4-6 wk to see maximum benefit
  - Longterm
    - Common recurrent of ventricular arrhythmia
    - Use for primary prevention of SCD in cardiomyopathy (high risk of SCD)

Class II

- B-blockers (> 3 days post MI)
  - ↓ mortality (~↓ 33%)
  - ↓ SCD (~↓ 33%)
- ACE inhibitors (CAD, HF)
  - ↓ mortality
  - ↓ SCD

Abbreviations: CAD, coronary artery disease; HF, heart failure; MI, myocardial infarction; SCD, sudden cardiac death

Class III

- Sotalol
  - ↓ VT / VF in 70%
  - Do not use in HF (heart failure)

Class Ib

- IV lidocaine
- po mexiletine

CLINICAL ALERTS

- Give the reason why lidocaine is not used prophylactically post-MI for PVC / NSVT.
  - Post-MI, lidocaine ↑ mortality (bradycardia)

- **Phynetoin**
  - IV loading dose, followed by po phenytoin for digitalis Induced ventricular arrhythmia

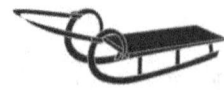

- Give the common adverse effects of IV lidocaine and po mexiletine.

- Lidocaine
  - CNS
    - Convulsion
    - Confusion
    - Coma
  - Lung
    - Respiratory arrest

- Mexiletine
  - CNS
    - Low dose
      - Tremor
      - Dizziness
      - Blurred vision
    - High dose
      - Nystagmus
      - Diploplia
      - Dysarthria

CLINICAL ALERTS

Do **not** use the following to treat VT

  - CCBs
    - Poor effect, no benefit
    - ↑ mortality post-MI (nifedipine

  - Class I
    - Flecainide, propafenone
    - ↑ mortality

  - Class IV
    - Poor effect, no benefit

Torsades de Pointes (TdeP)

  - Acute
    - IV magnesium sulfate 1-2 gm repeat 1-2 times
  - Chronic
    - Treat underlying cause
    - IV isoproterenol
      - ↑ HR to 90-120 bpm using 1-2 mcg / min
    - Pacing transvenous, temporary

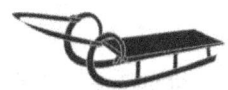

Ventricular Tachycardia with Structural Heart Disease

- ○ HF (heart failure) ⎫
- ○ IHD (ischemic heart disease) ⎬ β-blockers
- ○ Stable VT plus structural heart disease
- ○ Unstable VT arrhythmic drugs to ↓ ICD VF history

Clinical Caution

- Give the reason for the concern about ventricular tachycardia.

  - ○ VT (ventricular tachycardia) may lead to ↓ EF (ejection fraction), ↓ BP (blood pressure), syncope

  - ○ ↓ EF, ↓ BP, syncope → ↑ risk of SCD (sudden cardiac death)

Idiopathic Ventricular Tachycardia (VT)

- ○ Monomorphic
- ○ VT > 100 bpm
- ○ Clusters of VT brought on by
  - Exercise
  - Emotional stress
- ○ Originates from RV outflow tract
- ○ ECG
  - Runs of VT plus LBBB, positive in inferior leads
  - Differentiate IVT from ARVC / D (arrhythmogenic RV cardiomyopathy
- ○ Treatment
  - β-blockers on CCBs (calcium channel blockers)
  - Class I or III anti-arrhythmic agents (Na^+ or K^+ channel blockers, such as procainamide, lidocaine, flecainide; or sotalor, amiodarone, dronedarone)
  - Catheter ablation

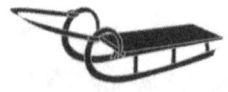

Inherited Arrhythmia Syndromes (aka "channelopathies")

- o Long QT syndrome
- o Short QT syndrome
- o Brugoda syndrome
- o CPVT (catecholaminergic polymorphic VT)
- o ARVC / D (arrhythmogenic right ventricular cardiomyopathy / dysplasia)

- ➤ Useful background
  - o Often present with syncope
  - o ↑ risk of SCD (sudden cardiac death)
  - o Generally treated with β-blockers and ICD (implantable cardioverter-defibrillator)

Arrhythmogenic Right Ventricular Cardiomyopathy / Dysplasia (ARVC / D)

- o Dysfunction of desmosomes
  - ↓ myocytes in RV (right ventricle) ⎱ ↓ function of RV and LV → ↑↑ risk
  - ⎰ of VT, SCD
  - ↑ fibrofatty infiltration
- o Diagnosis
  - ECG
  - Echocardiogram
  - CMR (cardiac magnetic resonance)
  - RV biopsy

Type	ECG	Triggers	Complication	Treatment
o Long QT syndrome	QT > 460 msec	Exercise Loud noise Sleep	SCD	β-blockers avoid drugs with ↑ QT interval ICD
o Short QT syndrome	QT < 350 msec		AF VT VF SCD	Quinidine ICD

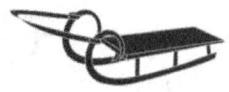

Type	ECG	Triggers	Complication	Treatment
o Brugada syndrome	J-point elevation ≥ 2 mm ST-segment ↑ and coved T-wave inversion	↑ Temp ↑ / ↓ K⁺ TCAs Alcohol Cocaine	VF SCD	ICD
o Catecholaninergic polymorphic VT	Polymorphic QRS	Exercise Emotional stress	SCD	β-blockers ICD
o ARVC /D	T-wave inversion in V1-V3 Epsilon wave ↑↑↑ PVCs		VT	β-blockers ICD

Abbreviations: ARVC /D, arrhythmogenic right ventricular cardiomyopathy / dysplasia; ICD, implantable cardioverter-defibrillator; PVCs, premature ventricular contractions; VT, ventricular tachycardia

Implantable Cardioverter-Defibrillator (ICD)

- o Markedly improves prognosis for ventricular tachyarrhythmias
- o Use for primary or secondary prevention
- o In presence of electromagnetic field (MR testing, airport security screening) → ICD shock capability is lost
- o ICDs may include biventricular pacemakers
- o Suspected infection of ICD or pacemaker
  - Blood cultures
  - TEE (transesophageal echocardiogram)
  - Remove devise plus leads
  - Do **not** aspirate site of erosion / abscess

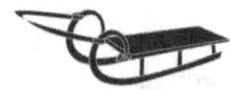

Dysrhythmias

- Perform a focused physical examination for risk factors for thromboembolism in non-rheumatic atrial fibrillation.

Clinical Risk Factors
- Heart failure
- Hypertension
- Age >75 years
- Diabetes mellitus
- Prior stroke
- Prosthetic heart valves
- Thyrotoxicosis Other high-risk clinical settings

Source: Ghosh AK. *Mayo Clinic Scientific Press* 2008, page 85.

Self Quiz

- There are many causes of sinus tachycardia (heart rate [HR]) greater than 120 bpm (beats per minute), give the causes of HR ≥ 140 bpm.
  - Atrial fibrillation (AF)
  - Atrial flutter
  - PAT (paroxysmal atrial fibrillation)

Using carotid massage, how can you distinguish between these 3 causes of HR > 140 bpm?
  - AF – no effect on HR
  - Atrial flutter – HR slowed temporarily
  - PAT – stops, or no effect

Syncope

- Associations
  - Prodrome
    - Warm
    - Sweating
    - Nausea

  - Position
    - Prolonged standing
    - Orthogenic

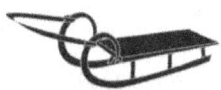

- o Provocation
  - – Pain
  - – Emotion
  - – Swallowing (or postprandial)
  - – Defecation
  - – Urination
  - – Coughing

Note: Orthostatic hypotension may be simple, but access for hypovolemia, drug effects, and disorders if the autonomic nervous system such as diabetes, parkinsonism

Palpitations

➢ Definition: sensations of a rapid or irregular heartbeat occurring in normal, healthy people during exercise and states of anxiety.

➢ Useful background

- o Only about 1 person in 6 with palpitations will have a cardiac arrhythmia.
- o Palpitations may be present only with exercise, especially if the basal heart rate is slow.

➢   Clinical

• Take a directed history for palpitations.

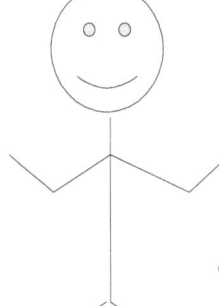

- o General
  - – Presyncope / syncope
  - – Malaise/fatigue
  - – Fever/chills/night sweats
  - – Diaphoresis

- o Heart
  - – Slow vs. rapid, regular vs. irregular
  - – Frequency of bouts
  - – Duration
  - – Nature of onset/offset

- o CNS
  - – Numbness/paresthesia
  - – Weakness
  - – Visual/ speech abnormalities

- o Lung
  - – Lung base crackles
  - – Dyspnea/orthopnea/PND
  - – Cough
  - – Chest pain

- o Ankles/ sacrum
  - – Edema

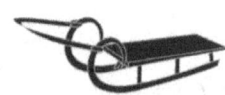

- ➤ Causes
  - o Heart disease causing
    - Tachycardia
    - Bradycardia
    - Extrasystole
  - o Causes of tachycardia
    - Fever
    - Exercise
    - Hyperthyroidism
    - Pheochromocytoma
    - Hypoglycemia
  - o Anxiety (da Costa syndrome, aka cardiac neurosis)
  - o Drugs
  - o Heart
    - Pericardial (pericarditis)
    - Myocardial (LVH, infarction, CHF, myxoma, ASD, amyloidosis)
    - Endocardial (infarction, sick sinus, valvular- MS/MR, AS/AR
  - o Lung
    - Asthma, COPD
    - Pneumonia
    - Pulmonary embolism
  - o Endocrine
    - Hyperthyroid
    - Pheochromocytosis
    - Hypoglycemia
  - o Drugs and Toxins
    - EtOH (binge or withdrawal)
    - CO poisoning
    - Stimulants (caffeine, theophylline, amphetamines, cocaine)
  - o Metabolic – electrolyte abnormalities
  - o Infection – sepsis

Abbreviations: ASD, atrial septal defect; CHF, congestive heart failure; CO, carbon monoxide; COPD, chronic obstructive pulmonary disease; CVA, cerebro vascular accident; ETOH, ethanol; LVH, left ventricular hypertrophy; PND, paroxysmal nocturnal dyspnea; TIA, transient ischemic attack

Adapted from: Jugovic PJ, et al. *Saunders/ Elsevier* 2004, pages 70 and 71.

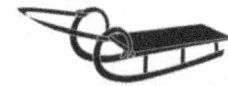

Mastering the Boards: Cardiology   A.B.R. Thomson

- Perform a focused physical examination for palpitations.

  o Head and neck
  – ↑ JVP
  – If JVP pulsations match the heart rate, especially with tachycardia, suspect AV nodal re-entrant trachycardia

  o Pulse
  – ↑ HR, ↓ HR, AF, MVE (irregular irregularity decreases with exercise)

  o Heart sounds
  – S$_1$ varies in intensity, and S$_2$ may be split in AF

  o Matched in murmur
  – Any associated cardiac conditions

Going for Gold !

- In a patient with a history of palpitations, perform a focused examination of the ECG.

  o P wave
  – Matched in II (AF)
  – Terminal wave > 0.04s negative (AF)

  o PR interval short, with delta waves – look for WPWS (Wolff – Parkinson – White syndrome)

  o Q wave
  – Present, suggests previous infarction, leading to possible non-sustained ventricular tachycardia
  – Deep Q waves (I, L, V4 to V6) suggesting LVH and possible HOCM

  o QT interval long, abnormal T wave morphology
  – Possible long QT syndrome

  o ↓ HR, HB
  – Look for long QT syndrome and torsade de pointes

Abbreviation: LVA, left ventricular hypertrophy; HOCM, hypertrophic obstructive cardiomyopathy; HB, heart block

Source: Baliga RR. *Saunders/Elsevier* 2007, pages 35 and 36.

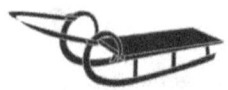

- Give the performance characteristics of palpation of the precordium.

Finding	PLR	NLR
o Hyperkinetic apical movement		
– Detecting associated mitral regurgitation or aortic valve disease in patients with mitral stenosis	11.2	0.3
o Sustained apical movement		
– Detecting severe aortic stenosis in patients with aortic flow murmurs	4.1	0.3
– Detecting moderate-to-severe aortic regurgitation in patients with basal early diastolic murmurs	2.4	0.1
– Detecting right ventricular peak pressure ≥ 50 mm Hg	3.6	0.4
– Palpable P_2		
■ Detecting pulmonary hypertension in patients with mitral stenosis	3.6	0.05
– Absence of palpable P2		0.05
o Varying intensity of S1, detecting AV dissociation in the presence of tachycardia	24.4 (prob-ability > 50%)	0.4
o Palpable P2, detecting PHT	3.6 (probability ~25% ↑)	
o Position of apical beat - Supine apical impulse lateral to MCL		
– Detecting cardiothoracic ratio >0.5	3.4	0.6
– Detecting low ejection fraction	10.1	0.6
– Detecting increased left ventricular end diastolic volume	8.0	0.7
– Detecting pulmonary capillary wedge pressure >12 mm Hg	5.8	NS
o Size of apical beat - Apical beat diameter ≥4 cm in left lateral decubitus position at 45 degrees		
– Detecting increased left ventricular end diastolic volume	4.7	NS

o Note

- A supine displaced apical impulse has a PLR < 2, and is not included here.

Abbreviations: AV, atrioventricular; EF, ejection fraction; PLR, positive likelihood ratio; NLR, negative likelihood ratio; MCL, midclavicular line; NS, not significant; PHT, pulmonary hypertension

Adapted from: McGee SR. *Saunders/Elsevier* 2007, Box 34-2, page 404.

Apical (pericardial) Impulse (PMI, point of maximal impulse)

o Double or even triple apical impulses occur in HOCM

o Pericardial impulse in mitral stenosis represents palpable S_1 and S_2 (from P_2 components), opening snap, and diastolic thrill (patient in left lateral deculoitus position).

o Precardial impulse in tricuspid regurgitation: palpable S_2 (from P_2 component) over pulmonic area, RV parasternal, pulsatile synchrony with each cardiac systole.

o Ectopic apical impulse (superior and medially): angina/previous MI, LV aneurysm, LV dyskimesia.

Adapted from: Mangione S. *Hanley & Belfus* 2000, page 201,202; Talley NJ, et al. *Maclennan & Petty Pty Limited* 2003, page 49 to 50; Filate W, et al. *The Medical Society, Faculty of Medicine, University of Toronto* 2005, Table 7 page 58.

• Give the performance characteristics of size and position of palpable apical impulse.

Finding	PLR
o Detecting cardiothoracic ratio >0.5	3.4
o Detecting low ejection fraction	10.1
o Detecting increased left ventricular end-diastolic volume	8.0
o Detecting pulmonary capillary wedge pressure >12 mmHg	5.8
o Detecting increased left ventricular end-diastolic volume	4.7

Abbreviation: PLR, positive likelihood ratio

Adapted from: McGee SR. *Saunders/Elsevier* 2007, Box 34-1, page 402.

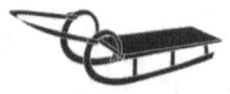

➢ Useful background: Performance characteristics for Atrioventricular Dissociation and Ventricular Tachycardia

Finding	Sensitivity (%)	Specificity (%)	PLR	NLR
o Varying arterial pulse	63	70	NS	NS
o Intermittent Cannon A waves, neck, veins	96	75	3.8	0.1
o Changing intesitity S_1	58	98	24.4	0.4

Source: McGee SR. *Saunders/Elsevier*, 2007, Table 14-1, page 149.

Sweet Nothing:

- o Pulsus parvus plus pulsus tardis (low amplitude plus slow upstroke) usually indicates the presence of aortic stenosis (AS).

- o Hyperkinetic pulse (rapid upstroke, high amplitude)
  - Wide pulse pressure
  - Aortic regurgitation.

- o Normal pulse pressure
  - Mitral regurgitation (MR)

"We are inherently critical as scientists, and inherently kind as physicians."

Grandad

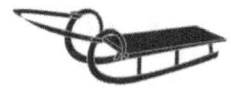

Mastering the Boards: Cardiology

A.B.R. Thomson

HEART SOUNDS

Normal

Systolic and Diastolic Normal Heart Sounds: S1 and S2

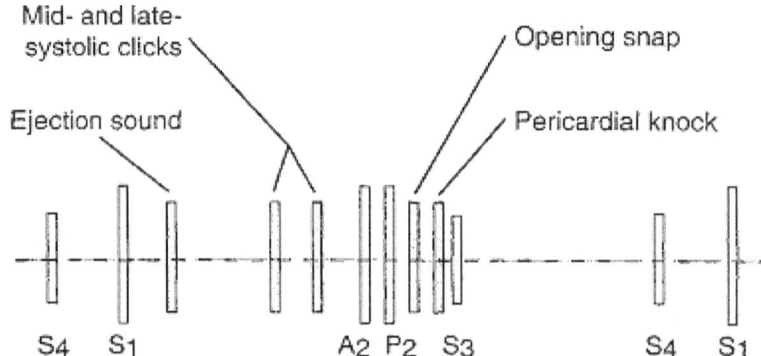

Adapted from: McGee S.R. *Saunders/Elsevier* 2007, Figure 38-1, page 445.

Sounds and extra sounds		Conventional teaching revisited
S1	↔	Still informative and valuable, albeit not as much as S2.
S2	↑	One of the most valuable sound, particularly in its variations of intensity and splitting.

Source: Mangione S. *Hanley & Belfus*, 2000, page 207

SO YOU WANT TO BE A CARDIOLOGY RESIDENT!

- In the context of listening to the heart sounds, give what is the Hamman Sign.

  - Crunching sound heard in time with systolic and diastolic components of heartbeat
  - This "mediastinal crunch" is due to air in the mediastinum
  - Seen after cardiac surgery, with a pneumothorax or aspiration of a pericardial effusion

Source: Talley NJ, et al. *Maclennan & Petty Pty Limited* 2003, page 59.

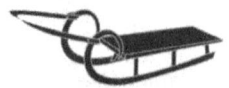

Useful background: The first (S_1) and second (S_2) heart sounds.

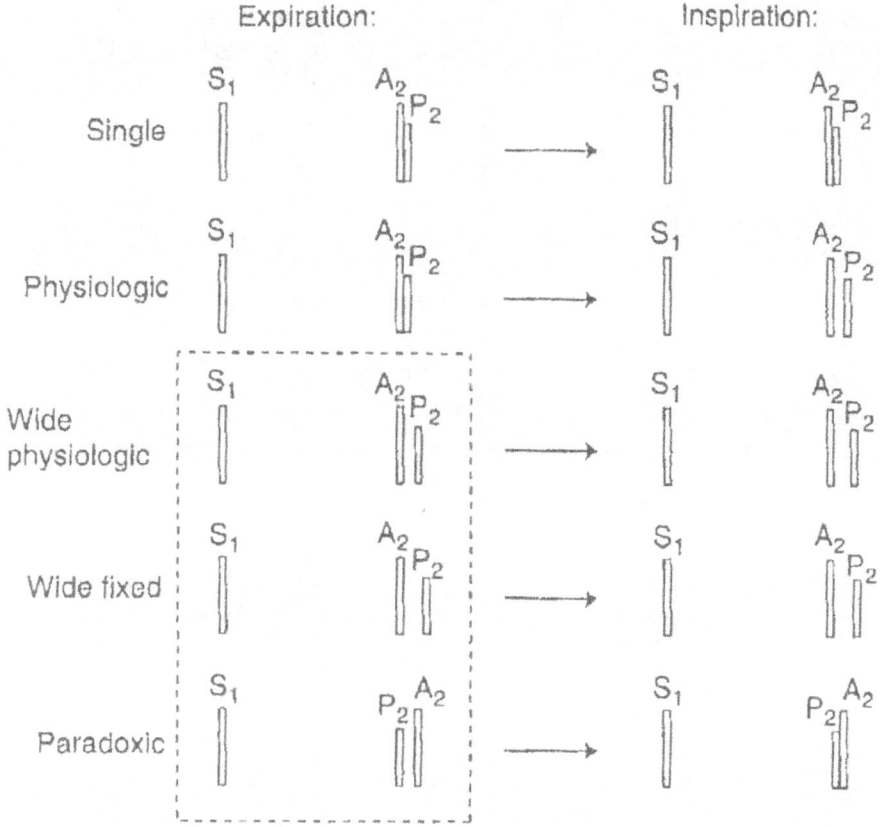

Adapted from: McGee SR. *Saunders/Elsevier* 2007, page 423.

- Give the special positions and maneuvers for optimal auscultation of heart sounds.

Position		Effect on heart sounds
o Sitting upright, leaning forward, holding exhalation		↑AS, AR, pericardial rubs
o Left lateral decubitus (LLD) (use bell of stethoscope)		S_3, S_4, MS
o Leg elevation	↑Venous return	↑Right sided murmurs, TR, PS

Maneuver	Physiological effect	Effect on heart sounds
o Fist clenching	↑Systemic arterial resistance	↑Some left-sided murmurs MR, AR, VSD; ↓ AS
o Squatting	↑Venous return, ↑vascular tone	↓MVP, HCM; ↑ AS
o Standing (opposite to squatting)		

Abbreviations: AS, aortic stenosis; AR, aortic regurgitation; HCM, hypertrophic cardiomyopathy; MR, mitral regurgitation; MS, mitral stenosis; MVP, mitral valve prolapse; PS. Pulmonary stenosis; TR, tricuspid regurgitation; VSD, ventricular septal defect

Adapted from: Filate W, et al. *The Medical Society, Faculty of Medicine, University of Toronto* 2005, Table 12, page 63.

Systolic		**Diastolic**	
Timing	Name	Timing	Name
• Early systolic	o Ejection sounds (aortic or pulmonary) o Click (mitral or tricuspid) o Aortic prosthetic valve sounds	• Early diastolic	o Opening snap (mitral or tricuspid stenosis) o Early S_3 o Pericardial knock o Tumour "plop"
• Mid-to-late systolic	o Click (mitral or tricuspid)	• Mid diastolic	o S_3 o Summation sound ($S_3 + S_4$)
		• Late diastolic (presystolic)	o S_4 o Pacemaker sound

Source: Mangione S. *Hanley & Belfus* 2000, page 217.

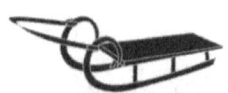

S_1 *Heart Sound*

➢ Clinical

- Perform a focused physical examination of the first heart sound (S_1). Explain what underlying cardiac abnormalities may be determined from this examination.

  - Caused by vibrations in cardiohemic system (chordae tendinae, ventricles, and blood)
  - Loudness varies beat-to-beat (strength of ventricular contraction, and position of AV leaflets at the onset of ventricular systole)
  - Loudness reflects strength of ventricular contractions
  - Mitral and tricuspid valve closure (MV before TV); synchronous with cardiac impulse beat or carotid impulse
  - Beginning of LV and RV systole
  - Loud in MS and TS, tachycardia, hypertrophy, 3° heart block;
  - Soft in MR, 1° HB, LBBB, CCF, shock; variation in intensity with any cardiac arrhythmia
  - Normally split in tricuspid area on inspiration
  - Splitting (wider on inspiration) – RBBB

- Give the disease processes associated with a loud, variable or soft intensity of heart sound.

  - Listen with diaphragm over apex for mitral component (M_1), and over epigastric/subxiphoid area for less important tricuspid component (T_1)
  - S_1 should be louder than S_2 in these locations
  - Normal closure of MV and TV
  - Sequence: mitral (M_1) and then tricuspid (T_1) close, pulmonary and then aortic valves open

  - Apex high pitched

  - ↑ S_1
    - ↑ HR
    - Hyperkinetic heart (eg. AR, PDA, AV fistulas, fever, anemia, thyrotoxicosis, beriberi, Paget's disease)
    - ↑ LAP (early MS)
    - ↓ PR interval (S_1 becomes softer with AV blocks; pre-excitation syndromes such as WPW [Wolff-Parkinson-White]
    - ↓ PR interval (<160 msec)
    - ↑ Thickness of AV or TV leaflets (when leaflets later become rigid or fixed, S_1 becomes softer or absent)
    - ↑ AV pressure gradient

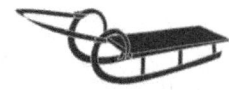

- o ↓ S$_1$
  - ↑ PR intermal (> 20 msec)
  - LV dysfunction
  - LBBB
  - 1st degree heart block
  - Calcified AV
  - Acute AI (premature closure of MV)
  - MI, TI
  - CHF

- o Variable S$_1$
  - AF
  - Conduction heart block
  - Progressive increase in duration of PR interval (Wenckeback phenomenon) with MS, MV prolapsed with regurgitation
  - MS
  - MV prolapsed with regurgitation

- o Split S$_1$: RBBB/LBBB

Abbreviation: AF, Atrial fibrillation; AI, aortic insufficiency; AV, atrio-ventricular; CHF, congestive heart failure; HB, heart block; LAP, left atrial pressure; MS, mitral stenosis; MV, mitral valve; PDA, patent ductus arteriosis; TV, tricuspid valve

Adapted from: Mangione S. *Hanley & Belfus* 2000, page 207.

- Give examples of conditions which change the intensity and splitting of S1.

  - o Changes of intensity
    - Second-degree heart block (type1 Wenckebach phenomenon, but S$_1$ progressively softens), S$_2$ remains of constant intensity,
    - Third-degree (complete) AV block (change in intensity of S$_1$ is random and chaotic; rhythm is slow and regular).
    - Soft intensity of S$_1$
      - Calcified mitral stenosis
      - Long P-R interval
      - L-HF
      - Severe aortic or mitral regurgitation
      - Myocardial infarction
      - LBBB

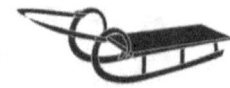

- o Splitting
  - - Wide splitting of S_1
    - ▪ Best heard over left lower sternal border
    - ▪ Usually from delayed closure of tricuspid valve (T_1), such as from RBBB
    - ▪ Wide splitting of S_2 may also occur with wide splitting of S_1

  - - Pseudosplitting of S_1
    - ▪ Normal S_1 proceeded by S_4 (heard only at apex, low-pitched, soft heard best with bell of stethoscope)
    - ▪ S_1 may be followed by early systolic ejection click (loudest over the base, high-pitched, loud heard best with diaphragm).

- • Reversed Splitting

- • Give 3 causes of reversed ("paradoxical") splitting of S_1.

- ➢ Definition P_1 before A_1; when LV systole is long or the LV is activated late (LBBB), the A_1 may be delayed and occur with or after P_1. If P_1 occurs with A_1 there will be only one sound during inspiration but two sounds are heard with expiration ($P_1 - A_1$)

- ➢ Causes

  - o Aortic stenosis (AS)

  - o Left bundle branch block (LBBB)

  - o Left ventricular failure (L-VF, aKa L-CHF)

  - o Fixed splitting of S_1 (A_1, P_1); i.e. delay in producing P1 component of S_1).
    - - RBBB
    - - Pulmonary stenosis
    - - R – CHF
    - - ASD
    - - PDA

Abbreviations: ASD, atrial septal defect; RBBB, right bundle branch block; PDA, patent ductus arteriosis; R-CHF, right-sided congestive heart failure.

Adapted from: Mangione S. *Hanley & Belfus* 2000, page 210-216; Talley NJ, et al. *Maclennan & Petty Pty Limited* 2003, pages 54 and 55.

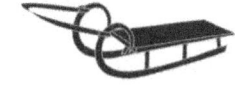

- Give disorders in which the intensity of A_1 and P_1 (S_1) is changed.

  - A1   ↑   - Hypertension
                        - Aneurysm

            ↓   - AS/AR
                        - L-HF
                        - Shock
                        - MS

  - P1   ↑   - Pulmonary hypertension (associated with narrow splitting of S_2)
            ↓   - Pulmonary hypertension (PS, R-CHF)

Abbreviations: AR, aortic regurgitation; AS, aortic stenosis; PS, pulmonary stenosis.

- Give the effects of inspiration on the peripheral pulse.

  - ↑ flow of blood in IVC
  - ↑ flow of blood into RV
  - ↑ blood in RV takes longer to expel
  - P valve closes after aortic valve (A-P)
  - ↑ pulse rate and volume

S_2 Heart Sound

- ➤ Definition   - Normal - ↑ split between A_2 and P_2 on inspiration
                  - Abnormal – effect of inspiration to increase the distance between A_2 and P_2 is lost.

- ➤ Causes   - ASD (atrial septal defect)
                  - VSD (ventricular septal defect)
                  - PR (pulmonary regurgitation)
                  - PS (pulmonary stenosis)
                  - RBBB (right bundle branch block)
                  - MR, VSD (mitral regurgitation)

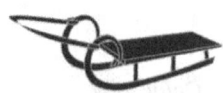

- ➢ General Concepts
  - ○ Heard best with the diaphragm over base of heart in the pulmonary area (Left 2ⁿᵈ /3ʳᵈ parasternal intercostals spaces).
  - ○ Produced by the sudden slowing of blood from with closure of the aortic (A_2) and then pulmonary (P_2) valves; P_2 canbe heard normally only a few centimetres to the left of the upper sternal border
  - ○ Splitting of S_2 and the various forms of splitting is not useful clinically; heard best (because of hearing P_2) at the 2-3 left interspace.
  - ○ Heard best a few centimetres to the left of the sternal border.
  - ○ Loudness: a loud A_2, or a loud P_2
    - Pulmonary or systemic or systemic hypertension
    - Correlation of the aorta
    - High-output states
    - a soft A_2, or soft P_2 – aortic or pulmonary valve stenosis
    - P_2 louder than A_2 – aortic or pulmonary valve stenosis
    - S_2 louder than S_1 at apex – pulmonary or systemic hypertention
  - ○ ↑ P_2
    - Pulmonary hypertension (e.g. MS, MR, L-CHF, PE, pulmonary fibrosis)
  - ○ ↑ A_2
    - Systemic hypertension, aortic slcerosis, arteriosclerosis, syphilitic aortitis; decreased in R-HF, hypotension, severe anemia
  - ○ Single splitting of S_2 (A_2 and P_2 cannot be heard as distinct sounds, so merge into a single sound)
    - Paradoxical (reversed) splitting (splitting in expiration)
    - Pulmonary hypertension
    - Emphysema (hyperinflatted lungs muffle P_2, so only A_2 is heart; P_2 is however still produced, so this is "pseudoparadoxical" splitting)

Adapted from: Mangione S. *Hanley & Belfus* 2000, page 210 to 216 and Talley NJ, et al. *Maclennan & Petty Pty Limited* 2003, pages 54 and 55.

- ➢ Clinical
  - ○ Aortic and pulmonary valve closure (AV closes before PV, but PV opens before AV) end of LV and RV systole, beginning of diastole
  - ○ Loud A_2 in HBP, loud P_2 in PHT; soft A_2 when AV calcified or in AR
  - ○ Normal splitting of S_2 on inspiration (A_2, P_2) especially in children; pathological splitting: PS, MR, RBBB, VSD, ASD
  - ○ P_2 > A_2 in youth; A_2 > P_2 in old age
  - ○ Fixed splitting of S_2 (not increasing normally on inspiration – ASD sudden opening of valve in MS or TS after S_2

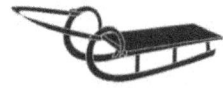

- o Loud narrowly split P2 in pulmonary hypertension
- o Soft widely split P2 in pulmonary stenosis
- o Paradoxically split P2 (narrows on inspiration) in LBBB and rarely in aortic stenosis and L and R shunts

- Give the performance characteristics of S_1 and S_2 findings.

  - o Paradoxic splitting is of no significance to detect aortic stenosis
  - o A loud P_2 is no significance to detect a mean pulmonary arterial pressure ≥ 50 mm Hg (pulmonary hypertension, PHT)
  - o S_1 of varying intensity has a positive likelihood ratio (PLR) of 24.4 to detect AV dissociation.
  - o S_2 with fixed wide splitting has a PLR of .6 for detecting ASD, whereas a palpable P2 has a PLR of 3.6 for detecting PHT.

Finding	PLR
• S_1	
o Varying intensity, Detecting AV dissociation	24.4
• S_2	
o Fixed wide splitting, detecting ASD	2.6
o Paradoxic splitting, detecting AS (peak gradient >50 mm Hg)	NS
o Loud P_2, detecting PHT (mean PAP $\geq$50 mm Hg)	NS
o Palpable P_2, detecting PHT	3.6

Abbreviations; AS, aortic stenosis; ASD, atrial septal defect; AV, Atrio ventricular; PLR, positive likelihood ratio; NLR, negative likelihood ratio; PAP, pulmonary arterial pressure; PHT, pulmonary hypertension; S1, first heart sound; S2, second heart sound

Adapted from: McGee SR. *Saunders/Elsevier* 2007, Box 36.1, page 420.

- RV – S_4
  - o PHT, PS ($\downarrow$ RV compliance)

- $S_3 + S_4$
  - o Summation gallop (when HR > 120 bpm)

- Artificial
  - o Prosthetic heart valves, pacemaker sounds

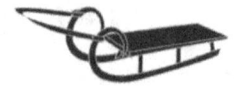

- Perform a directed physical examination of abnormal S_2 splitting to detect the presence of associated pathological abnormalities.

Splitting and pathogenesis	Associations
o Wide physiologic	
- P_2 late	
▪ Electrical delay of RV systole	RBBB LV paced or ectopic beats PS
▪ Prolongation of RV systole	Acute cor pulmonale Dilation of PA
▪ Increased hangout interval	MR
o A_2 early	
- Shortening of LV systole	
o Wide and fixed	
- Increased hangout interval or prolongation of RV systole	ASD
- Prolongation of RV systole	R-CHF
o Paradoxic	
o A_2 late	
- Electrical delay of LV systole	LBBB RV paced or ectopic beats AS IHD
- Prolonged LV systole	

Abbreviations: AS, aortic stenosis; ASD, atrial septal defect; IHD, ischemic heart disease; LBBB, left bundle branch block; L-HF, left side heart failure; LV, left ventricular; MR, mitral regurgitation; RBBB, right bundle branch block; PA, pulmonary artery; PS, pulmonary stenosis; R-HF, right side heart failure; RV, right ventricular; RV systole and LV systole refer to the duration of right and left ventricular contraction.

Printed with permission: McGee SR. *Saunders/Elsevier* 2007, page 426.

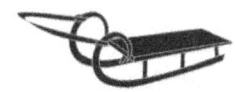

SO YOU WANT TO BE A CARDIOLOGIST!

- If there is splitting of S2 during expiration, give why you sit the patient up and listen again.
  - Splitting of S2 in expiration which disappears on sitting is normal, where as if splitting of S2 in expiration persists on sitting, then the wide, fixed or paradoxical splitting of S2 is abnormal.
  - Inspiration – normal
  - Inspiration plus expiration $\rightarrow$ slowing of RV ejection
  - Expiration (reversal splitting)

- Give the causes of fixed splitting of S2 (splitting in both supine and sitting position).
  - Severe HF
  - ASD
  - VSD plus PHT (pulmonary hypertension)
  - PS (pulmonary stenosis), PHT
  - Massive PE

Adapted from: Mangione S. *Hanley & Belfus* 2000, pages 214 and 215.

- Give when a soft S_2 occurs in AS due to causes other than valvular stenosis.
  - When the aortic valve is stenotic and is also calcified
  - If the leaflets remain mobile, S_2 may be soft but the stenosis is not valvular.

- Distinguish between RBBB and LBBB, by listening to the heart sounds(!)
  - RBBB: A_2-P_2 – when moving stethoscope from cardiac base to apex, the second component of S_2 dissappears; associated with wide splitting of S_2.
  - LBBB: P_2-A_2 – first component of S_2 becomes softer when moving stethoscope from the base to the apex of the heart (A_2 and not P_2 is heard at the apex).

- Give how it is possible to distinguish between a mitral opening snap (OS) and a split P_2.

  - OS is maximal internal to the apex, and becomes louder with expiration.

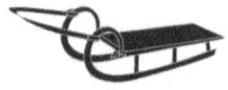

- Perform a focused physical examination for wide splitting of S_2.

  - Early closure of aortic valve
    - Mitral regurgitation (severe)
    - VSD
    - CHF (severe)
    - Pericardial temponade

  - Late closure of pulmonary valve
    - Cor pulmonale complicated by R-CHF
    - ASD
    - Massive pulmonary embolus
    - In associated with RBBB

Adapted from: Talley NJ, et al. *Maclennan & Petty Pty Limited* 2003, page 55 and Mangione S. *Hanley & Belfus* 2000, page 211.

- Perform a focused physical examination for the causes of fixed splitting of S_2 (splitting of S_2 which persists on supine $\rightarrow$ expiration).

  - Listening
    - Diaphragm
      - High pitched, high pressure gradient across a small surface (AR)
    - Bell
      - Low pitched, low pressure gradient across a wide surface (MS)

  - Disorders
    - ASD, VSD with pulmonary hypertension
    - Pulmonary stenosis
    - Pulmonary hypertension
    - Massive pulmonary embolism

Adapted from: McGee SR. *Saunders/Elsevier*, 2007, page 426, 427; Mangione S. *Hanley & Belfus*, 2000, pages 210 to 216.

➤ Pansystolic murmurs

  - MR, TS; VSD (L-4th ICS); PDA) L-2nd ICS)

Abbreviations: A_2, aortic part of S_2; AI, aortic incompetence; AR, aortic regurgitation; ICS, intercostal space; MR, mitral regurgitation; TS, tricuspid stenosis; VSD, ventricular septal defect

Adapted from: Mangione S. *Hanley & Belfus* 2000, page 210-216; Talley NJ, et al. *Maclennan & Petty Pty Limited* 2003, pages 54 and 55.

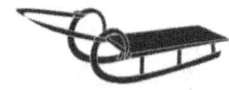

Mastering the Boards: Cardiology

A.B.R. Thomson

THIS IS A REAL CARDIOLOGY DEAL-BREAKER!

- Give the pathophysiological explanation for the cause of a widely split S_2 in the following conditions:

  o ASD, VSD, PR   - ↑ RV volume

  o PS   - ↑ RV pressure

  o RBBB   - ↓ RV conduction

  o MR, VSD   - Early LV emptying

Abbreviations: ASD, atrial septal defect; LV, left ventricle; MR, mitral regurgitation; PR, pulmonary regurgitation; PS, pulmonary stenosis; RBBB, right bundle branch block; RV, right ventricle; VSD, ventricular septal defect;

Adapted from: Baliga RR. *Saunders/Elsevier* 2007, pages 72 and 73.

- Give what the S_2 tells us in aortic stenosis (AS).

  o Normal
    - Strong evidence against the presence of critical aortic stenosis.
  o Soft S_2
    - Valvular stenosis (except in calcific stenosis of the elderly, where the margins of the leaflets usually maintain their mobility)
  o Single
    - Second heart sound may be heard when there is fibrosis and fusion of the valve leaflets
  o Reversed
    - Splitting of the second sound: Indicates mechanical or electrical prolongation of ventricular systole.

Source: Baliga RR. *Saunders/Elsevier* 2007, page 19.

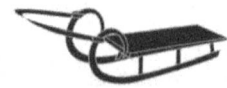

Pathological Heart Sounds

S3 Heart Sound

➢ Useful backgroung about S_3
  - ○ < 40 years
    - May be physiologic (these persons are lean, with rapid early dibstolic filling), or with tachycardia, fever, excercise, anemia, hyperthyroidism, pregnancy, anxiety.
  - ○ 40 years, S_3 represents ↓ejection fraction (dilated cardiomyopathy, ↓cardiac output), ↑atrial pressure
  - ○ Caused by sudden and abnormal deceleration in left ventricular flow at the end of its rapid filling phase, reflecting early and passive LV filling.
  - ○ A pathologic S_3 "keeps bad company"
  - ○ Ken-tu'-cky: S_3 gallops (S_3+S_1/S_2); Ten-ne-ss'es: S_4 gallop (S_4+S_1/S_2)
  - ○ Pathological S_3 is due to diastolic overload (increased LV preload), decreased myocardial contractility, or loe ejection fraction (low-output failure)
  - ○ An S3 (pathologic) plus an early diastolic rumble suggests sudden increased flow across the mitral valve.
  - ○ The pressure of S_3 rules out mitral stenosis; opening sanp of MS is left sterna border, S_3 loudest at apex.
  - ○ S3 predicts post-surgical development of CHF, predicts cardiac risk during non-cardiac surgery, and predicts response to digitalis in treatment of CHF hypertension.
  - ○ Increased LV preload (diastolic overload): VSD, PDA (S_3 softens with the development of increased pulmonary mitral regurgitation)

Source: Mangione S. *Hanley & Belfus* 2000, pages 221 to 224; McGee SR. *Saunders/Elsevier* 2007, page 436.

SO YOU WANT TO BE A CARDIOLOGY RESIDENT!

- Give the mechanism of the production of S_3 heart sound.

  - ○ Rapid ventricular filling in early diastole

Source: Baliga RR. *Saunders/Elsevier* 2007, page 39.

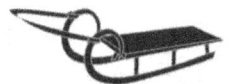

Mastering the Boards: Cardiology　　　　A.B.R. Thomson

Sounds and extra sounds		Conventional teaching revisited
o S3	↑	The most clinically valuable cardiac extra sound.
o S4	↔	Most important for what it sounds like without being it (e.g. an S4 is important for *not* being an S3).
o Pericardial friction rub	↑	One of the most valuable extra sounds (probably at the top of the list with S3)
o Early systolic (ejection) click	↑	Valuable and not too much uncommon; should not be missed.
o Mid-to-late systolic click	↑	As above
o Open snap	↔	Important, but its prevalence is rapidly fading.
o Pericardial knock	↓	Need to think of it, but it is a "canary"
o Tumor "plop"	↓	As above

Source: Mangione S. *Hanley & Belfus* 2000, page 207.

SO YOU WANT TO BE A CARDIOLOGIST!

- In the context of splitting hairs, give what causes splitting of the second heart sound (S2, comprised of A2 and P2).
    - o Physiologic
    - o Delayed A2 (delayed closure of Aortic valve) from
        - Atrial septal defect (ASD)
        - Severe MR (mitral regurgitation),
        - Severe CHF,
        - Severe pericardial tamponade

    - o Delayed A2 and P2
        - Delayed P2 (delayed closure of pulmonic valve)
        - Right bundle branch block (RBBB)
        - Severe impedence of the emptying of RV
            - PS (pulmonary stenosis)
            - Cor pulmonale + R-HF
            - ASD (atrial septal defect)
            - Massive PE (pulmonary embolus)

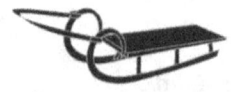

XXX

SO YOU WANT TO BE A CARDIOLOGIST!

- Does S2 reflect the prognosis of the underlying condition?

  o A delayed P2 will cause splitting of S2; when there is expiratory splitting of S2, there has usually been a massive pulmonary embolism leading to the development of acute cor pulmonale.

S_3 and S_4 Heart Sounds

  o S_3/S_4 are best heard and felt at the apex (or PMI) with patient in left lateral decubitus position and accentuated by sitting, standing, exercise, leg elevation, abdominal pressure.
  o Early diastolic snap of MS/TS; opening plop of myxoma of mitral or tricuspid valve; (varies from cycle to cycle) and pericardial knock

Timing and mechanism of production of third and fourth heart sounds (S_3 and S_4)

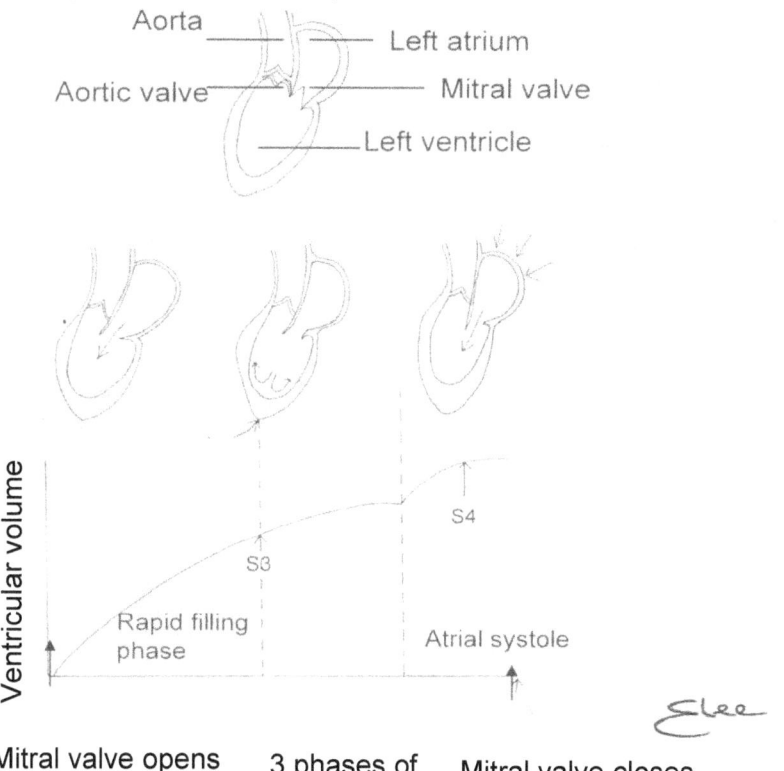

Adapted from: McGee SR. *Saunders/Elsevier* 2007, Figure 37.1, page 435.

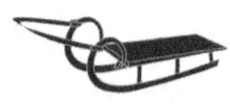

LV – S₃ Heart Sounds

- o Mild diastolic gallop,
- o Louder on expiration
- o Maybe: physiological; in young persons due to rapid diastolic filing;
- o Pathological: ($\downarrow$ RV compliance) LVF, AR, MR, VSD, PDA

- ➢ Mechanism
  - o Early, rapid filling of ventricles, resulting in sudden distention of walls of LV
  - o Turbulent flow across the mitral valve

- ➢ Clinical
  - o Just internal to apex
  - o Loudest at end of expiration
    - - Patient on left side
    - - Not heard when atrial fibrillation is present

- ➢ Causes
  - o Myocardial infarction
  - o Mitral or tricuspid regurgitation
  - o R-/L-HF
  - o Constrictive pericarditis
  - o Ventricular septal defect (VSD)

Trick Question

- • An S₃ is auscultated in a patient with a systolic murmur. There are no signs of associated HF. Give the prognostic value the S₃ has in terms of ventricular systolic dysfunction or increased filling pressure.

  - o In AS, but not in MR, S₃ reflects ventricular systolic dysfunction or increased filling pressure.

Abbreviations: AS, aortic stenosis; HF, heart failure; MR, mitral regurgitation

---

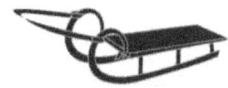

RV-S$_3$ Heart Sounds

- o Right ventricular S$_3$ in
    - Right ventricular failure
    - Tricuspid regurgitation

SO YOU WANT TO BE A CARDIOLOGIST!

- Give the implications of the S3 sound in patients with valvular heart disease.
    - o In patients with mitral regurgitation, they are common but do not necessarily reflect ventricular systolic dysfunction or increase filling pressure
    - o In paietns with aortic stenosis, third heart sounds are uncommon but usually indicate the presence of systolic dysfunction and raised filling pressure

- Give the causes of the third heart sound (S$_3$).
    - o Physiological: in normal children and young adults
    - o Pathological
        - Heart failure
        - Left ventricular dilatation without failure
            - Mitral regurgitation (MR)
            - ventricular septal defect (VSD)
            - patent ductus arteriosus (PDA)

- Does the fourth heart sound (S$_4$) denote heart failure, like the S$_3$ gallop does?
    - o No

S$_4$ Heart Sound

- ➤ LV – S$_4$
    - o Late diastole, from atrial contraction (disappears in AF)
    - o AS, MR, HBP, CAD, old age
    - o Late diastolic, low-pitched extra sound due to progressive loss of compliance of ventricles, corresponding to atrial and sudden tension of the AV valve ventricle with atrial contraction and stronger atrial boost, with an increased LV diastolic pressure

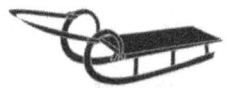

➤ Mechanism
  o Constriction of the atria at the end of diastole, but reduced filling of the ventricles.

➤ Causes
  o L-HF
  o Finding an S_4 suggests the presence of heart disease, but does not suggest a cause
  o Systemic or pulmonary hypertension
  o Aortic stenosis, particularly with a high gradient
  o Coarctation of the aorta cardiomyopathy
    - Ischemic
    - Hypertrophic (almost always associated with S_4)

Source: Mangione S. *Hanley & Belfus* 2000, pages 223 to 225.

SO YOU WANT TO BE A CARDIOLOGIST!

• Give the causes of the fourth heart sound (S_4).

  ➤ Normal: in the elderly
  ➤ Pathological:
    o Acute myocardial ischemia / infarction (~ 90%)
    o Aortic stenosis (the presence of S_4 in individuals below the age of 40 indicates significant obstruction)
    o Hypertension
    o Hypertrophic cardiomyopathy
    o Pulmonary stenosis

Adapted from: McGee SR. *Saunders/Elsevier* 2007, pages 217-225 and 434-437.

Note: When there is ↑ HR, the S_3 and S_4 cannot be identified separately, and the combined sound is the "summation gallop"

➤ S_3 and S_4
  o S_3/S_4 are best heard and felt at the apex (or PMI) with patient in left lateral decubitus position and accentuated by sitting, standing, exercise, leg elevation, abdominal pressure.
  o Early diastolic snap of MS/TS; opening plop of myoxoma of mitral or tricuspid valve; (varies from cycle to cycle) and pericardial knock

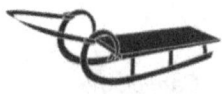

- Give the performance characteristics of the third (S_3) and fourth (S_4) heart sounds.

  - S_3 has good performance characteristics in terms of its positive likelihood ratio for detecting or predicting a range of cardiac abnormalities ranging from ↑ LV filling pressures or reduced ejection fraction, to predicting a myocardial infarction or postoperative cardiac death.
  - In contract, the S_4 does not have a significant use to detect ↑ LV filling pressure or aortic stenosis, but has a PLR of 3.2 for predicting 5 - year mortality in patients after a myocardial infarction.

Finding	PLR
○ The third heart sound – S_3	
- Detecting ejection fraction < 0.5	3.4
- Detecting ejection fraction < 0.3	4.1
- Detecting elevated left heart filling pressures	5.7
- Detecting elevated BNP level	10.0
- Detecting myocardial infarction in patients with acute chest pain	3.2
- Predicting postoperative pulmonary edema	14.6
- Predicting postoperative myocardial infarction or cardiac death	8.0
○ The fourth heart sound – S_4	
- Predicting 5-year mortality in patients after myocardial infarction	3.2
- Detecting elevated left heart filling pressures	NS
- Detecting severe aortic stenosis	NS

Adapted from: McGee SR. *Saunders/Elsevier* 2007, Box 37-1, page 438.

SO YOU WANT TO BE A CARDIOLOGIST!

- S_4 does not wax and wane, but give when S_4 may disappear.
  - When AF (atrial fibrillation)
  - Atrial flutter or L-HF develop.

- Give what the fourth heart sound (S_4) indicates.

  - An audible S_4 may be physiologic, but a palpable S_4 is always pathological

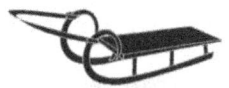

Other Pathological Heart Sounds

Opening Snap (OS)

- o Sudden opening of the mitral valve as the result of increased left atrial pressure causes a high pitched sound at the left sternal edge in persons with mitral stenosis (MS).
- o The earlier the opening snap (OS) of mitral stenosis, the worse the stenosis; tachycardia also makes the OS earlier
- o Softening in intensity of the opening snap
  - Severe mitral stenosis (OS is present in 75-90% of MS)
  - CHF
  - Large right atrium (eg. pulmonary hypertention)
  - P_2 is loudest at the base, OS is loudest at the apex: if you think you hear an OS at the base, it's likely a P_2 (split S_2); if the sound becomes wider and louder on breathing out, you are probably hearing an OS, not a split S_2 or loud P_2 from PHT
- o OS is loudest in expiration, helping to distinguish it from a split P_2

SO YOU WANT TO BE A CARDIOLOGIST!

- How is it possible to distinguish between a mitral opening snap (OS) and a split P_2?

  - o OS is maximal internal to the apex, and becomes louder with expiration.

- o Indicates mobile AV valve and LA pressure
- o Mitral opening snap in mitral stenosis is maximal internal to apex, louder during expiration, thereby differentiated from split P2

Adapted from: Mangione S. *Hanley & Belfus* 2000, page 210-216; Talley NJ, et al. *Maclennan & Petty Pty Limited* 2003, pages 54 and 55.

- Perform a focused physical examination for **pulmonary hypertension**.
  - o Loud (even palpable) P_2 over pulmonic area
  - o Loud S_4, right side
  - o Pulmonary ejection sound
  - o Tricuspid regurgitation
  - o Inspiration widens the interval between closure of aortic and pulmonary valves

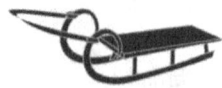

- Inspiration increases the distance between A_2 and P_2, and thus causes physiological (normal) splitting of S_2.
- Physiological splitting of S_2 is increased by lying down. Physiological splitting of S_2 occurs in about half of adults.
- Paradoxical splitting of S_2: A split S_2 in the sitting/standing patient who breaths out (expiratory) is likely to be pathological (i.e. not physiological); however wide splitting of S_2 may be normal in young adults.

Gallop Rhythm

➢ Definition   o S_3 or S_4 plus tachycardia

➢ Pathophysiology

- S_3 – rapid filling of ventricles in early diastole
- S_4 – rapid emptying of atria in late diastole

➢ Clinical   o   With bell for low pitched sound
       o   "Kentucky" came before "Tennessee": S_3 before S_4
       S_3 sounds like "Kentucky" S_4 sounds like "Tennessee"

       o   Where

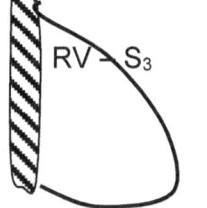

LSE

RV S_3

LV – S_3

Abbreviation: LSE, left sterna edge; RV, right ventricle; LV, left ventricle
Figuring Out S_3 and S_4

➢ Causes

	S_3	S_4
o Normal	- Young persons	- Old persons

o Abnormal	- CHF (L or R)
	- LVD (No CHF)
	- Murmurs
	  ▪ MR
	  ▪ AS
	  ▪ TR
	  ▪ VSD
	  ▪ PDA
		- Acute MI
		- Systemic hypertension
		- Murmurs
		  ▪ AS
		  ▪ PS
		  ▪ HOCM
		- Not seen in CHF

Abbreviation: AS, aortic stenosis, CHF, congestive heart failure; HOCM, hypertrophic cardiomyopathy; LVD, left ventricular dilation; MR, mitral regurgitation; PS, pulmonary stenosis; TR, tricuspid regurgitation; VSD, ventricular septal defect.

SO YOU WANT TO BE A CARDIOLOGIST

- Give the expression used when both the third and fourth heart sounds (S_3 and S_4) are heard with tachycardia.

    o The summation gallop
    o Sometimes be mistaken for a diastolic rumbling murmur

- Give the expression used when both the third (S_3) and fourth (S_4) heart sounds are heard with tachycardia.

    o The summation gallop
    o Sometimes be mistaken for a diastolic rumbling murmur

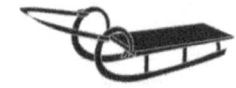

Mitral or Tricuspid Valve Myxoma

- o Diastolic prolapsed of a left atrial myxoma through an open valve, or a right atrial prolapsed through an open tricuspid valve
- o Vary in intensity and quality from cycle to cycle

Ejection Sounds

- o Sudden early ventricular systolic distention of aorta or pulmonary artery
- o Best hear at apex, sitting position or expiration
- o Hyperdynamic heart syndrome – fever, anemia, pregnancy, shunts, hyperthyroidism
- o Stenosis semilunar valve (valvular, not sub – or supraventricular aortic or pulmonary stenosis) or biscuspid valve
- o Ejection sound plus an ejection murmur occurs with stenosis of semilunar bicuspid valve with post stenosis dilation of aorta or root of pulmonary artery

Sound	Location, pitch	Pathology
o Early ejection sound	- Aortic: apex & base - Pulmonic: base (high pitched)	▪ Congenital AS, bicuspid AV, congenital PS, Ao. Root or PA dilation, physiologic (flow murmur)
o Mid to late ejection click	- Mitral: apex - Tricuspid: LLSB (high pitched)	▪ MV or TV prolapse

Abbreviations: AF, arterial fibrillation; AS, aortic stenosis; AV, aortic valve; HR, heart rate; LAP, left arterial pressure; LBBB, left bundle branch block; LLSB, left lower sternal border; MS, mitral stenosis; MV, mitral valve; PA, pulmonary artery; PR, pulse rate; PS, pulmonary stenosis; RBBB, right bundle branch block; TV, tricuspid valve

Source: Filate W, et al. *The Medical Society, Faculty of Medicine, University of Toronto* 2005, Table 8, pages 59 and 60.

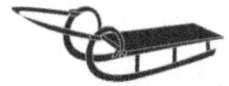

Mastering the Boards: Cardiology　　　　A.B.R. Thomson

SO YOU WANT TO BE A CARDIOLOGIST!

- Give how to differentiate between the fourth heart sound (S_4), a split first heart sound (S_1), and an ejection click.

  - The fourth heart sound is not heard when pressure is applied on the chest piece of the strethoscope, but pressure does not eliminate the ejection sound or the slitting of the first heart sound.

SO YOU WANT TO BE A CARDIOLOGY RESIDENT!

- Give the relationship between the intensity of S_4 and the severity of HF.

  - S_4 is not associated with HF. If an elderly person has an S_4 plus CHF, the S_4 is a normal finding in old age.

- Give the mechanism of the production of S_3 heart sound.

  - Rapid ventricular filling in early diastole

Source: Baliga RR. *Saunders/Elsevier* 2007, page 39.

SO YOU WANT TO BE A CARDIOLOGIST

- Give the difference between "a snap", "a click", "a knock" and "a rub".

  - "Snap" – diastole, abnormal opening of the leaflets.
  - "Click" – systole, prolapse and backward ballooning of valve leaflet(s).
  - "Knock" (pericardial) - Louder and higher-pitched form of S3 (caused by early ventricular filling), and sudden stretching of the LV against a thick, calcified pericardium, or also heard in constrictive pericarditis. Occur in chronic calcified or constrictive pericarditis
  - "Rub" (pericardial) - High-pitched, scratchy systolic and diastolic sounds, best heard with firm pressure of diaphragm, heard best at lower (3/4 interspaces) sterna border during inspiration, due to acute pericarditis

Source: Mangione S. *Hanley & Belfus* 2000, pages 225 to 236.

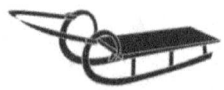

ENDOCARDIAL DISORDERS

Infective Endocarditis

➢ Definition: Infective endocarditis (IE) is a life-threatening infection of the cardiac endothelium associated with significant morbidity and mortality.

➢ Causes / associations
  o Injury or trauma to the cardiac andothelial surface, e.g.
    - Turbulent blood flow
    - Fibrin deposition
    - Bacterial adherence

➢ Complications
  o Heart
    - HF (heart failure)
    - Peri-annular abscess
  o Vessels
    - Aneurysm
  o Kidney
    - Glomerulonephritis
  o Embolization

Gin AS, et al. Chapter 113. In: Therapeutic Choices. Grey J, Ed. 6th Edition, *Canadian Pharmacists Association* 2012, page 1474.

➢ Common   o Streptococci
  pathogens   o Staphylococci
                 o Enterococci

➢ Clinical

• Perform a focused physical examination to detect evidence of peripheral embolisation to limbs or central nervous system.

  o Systemic   - Fever
    disease   - Pallor (anemia)
                    - Weight loss
                    - Fever, tachycardia, arthralgia, pallor with café au lait complexion

  o Hands   - Splinter hemorrhages
                    - Clubbing (within six weeks of onset)
                    - Osler nodes
                    - Janeway lesions
                    - Clubbing

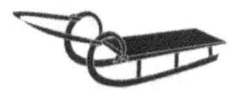

- o Eyes
  - Pale conjunctivae (anemia)
  - Retinal or conjunctival hemorrhages (Roth's spots are fundal vasculitic lesions with a yellow centre surrounded by a red ring).
  - Roth spots
  - ↓ visual acuity
  - Conjunctival petechiae

- o Arms
  - Evidence of intravenous drug use

- o Mucosal surfaces
  - Petechiae

- o Vasculitis
  - CNS – CVA (embolic)
  - Eye – Roth spots
  - Heart
    - New, or change in pre-existing murmur
    - HF (heart failure)
    - Conduction defects
    - Pericarditis
    - Endocarditis
    - Infection of prosthetic valves
      - Valve dysfunction
      - Structural or non-structural dysfunction
      - Endocarditis
  - Artery
    - Mycotic aneurysm
    - Rupture of aneurysm
  - Skin
    - Finger clubbing splinter hemorrhages in beds of nails
    - Osler nodes
    - Janeway lesions
    - Petechiae
  - GI – ischemic bowel disease

- o Skin
  - Splinter hemorrhages
  - Osler nodes

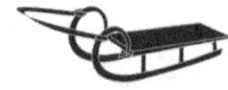

- o Lung
  - Pulmonary edema
  - Pleuritic rub

- o CNS
  - Numerous defects

- o Spleen
  - Splenomegaly

- o Immune changes
  - MSK
    - Arthralgias
    - Clubbing
    - Anemia

- o Acute damage
  - Cusps
  - Chordae tendinae
  - Endo cardium
    - Pneumococcus, haemolytic streptococcus, staphylococcus, gonoccus
  - Pericardium
    - Pneumonia
    - Strep'
  - Myocardium
    - Staph'
  - Affects either a previously normal or abnormal valve

- o Subacute damage
  - Cusps, chordae tendinae, endocardium, aorta
  - Usually affects a previously abnormal valve
  - New murmur, or changing murmur
  - Fever
  - Joint pain and tenderness
  - Anemia
  - Petechial haemorrhage
  - Embolism
  - Clubbing

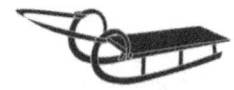

o Complications - Heart
- Signs of underlying heart disease
  - Acquired (mitral regurgitation, mitral stenosis, aortic stenosis, aortic regurgitation)
  - Congenital (patent ductus arteriosus ventricular septal defect, coarctation of the aorta
  - Prosthetic valves
  - R- HF or other endocardial damage
- HF
- Conduction defect
- Valve damage
- Coronary artery embolization
- Infection of
  - Valve ring (abscess)
  - Myocardium
  - Fungal endocarditis
  - Pericarditis
  - Aortic root
  - Fistula in sinus valsalva
- Arteries
  - Septic emboli to vasa vasorum
  - Mycotic aneurysms
  - Rupture of aneurysms (eg cerebral vessels, and hemorrhage)
- CNS
  - Brain abscess
  - Fungal endophthalmitis
- Spleen – infarcts
- GI tract – mesenteric ischemia
- Kidney – diffuse or focal glomerulonephritis

➢ Diagnosis
  o Use the Duke clinical criteria (MKSAP 16 2012, Cardiology, Table 36, page 81).
  o Use "Duke" criteria
    - 2 major, or
    - 1 major plus minor criteria

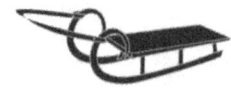

Major	Minor
o New murmur (regurgitation)	- IVDU or previous / predisposing heart abnormality
o ECG abnormal	- Fever
o Blood cultures positive x2 for endocarditis	- Blood culture positive x1 "not meeting major criteria"
	- Vascular emboli
	- Glomerulonephritis / RF (rheumatoid factor)

- Give 2 explanations for endocarditis diagnosed positive by Duke criteria, but blood cultures negative.

  o Recent antibiotic treatment before blood cultures taken

  o HACEK organisms
    - Haemophilus aphrophilus
    - Actinobacillus actinomycetemcomitans
    - Cardiobacterium hominis
    - Eikenella corrodens
    - Kingella kingae

➤ Differential

  o SBE (subacute bacterial endocarditis)

  o Non-bacterial endocarditis

  o Atrial myxoma

  o SLE (systemic lupus erythematosus)

  o Sickle cell disease

➤ Clinical

- Perform a focused physical examination for IE (infectious endocarditis)

  o Teeth — Possible source of infection usually microscopic

  o Renal — Hematuria (from small renal infarcts)

  o CNS — Roth spots (hemorrhagic lesion of the retina)
    - Septic emboli → focal neurological signs

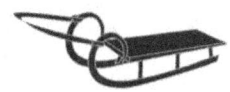

Mastering the Boards: Cardiology   A.B.R. Thomson

- o CVS
  - – New murmur
  - – Changing murmur
  - – New onset of
    - ▪ Cardiac murmur
    - ▪ HF (heart failure)
    - ▪ ECG condition abnormality

- o Skin
  - – Splinter hemorrhages under fingernails
    - ▪ Shunt
    - ▪ Red /brown
    - ▪ Linear
    - ▪ Non-blanching
  - – Petechiae
  - – Clubbing
  - – Café-au lait spots

- o Osler nodes
  - – Present in pulp of fingers and toes
  - – Small red / purple
  - – Painful
  - – Papules / pustules
  - – Circumscribed
  - – Arise from inflammation around infected embolization

- o Janeway lesions
  - – Red, non-tender flat lesions on palms of hands and soles of feet
  - – Blanch on pressure
  - – Arise from septic emboli or sterile vasculitis in endocarditis (with or without bacteremia, gonococcal sepsis, or lupus (SLE).

- – In a person with suspected bacterial endocarditis, perform a focused physical examination to distinguish between Osler nodes, and Janeway lesions.

Finding	Osler nodes	Janeway lesions
▪ Small	✓	✓
▪ Red	✓	✓
▪ Tender	✓	No
▪ Nodules	✓	Flat lesions
▪ Blanch	No	✓
▪ Finger tips	✓	No
▪ Palms/ soles	No	✓

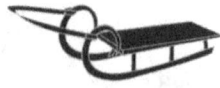

- o Lung
  - Septic emboli →
    - Multiple
    - Bilateral
    - Patchy
    - Poorly defined

- o Hematology
  - Splenomegaly
  - Anemia

- o GU
  - Hemauria
  - ↑ WBC

> Risk factors

- Give risk factors for infectious endocarditis (IE).

  - o High risk patient
    - IVDU (IV drug use)
    - Previous IE
    - Valve disease in heart transplant patient

  - o High risk heart
    - Cyanotic congenital heart disease (unrepaired)
    - Prosthetic
      - Left-sided
      - Valve
      - Intravascular
      - Prosthetic Intracardiac material
      - Shunt
      - Material for repair

  - o Other high risk situations

Site	Procedure
o Mouth	– Dental, causing bleeding
o Skin	– Infected – Palms and soles – Red macules – Painless
o Lung	– Incision / biopsy of respiratory mucosa
o GI / GU	– Infected GI / GU tract
o MSK	– Infected muscle

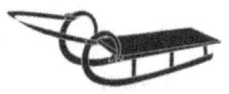

- Give the stratification of the risk of having bacterial endocarditis.

- High Risk Factors
  - Rheumatic fever
  - Artificial valves
  - Previous IE
  - IV drug users
  - Intravascular devices (e.g. arterial lines)

- Moderate risk factors
  - Most congential heart
  - Malformations
  - Valvular dysfunction
  - HCM
  - MVP with MR

- Ask the patient about:
  - Prosthetic heart valves
  - Recent surgeries
  - Indwelling catheters or hemodialysis
  - Recent IV drug use

- Peripheral signs
  - Petechiae
  - Conjunctivae
  - Buccal mucosa
  - Palate
  - Splinter hemorrhages: linear dark red streaks (nails)
  - Janeway lesions: ~ 5mm non-tender hemorrhagic macules on palm and soles
  - Osler's nodes: small painful nodules on fingers, toe pads, lasing hours-days
  - Roth spots: retinal hemorrhage with pale center near optic disc

- Constitutional risk factors
  - Fever
  - Chills
  - Malaise
  - Night sweats
  - Anorexia
  - Arthralgias

- Cardiac risk factors
  - Murmur
  - Palpatation
  - CHF

- Pulmonary risk factors
  - Septic pulmonary embolism

- Neurological risk factors
  - Immune mediated phenomena
  - Focal deficit
  - Headache
  - Meningitis

- MSK
  - Splenomegaly
  - Synovitis
  - Vasculitis
  - Glomerulonephritis

- Metastatic infection
  - Organ infarction
  - Embolic manifestations

Abbreviations: R-CHF, right side congestive heart failure; HCM, hypertrophic cardiomyopathy; IE, infectious endocarditis; MR, mitral regurgitation; MVP, mitral valve prolapse.

Adapted from: Burton JL. *Churchill Livingstone* 1971; Filate W, et al. *The Medical Society, Faculty of Medicine, University of Toronto* 2005, page 66.

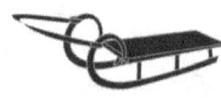

- o Patient
  - Prosthetic valves*
  - Previous endocarditis*

- o Valves
  - Mitral or aortic regurgitation (MR, AR)*
  - Ventricular septal defect (VSD)*
  - Patent ductus arteriosus (PDA)*
  - Aortic stenosis (AS)
  - Hypertrophic cardiomyopathy
  - Atrial septal defect (ASD)
  - Pure mitral stenosis (MS)

*high risk

Adapted from: Davey P. *Wiley-Blackwell* 2006, page 166.

➢ Diagnosis

- Definitive infective endocarditis
  - o Pathological criteria
    - Microorganisms demonstrated by culture or histological examination of a vegetation
    - A vegetation that has embolized
    - An intracardial abcess specimen
    - Pathological lesions
    - Vegetation or intracardiac abscess confirmed by histological examination showing active endocarditis

  - o Clinical criteria
    - 2 major criteria; or
    - 1 major criteria and 3 minor criteria; or
    - 5 minor criteria

- Possible infective endocarditis
  - o 1 major criterion and 1 minor criterion; or
  - o Minor criteria

- Rejected diagnosis of infective endocarditis
  - o Firm alternative diagnosis explaining evidence of IE; or
  - o Resolution of IE syndrome with antibiotic therapy for ≤ 4 days; or
  - o No pathological evidence of IE at surgery or autopsy, with antibiotic therapy for ≤ 4 days; or
  - o Does not meet criteria for possible IE as above

Reproduced with permission: Therapeutics Choices. Sixth Edition. Ottawa, Canada: *Canadian Pharmacist Association* 2012, page 1476.

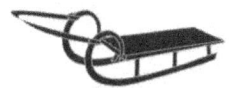

Definition of terms used in **Modified Duke Criteria** for the diagnosis of infective endocarditis

➢ Major criteria
  ○ Blood culture positive for IE
    – Typical microorganisms consistent with IE from 2 seperae blood cultures: Viridans streptococci, Streptococcus bovis, HACEK group, Saphylococcus aureus; or community-acquired enterococci in the absence of a primary focus; or
    – Microorganisms consistent with iE from persistently positive blood culture defined as follows: At least 2 positive cultures of blood samles drawn > 12 hour apart; or all of 3 or a majority of ≥ 4 separate culture of Coxiella burnetii or anti-phase 1 IgG antibody titer > 1:800
  ○ Evidence of endocardial involvement
  ○ Echocardiogram positive for IE (TEE recommended for patients with prosthetic valves, rated at least "possible IE" by clinical criteria, or complicated IE (paravalvular abscess); TE as first test in other patients) defined as follows:
    – Oscillating intracardiac mass on valve or supporting structures, in the path of regurgitant jets, or on implanted material in the absence of an alternative anatomic explanation; or abscess; or new partial dehiscence of prosthetic value.
  ○ New valvular regurgitation (worsening or changing or pre-existing murmur not sufficient)

Reproduced with permission: Therapeutics Choices. Sixth Edition. Ottawa, Canada: *Canadian Pharmacist Association* 2012, page 1476.

➢ Prophylaxis

• Give the current indications for endocarditis prophylaxis, and the appropriate antibiotic regimens.

  ○ Prophylactic antibiotics
    – Indications
    – Use of prophylactic antibiotics prior to low risk procedures such as dental procedures is no longer recommended
    – High risk setting where prophylactic antibiotics are recommended
      ▪ Patient history
        - Past history of infective endocarditis
      ▪ Valve
        - Prosthetic heart valve
        - Valvulopathy after cardiac transplantation
        - Congenital heart disease (CHD)
          ▪ Cyanotic CHD
          ▪ For 6 mon after repair of CHD abnormality using prosthetic material

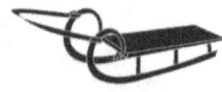

Suggested antibiotic regimen for endocarditis prophylaxis in dental procedures

Drug	Adult dose	Pediatric dose
o Standard regimen		
- Amoxicillin	2 g Po	50 mg/kg
- Unable to take oral medications		
▪ Ampicillin	2 g IM or IV	50 mg/kg IM or IV
▪ Cefazolin	1 g IM or IV	50 mg/kg IM or IV
▪ Ceftriaxone	1 g IM or IV	50 mg/kg IM or IV
- Allergic to Penicillins		
▪ Cephalexin	2 g po	50 mg/kg
▪ Clindamycin	600 mg po	20 mg/kg
▪ Azithromycin	500 mg po	15 mg/kg
▪ Clarithromycin	500 mg po	15 mg/kg

o Allergic to penicillins and unable to take oral medications

- Cefazolin	1g IM or IV	50 mg/kg IM or IV
- Ceftriaxone	1g IM or IV	50 mg/kg IM or IV
- Clindamycin	600 mg IM or IV	20 mg/kg IM or IV

Reproduced with permission: Therapeutics Choices. Sixth Edition. Ottawa, Canada: *Canadian Pharmacist Association* 2012, page 1482.

- Active treatment
  - o Antibiotics
    - 0.5-1 hr before, or up to 2 hr after procedure
  - o Compensated (no complications)
    - Empiric antibiotics → selected antibiotics based on blood cultures

Type of IE	In antibiotic combinations
o Community acquired	- Vancomycin or ampicillin-sulbactam plus gentamycin
o Health-care associated facility	- Vancomycin, gentamycin, rifampin plus anti-pseudomonal β-lactam
o Prosthetic valve	- Vancomycin, gentamycin plus rifampin

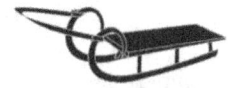

Type of IE		In antibiotic combinations	
○ Not allergic to penicillin / ampicillin	PO	Amoxicillin	2g
	IM / IV	Ampicillin, or Cefazolin /	2 g
		Ceftriaxone	1 g
○ Allergic to penicillin / ampicillin	PO	Cefphalexin, or	2 g
		Clindamycin, or	600 mg
		Clarithromycin / Azithromycin	500 mg
	IM / IV	Cefazolin / Ceftriazone or	1 g
		Clindamycin	600 mg

Adapted from MKSAP 16, Infectious disease 2012, page 85.

- ○ Bacteremia → organisms (e.g. Staphylococcus aureus) attach to
  - Endocardium of native valve
  - Prosthetic valve
  - Cardiac device
  - TEE (transesophageal echocardiography)

- ○ Surgery
  - Large vegetation
  - Persistent bacteremia despite antibiotics
  - HF (heart failure)
    - Left-sided
      - Valve regurgitation
      - Fistula
  - Prosthetic valve
    - Mechanical valve
      - Patient < 65 yr (mechanical valve is more durable)
      - ASA plus warfarin
    - Biological prosthetic value
      - Patient > 65 yr
      - Cannot take (contraindication) to anti-coagulation
      - ASA

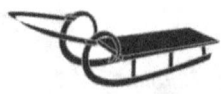

Site	Name – "SOJ"

- o Fingernails   - Sphincter hemorrhages
- o Fingers and toes   - Osler notes (painful)
- o Palms and soles   - Janeway lesions (painless)

- o Hypertrophic Osteoarthropathy

Hypertrophic osteoarthropathy is comprised of clubbing of the digits, plus

- o Synovia   - Effusions
- o Bones   - Painful periostosis of long bones
                - Perioteal formation of new bone
- o Skin   - Edema

- There are many causes of clubbing, but give the commonest causes of hypertrophic osteoarthropathy.

  - o Lung   - Cancer
                - Chronic infection (e.g. bronchiectasis)
  - o Heart   - Pulmonary (R)-to-systemic (L) heart shunts

SO YOU WANT TO BE A CARDIOLOGIST!

- In the context of the patient with suspected SBE (subacute bacterial endocarditis), give how to differente Roth spots from other types of red lesions of the retina?

Red lesions of the retina are caused by
  - o Microaneurysm
  - o Blot an dot hemorrhages
  - o Flame and splinter hemorrhages
  - o Preretinal hemorrhages, including subhyaloid hemorrhages space
  - o Roth spots are hemorrhages with a fibrinous centre which gives them a white spot with a red halo.
  - o White- Centered hemorrhages are associated with
      - SBE
      - Diabetes
      - Intracranial hemorrhage
      - Leukemias
      - Various infectious processes

Adapted from: Mangione S. *Hanley & Belfus* 2000, page 99.

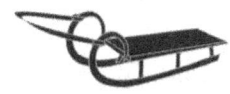

Mastering the Boards: Cardiology   A.B.R. Thomson

PERICARDIAL DISEASES

Pericarditis

➤ Causes (see also pericardial tamponade)

- Acute
  - o Idiopathic
    - Endomyocardial fibrosis (EMF)
  - o Infection
    - Viral
    - Bacterial (pyogenic or TB)
    - Mycotic
    - Parasitic
    - Post – purulent constriction
  - o Post - myocardial infarction (Dressler syndrome; pericarditis may be focal)
  - o Inflammatory (autoimmune)
    - Connective tissue disease
  - o Ischemic
    - Early
      - Acute myocardial infarction)
    - Late
      - Dressler syndrome
  - o Drugs
    - Hydralazine
    - Minoxidil
  - o Recent cardiac / thoracic surgery / trauma
  - o Dissecting aneurysm
  - o Metastatic disease to pericardium

- Take a directed history for the causes of pericarditis.
  - o Metabolic
    - Rh. Fever
    - Uremia
    - Myxedema
  - o Trauma
    - Post – surgery
  - o Drug (phenylbutazone)
  - o Injury
  - o Infiltration (cancer)
    - Breast
    - Lung
    - Leukemia
    - Lymphoma

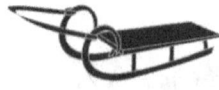

- o Iatrogenic (drug, radiation)
- o Aortic dissection
- o Takotsubo cardiomyopathy (stress related)
- o Note:

    All of these causes apply to both pericarditis and pericardial effusion

    An additional cause of pericardial effusion is hypothyroidism

Abbreviations: EMF, endomyocardial fibrosis; TB, tuberculosis

Adapted from: Burton JL. *Churchill Livingstone* 1971, page 18; Baliga RR. *Saunders/Elsevier* 2007, page 96.

Please see a Standard Internal Medicine textbook, or a recent review, such as MKSAP 16 2012, Cardiology, Table 27, page 62-63)

➢ Clinical

- o Elevated jugular venous pressure (JVP), hepatomegaly, ascites and ankle edema are signs of right-sided heart failure, which occur in constrictive pericarditis as well as other causes of R-HF.

- o Sharp substernal chest pain
    - ↑ with inspiration
    - ↓ with leaning forward

- o Differentiate chest pain from
    - AMI (acute myocardial infarction)
    - PE (pulmonary embolus)
    - AD (aortic dissection)

- o Chest pain of pericarditis
    - Sharp, pleuritic
    - Left sternal border, or retrosternal
    - ↓ leaning forward
    - ↑ recumbent position

- o Triad
    - Pericarditis chest pain
    - Pericardial friction rub
    - Diffuse on ECG (all leads except aVR)

    If idiopathic pericardial effusion on echocardiogram, then only 1 of these 3 is needed

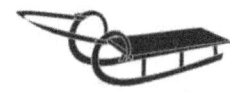

Mastering the Boards: Cardiology   A.B.R. Thomson

- o Recurrence
  - – 30% of persons with pericarditis have recurrent episodes of pericarditis
  - – ↑ risk of recurrent pericarditis
    - ▪ Poor response to ASA / NSAIDs
    - ▪ Need for corticosteroids
  - – May be associated with
    - ▪ Fever
    - ▪ Inflammatory markers
  - – Pericardial effusion

- o Possible pathognomic sign
  - – Pericardial friction rub

    3 sound, "squeak, scratch, swoosh"

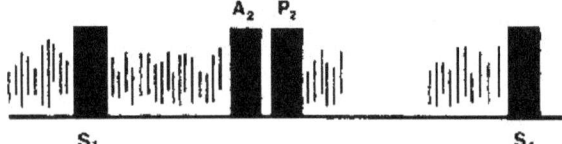

Abbreviations:
JVP, jugular venous pressure;
PP, pulse pressure;
PR, pulse rate;
SBP, systolic blood pressure

- ➤ Pulse
  - o PR ↑
  - o PP (pulsus paradoxicus) ↓
- ➤ Blood pressure
  - o SBP ↓ (↓ PP and ↓ BP with tamponade)
- ➤ JVP
- ➤ HEART
  - o Percussion
    - – Enlarged, with effusion
  - o Auscultation
    - – Friction rub
    - – Heart sounds may be reduced

Source: Mangione S. *Hanley & Belfus* 2000, page 246-251; pages 74 and 75.

- Perform a focused clinical examination to distinguish between R-sided heart failure from constrictive pericarditis versus other R-HF.

Physical signs	Right-sided heart failure	
	Constrictive pericarditis	Other causes of R-HF
↑ JVP with pronounced Y descent	+	-
↓ JVP on inspiration (Kussmaul sign)	No / ↑	Yes
Early, loud, high-pitched S3 (pericardiac knock)	+	-

➢ Diagnostic testing

While the presence of constructive pericarditis may be suspected in the person with signs of right-sided heart failure plus ↑ JVP with prominent Y descent, Kussmaul sign, and pericardiac knock, a variety of diagnostic imaging and laboratory measurements are needed to be more certain if this etiological distinction.

Pericardial Friction Rubs

➢ Clinical
  o Systolic as well as diastolic components (one near S3, early in diastole; the second diastolic component is at time of S4)
  o May resemble a S3 gallop
  o Best heard 3/4th LSB (left sterna boarder); sitting up, leaning forward, holding breath in inspiration

  o Softening of rub suggests development of pericardial effusion
  o May be diffuse or localized (eg. MI, trauma, metastatic tumor)
  o Effect of breathing:
    - Pericardial rub persists in inspiration, expiration, or both.
    - Pleural rub disappears when breathing held in either inspiration or expiration
  o The "Big 3" for the diagnosis of chest pain, pericardial rub, characteristic ECG changes

Adapted from: McGee SR. *Saunders/Elsevier* 2007, page 510 to 512 and Mangione S. *Hanley & Belfus* 2000, page 234.

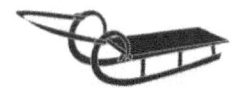

➢ Cause
  ○ All of pericardium
    - Viral
    - Lupus
    - Uremia
  ○ Focal pericarditis
    - Myocardial infarction
    - Tumor

Source: Mangione S. *Hanley & Belfus* 2000, page 272 to 273.

➢ Treatment

  ○ Consider need for hospitalization

  ○ Treat underlying causes

  ○ ASA (aspirin); consider need for PPI (proton pump inhibitor) gastroprotection

  ○ Colchicine plus ASA, if poor response to ASA

  ○ Corticosteroids, if poor response to ASA, alone

  ○ Treat complications
    - Tamponade
    - Hemodynamic instability
    - Poor pain relief
    - Effusion ≥ 1 cm
    - Myocarditis
    - Pyogenic infection / sepsis
    - Coagulopathy
    - Suspicion of malignancy as a cause
      ▪ Breast
      ▪ Lung
      ▪ Leukemia
      ▪ Lymphoma

• Give the rationale for choosing colchicine plus ASA versus corticosteroids for recurrent pericarditis, after initial treatment ASA / NSAIDs

  ○ Steroid use for short term (2-3 days) is associated with even more recurrence

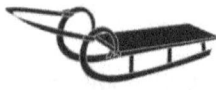

Clinical Cautions for pericarditis associated with acute myocardial infarction (AMI)
- o NSAIDs
  - Effective in treatment of pericarditis, but
  - Dangerous if pericarditis is associated with AMI (acute myocardial infarction) because of
    - ↓ formation of fibrosis
    - ↑ risk of rupture of ventricle
- o Anticoagulation
  - Not used if pericardial effusion develops post-MI
- o Pericardiectomy
  - Not used for acute or recurrent pericarditis

- o Recurrence
  - ASA plus colchicine, or
  - NSAID plus colchicine

Constrictive and Restrictive Pericarditis

➤ Pathophysiology: Pericarditis from any cause may evolve into a stiff pericardium which reduces filling because the ventricles cannot expand normally during diastole.

➤ Causes
- o Ideopathic
  - Viral
- o Infection
  - Tuberculosis (<15% of patients)
  - Postpurulent pericarditis
  - Histoplasmosis or pyogenic infection
- o Infiltration
  - Neoplasm
  - Lymphoma
  - Metastases
    - Lung
    - Breast
- o Immune
  - Connective tissue disease (especially rheumatoid arthritis)
- o Radiation
  - Often years earlier
- o Surgery
  - Hemopericardium
  - Cardiac operation or trauma
- o Chronic renal failure

Adapted from: Baliga RR. *Saunders/Elsevier*, 2007, page 96.

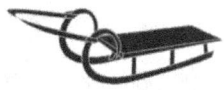

➢ Clinical
- ○ General
  - Dyspnea
  - Cachexia
- ○ JVP
  - Prominent x and y descents
  - Kussmaul's sign (↑ JVP with inspiration)

- ○ Pulse
  - 1/3 have AF
  - Pulsus paradoxus > 10 mm Hg fall in the arterial pulse pressure on inspiration, because increased right ventricular filling compresses the left ventricle)

- ○ Apex beat
  - Not palpable
  - Auscultation: Heart sounds, early S3, early pericardial knock (rapid ventricular filling abruptly halted)
- ○ LSE
  - Early diastolic knock which ↑ with inspiration
  - Differentiate from
    - ↑ P2
    - S3 gallop
    - OS of MS
    - Pericardial sound
    - Atrial myxoma (tumor "plop")
  - No pericardial rub
- ○ Lungs
  - Associated pleural effusion

- ○ Abdomen
  - Hepatomegaly
  - Ascites

- ○ Lower legs
  - Pitting edema

Abbreviations: AF, atrial fibrillation; JVP, jugular venous pressure; LSE, left sterna edge; MS, mitral sternosis; OS, perning snap

- ○ Atrial fibrillation (20%)
  - May be signs of effusion ("effusive-constrictive pericarditis)
- ○ Note: use ECG, chest x-ray, echo', CMR /CT and hemodynamic right and left heart catheterization studies (please see MKSAP 16 2012, Cardiology, Table 32, page 69 for further details)

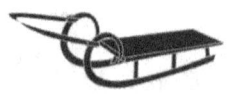

- Give a distinction constrictive pericarditis from restrictive cardiomyopathy.

Finding	Constrictive pericarditis	Restrictive Cardiomyopathy (RCM)
o Ventricular interdependence	+	-
o Septal bounch	+	-
o Abnormal pericardium	+	-
o Abnormal myocardium	-	+
o Abnormal myocardium	-	+
o Doppler velocity	N / ↑	↓
o Pulmonary pressure	N / ↑	↑
o LVEDP-RVEDF	< 5 mmHg	> 5 mmHg
o RVEDP / RVSP	> 1/3	< 1/3
o BNP	< 200	> 200

Abbreviations: BNP, brain naturetic peptide; LVEDP, left ventricular end-diastolic pressure; RVEDP, right ventricular end-diastolic pressure; RVSP, right ventricular systolic pressure

Adapted from: Shah J and Lindman BR. The Washington Manual of Medical Therapeutics, Edited by Godara H, et al., 34th Edition, 2014. Wolters Kluwer. Chapter 6, pages 194-219.

Clinical Gem and Pearl

- A patient with pericarditis develops an effusion The effusion is adequately drained, but dyspnea persists. Give the likely complication which has developed.

  - The patient has effusive-constrictive pericarditis, with the constriction becoming apparent after the pericardiocentesis

- Give the method used to determine if a mild degree of constriction is present.

  - Right-heart catheter studies are normally at rest, but become abnormal with an infusion of saline performed at the time of catheterization.

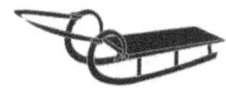

➤ Treatment
  o Treat underlying causes (e.g. autoimmune disease, TB)
  o Loop diuretic
    - Use **cautiously**, so as not to reduce filling pressure, and thereby SV (stroke volume) and CO (cardiac output)
  o Rate response if there is associated AF
    - Use cautiously so as not to cause bradycardia
  o Anti-inflammatory trial for 2-3 mon
  o Pericardiotomy (NYAA class II or III symptoms)

Radiation Cardiotoxicity

- For the patient who has received thoracic radiation therapy for cancer, give potential cardiac complications for which they will need to be followed long-term.

o Pericardium	-	Pericarditis
	-	Effusion
	-	Fibrosis
	-	Constriction
o Valves	-	Fibrosis
	-	Regurgitation
o Myocardium	-	Ischemia (accelerated coronary atherosclerosis)
	-	Cardiopathy
	-	Heart
o Conduction system	-	Dysrhythmias

Pericardial Effusion / Pleural

➤ Causes

o Exudates	-	Acute pericarditis
	-	Metastatic malignancy
o Transudates	-	CHF
	-	Liver failure
	-	Nephrotic syndrome
	-	Myxedema
o Hemopericardium	-	Aortic dissection
	-	Trauma

Source: Davey P. *Wiley-Blackwell*, 2006, page 163.

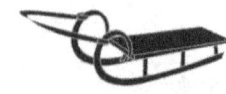

- o Common causes of malignant pleural or pericardial effusion
  - Breast cancer
  - Lung cancer
  - Lymphoma
- o Percardium
  - Thick, echogenic
- o Septum
  - Bounce
- o Mitral valve
  - N/ ↑ Doppler velocity through mitral annulus
  - Mitral flow velocity curves vary with inspiration
- o Hepatic vein
  - Flow reverses upon expiration
- o Cardiac catheterization
  - Measurements
    - RA (right atrium) pressure
    - RVEDP (right ventricular end diastolic pressure)
    - PA (pulmonary artery) pressure
    - LVEDP (left ventricular end diastolic pressure
    - CO, cardiac output
    - CI, cardiac index

- o Gated CT, MRI
  - Ventricular interdependence
  - Enlarges IVC, hepatic veins
  - Tumor, lymph nodes

- ➤ Clinical

- • Perform a focused physical examination to determine if a patient's pericardial rub has progressed to the development of a pericardial effusion.

- • Rub
  - o Transient
  - o Localized
  - o Present in both systole and diastole
  - o Louder when
    - Sitting forward
    - Pressing more firmly with stethoscope

- • Effusion
  - o Pulsus paradoxicus (inspiration decreases rather than the normal increase in pulse rate & volume).
  - o Dullness, 2nd left ICS (intercostals space)
  - o 2nd L. ICS dullness disappears on sitting.
  - o Collapse of base of L. lung

Note: At lease 250 mL of fluid is necessary in pericardial sac before a clinical diagnosis of effusion can be made.

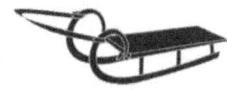

➤ Diagnosis

  o Pericardial effusion
  o Pleural effusion
    - Chest X-ray
    - CT chest
    - Pleural tap

  o Heart   - Chest X-ray
                   - ECG-low voltage QRS complexes
                   - Echocardiogram

➤ Treatment
  o Pericardial effusion

    - Underlying cause
    - Surgery
      ▪ Cardiocentesis
      ▪ Atrial pericardiectomy
      ▪ Placement of pericardial window
      ▪ Percutaneous / surgical decompression
    - Radiochemotherapy
    - Drainage (pericardiocentesis) for effusion causing hemodynamic
      compromise
    - Empiric antibiotics
    - Sclerosis

  o Pleural effusion

    - Maximum thoracentesis volume of 1500 mL, or 20 mL/kg
    - Recurrence
      ▪ Chest tube / indwelling catheter
      ▪ Pleurodesis

• Give circumstances under which surgical drainage of a pericardial effusion is
  recommended over pericardiocentesis.

  o Mechanical ventilation with high PEEP → ↓ venous return, thereby further
    decreasing filling, stroke volume and cardiac output
  o Deep sedation needed for the mechanical ventilation → ↓ sympathetic
    drive → ↓ BP

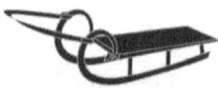

Mastering the Boards: Cardiology   A.B.R. Thomson

Pericardial tamponade

➢ Definition
   - Rapid accumulation of fluid in the space between the visceral and parietal layer of the pericardium reduces cardiac filling → ↓ CO (cardiac output)
   - Even a small effusion may have an important hemodynamic impact, but a large circumferential effusion will also cause this medical emergency

➢ Pathophysiology
   - Rapid collection of fluid around heart → compression of R/L A (trial) / V (ventricles) → ↑ pericardial pressure
      - ↓ SV (stroke volume)
      - ↓ CO (cardiac output)
   - Local (loculated) effusion may cause local tamponade
   - Note
      - It is the hemodynamic effect which is important, not the amount of pericardial fluid (effusion)

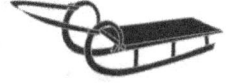

➢ Causes

Useful background: when thinking about possible pericardial tamponade, consider the clinical setting, and the cause of pericardial disease:

- o Infection   - Bacterial
                        - Viral

- o Immune   - Connective tissue disease

- o Recent cardiac / thoracic surgery / trauma

- o Dissecting aneurysm

- o Metastatic disease to pericardium

➢ Clinical
  - o In the context of cardiac tamponade, give the components of the Beck triad
    - ↑ JVP (jugular venous pressure)
    - ↓ SBP (systolic blood pressure)
    - Distant heart sounds

Pericardial tamponade is a life-threatening condition, and must be rapidly suspected on physical examination.

- Give the physical findings of pericardial tamponade.

  - o Inspection

  - o Tachypnea
    - Anxiety
    - Restlessness
    - Syncope

  - o JVP ↑, Kussmaul sign, prominent x but absent y descent

  - o Pulse and blood pressure
    - Rapid pulse rate
    - Pulsus paradoxus
    - Hypotension

  - o Apex beat: not palpable

  - o Auscultation: reduced heart sounds

  - o Lungs: dullness and bronchial breathing at the left base (due to lung compression by the distended pericardial sac).

Abbreviation: JVP, jugular venous pressure

Adapted from: Talley NJ, et al. *Maclennan & Petty Pty Limited* 2003, page 69.

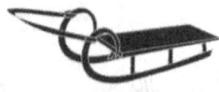

- Give additional physical findings, which suggest cardiac tamponade.

  o Pulsus paradoxus > 10 mmHg
  o Tachycardia
  o Signs of shock

- Perform a focused physical examination to distinguish between the jugular venous pulse and the carotid artery pulse.

Kussmaul signs

  o Paradoxical elevation of CVP during inspiration
  o In addition to causing an elevated CVP, venoconstriction probably also contributes to the positve abdominojugular test and Kussmaul sign, two signs that often occur together
  o Most patients with constrictive pericarditis and Kussmaul sign also have a notably positive abdominojugular test

Source: McGee SR. *Saunders/Elsevier* 2007, page 382.

SO YOU WANT TO BE AN HCM CARDIOLOGIST!

- Give the most useful clinical signs for the emergency diagnosis of acute cardiac tamponade include
  o ↑ jugular venous pressure (JVP)
  o Pulsus paradoxicus

- Give the circumstances may the patient have cardiac tamponade, yet those physical signs are absent.

  o ↑ JVP does not occur if
    - The pericardial effusion collects slowly, providing time for the pericardium to stretch, so there is no ↑ pericardial pressure ("low-pressure tamponade")
    - There is severe hypovolemia
  o Pulsus paradoxicus
    - False-positive
      Respiratory distress
    - False-negative
      ▪ ASD (atrial septal defect)
      ▪ PHT (pulmonary hypertension)
      ▪ AR (aortic regurgitation)
  o Severe LV dysfunction (especially those with uremic pericarditis), regional tamponade (tamponade affecting 1 or 2 heart chambers, such as following heart surgery), severe hypotension

---

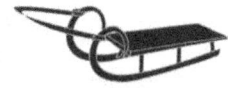

- Perform a focused physical examination to distinguish a chronic constrictive pericarditis (CP) from acute cardiac tamponade (CT).

Vital Signs		CT	CP
o Pulse and blood pressure	Pulsus paradoxus	✓	✓
	Pulse rate	↑	✓
o Respiratory Rate		↑	↑
o Kussmaul Sign		✓	↑
o JVP	↑x, absent y descent	+	+
o Apex Beat	Impalpable	✓	✓
o Heart sounds	Loudness	↓	↓
	S3	-	-
	Pericardial knock	-	-
o Lungs	Left base dull	✓	-
	Bronchial breathing	✓	-
o Abdomen	Hepatomegaly	-	+
	Splenomegaly	-	+
o Lower leg Edema		-	+

Adapted from: Talley NJ, et al. *Maclennan & Petty Pty Limited* 2003, page

- Perform a focused physical examination for constrictive pericarditis (CP) and cardiac tamponade (CT).

Physical finding	Frequency (%)	
	CP	CT
o JVP ↑		
- ↑ y descent	98	100
- Friedrich sign	57-94	-
- Kussmaul sign	50	0

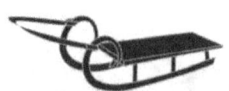

Mastering the Boards: Cardiology A.B.R. Thomson

Physical finding	Frequency (%)	
	CP	CT
o Pulse		
- AF tachycardia > 100 bpm	36-70	0
o BP		
- Pulsus > 10 mmHg	17-43	81-100
- Paradoxicus	>20	98
	>30	78
	>40	49
		38
o Auscultation of precordium		
- Pericardial knock	28-94	23
- Rub	4	
- ↓ heart sounds	-	36-84
o Others		
- Hepatomegaly	87-100	58
- Edema	63	27
- Ascites	53-89	-

Abbreviations: AF, arterial fibrillation; BP, blood pressure; CP, constrictive pericarditis; CT, cardiac tamponade; JVP, jugular venous pressure

Adapted from: McGee SR. *Saunders/Elsevier* 2007, pageS 513 and 514.

xxxxxxxxxxxxxxxxxxxxxxxxxxxxxxxxxxxxxxxxxxxxxxxxxxxxxxxx

SO YOU WANT TO BE A CARDIOLOGY RESIDENT!

- Which cause of constrictive pericarditis does not usually cause cardiomegaly, murmurs or atrial fibrillation (AF).

    o Tuberculous pericarditis

- In the context of the patient with constrictive pericarditis, give what is the Broadbent sign.

    o Intercostal indrawing during systole.

- In the context of cardiac tamponade, give what is the Beck triad.

    o Low arterial blood pressure
    o High venous pressure
    o Absent apex in cardiac tamponade is known as Beck's triad

Source: Baliga RR. *Saunders/Elsevier* 2007, page 100.

xxxxxxxxxxxxxxxxxxxxxxxxxxxxxxxxxxxxxxxxxxxxxxxxxxxxxxxx

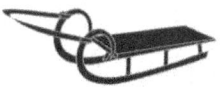

Mastering the Boards: Cardiology   A.B.R. Thomson

```
SO YOU WANT TO BE A CARDIOLOGY RESIDENT!
```

- Give which causes of pericardial rub do **not** usually progress to a pericardial effusion.

    - Pericardial rub caused by
        - Myocardial infarction
        - Uremia.

- Give what are the ECG changes which suggest that a rub has progressed to an effusion.
    - Low voltage
    - ↑ ST
    - Changes occur in all limb leads

- Give the easy way to distinguish between the ECG changes of a myocardial infarction (MI) versus pericardial effusion.

    - Low voltage and ST changes do not occur in all limb voltages

➢ Diagnosis
  o ECK
    - ↓ voltage
    - ↑ HR (tachycardia)
    - Electrical alternans

  o Transthoracic echocardiogram (TTE)
    - Identify location and nature of effusion (free flowing, loculated) for echocardiogram guided percutaneous pericardiocentesis
    - Determine if effusion is hemodynamically significant, and should be drained

- Give features on TTE (transthoracic echocardiogram) that a pericardial effusion is hemodynamic significant and should be drained urgently because of cardiac tamponade.

o IVC	- Dilated
	- Non-compressible
o TV / MV	- Inflow velocities vary with respiration
o RV	- Diastolic collapse
o RA	- Systolic collapse

Abbreviations: IVC, inferior vena cava; MV, mitral valve; RA, right atrium; RV, right ventricle; TV, tricuspid valve

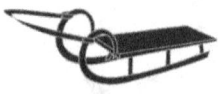

Mastering the Boards: Cardiology   A.B.R. Thomson

- o Transesophageal echocardiogram (TEE)
  - Higher sensitivity than TTE, especially for loculated effusion near atria, posteriorly

- o CT, MRI
  - Higher sensitivity for loculated effusion
  - May show associated pathology, e.g. tumor
  - Remember
    - As always, CT /MRI may not be safe to do in patient who is not stable
- o Right heart catheterization (RHC)
  - Measure LVEDP, RVEDP, RVSP

➢ Diagnostic imaging

- Give the findings on echocardiography, which suggest the diagnosis of pericardial tamponade.

  - o Diastolic collapse (invagination of wall of RV or atria in diastole)

  - o ↑ inflow velocity across MV / TV during inspiration

  - o ↓ fall in IVC diameter during inspiration

  - o ↑ intrapericardial pressure
  - o Echocardiogram
    - Peak transvalvular velocities
    - ↑ respiratory
    - Fluctuations

Abbreviation: IVC, inferior vena cava; JVP, jugular venous pressure; MV, mitral valve; PR, pulse rate; TV, tricuspid valve

➢ Treatment

- o IV fluids to maintain filling pressures

- o May require intubation

- o Pericardiocentesis
  - Percutaneous
  - Open

- o Hypotension
  - IV fluid (volume) replacement
  - Vasopressors

- o ↓ ventricular function
  - Inotropes, and/or
  - Intra-aortic balloon pump

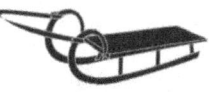

- o Drain effusion
  - Drainage of pericardial fluid (for hemodynamic instability, such as in presence of pulsus paradoxicus)
  - Percutaneous pericardiocentesis
  - Pericardiectomy for NYHA II or NYHA III (<u>not</u> for I and IV)
  - Caution: **extreme caution** with use of diuretics, which may reduce the preload, and further decrease cardiac output

---

CLINICAL CAUTION

The patient with cardiac tamponade will understandably have anxiety with their dyspnea, and the dyspnea may be sufficiently severe to require intubation of the patient.

- Give the reason why the pericardiocentesis needle must be at the bedside when the patient is given sedation prior to their intubation.

  - o The sedation may cause venodilation → ↓ preload → further ↓ cardiac filling and further ↑ cardiac output

---

Myopericarditis

- o ↑ ST segment with downward concave component
- o LV dysfunction
- o ↑ cardiac enzymes

Acute Myocarditis

- o Usually due to viral infection
- o Possible autoimmune injury
- o Curiously, prognosis is better with fulminant S-HF (systolic heart failure)
- o No specific treatment: supportive care and usual treatment for S-HF

Giant Cell Myocarditis (GCM)

- o Rapid onset of severe HF (heart failure) and refractory ventricular arrhythmias
- o Often fatal unless with
  - Insertion of VAD (ventricular assist device, or cardiac transplantation
- o GCM may recur in transplanted heart

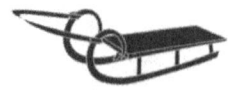

Clinical Alert

- o Anti-coagulation during pregnancy
  - High risk pregnancy evaluation
  - Avoid warfarin
    - T1 embryopathy
    - Before delivery
    - Intracranial hemorrhage with vaginal delivery

- o β-blockers
  - Monitor heart rate of mother and baby
  - Monitor blood sugar of baby

- o Cardiac Drugs to Avoid in Pregnancy
  - Pregnancy
    - ACE inhibitors (ACEIs)
    - ARBs
    - Amiodarone
    - Sodium nitroprusside
    - Phenytoin

  - Lactation
    - Amiodarone
    - Atenolol
    - Sodium nitroprusside

"Let's see if there is mechanistic information that
we can tease out."

Grandad

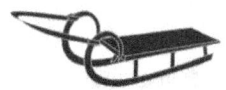

CARDIOMYOPATHY

- o Peripartum cardiomyopathy: symptoms / signs of HF, LVEF < 45%, occurring any time between 1 month before and 5 months after delivery
  - Treatment
    - Dilated
    - Early delivery
    - Avoid future pregnancies (↑ risk of recurrence)
    - If peripartum cardiomyopathy develops prepartum, do <u>not</u> use ACEI / ARBs (fetal renal agenesis)

- ➢ Causes
  - o Primary
    - Idiopathic
    - Endomyocardial fibrosis or fibro-elastosis
    - Hypertrophic obstructive cardiomyopathy (HOCM)
    - Pregnancy and puerperium

  - o Infection
    - Viral (Coxsachie)
      - Toxoplasmosis
      - Schistosomiasis
      - Chagas disease (trypanosoma)
      - Sarcoidosis
      - TB

  - o Infiltration
    - Amyloidosis
    - Hemochromatosis
    - Glycogen storage disease
    - Leukemia
    - Sarcoidosis
    - Fat
    - Carcinoid

  - o Inherited
    - Obstructive Endomycardial Fibrosis
    - Fibroelastosis Puerperal Idiopathic
      - Friedreich ataxia
      - Muscular dystrophies
      - Gargoylism

  - o Nutritional
    - Starvation
    - Beriberi
    - Kwashiorkor
    - Anemia

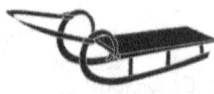

- o   Toxic   - Alcohol
                              - Drugs
                              - Cobalt or antimony poisoning

- o   Immune   - Rheumatoid arthritis
                              - SLE
                              - Scleroderma

- o   MSK   - Polyarteritis nodosa
                              - Myasthenia gravis

- o   Endocrine   - Myxedema
                              - Acromegaly
                              - Pheochromocytoma
                              - Thyrotoxicosis
                              - Hypoadrenalism
                              - Porphyria
                              - 'Collagen-vascular' disease
                                - SLE
                                - Arteritis
                                - Systemic sclerosis
                                - Rheumatoid disease
                                - Ankylosing spondylitis
                              - Neuromuscular
                                - Friedreich ataxia
                                - Myopathies (eg dystrophia myotonica, Duchenne)

Abbreviations: HOCM, hypertrophic obstructive cardiomyopathy; SLE, systemic lupus erythematosus; TB, tuberculosis

Adapted from: Davies IJT. *Lloyd-Luke LTD* 1972, Table III, page 84; Burton JL. *Churchill Livingstone* 1971

- ➤ Types
  - o Hypertrophic cardiomyopathy (HCM): symptoms / signs of HF "…. Characterized by diffuse or focal myocardial hypertrophy disproportionate to loading conditions" (board Basic 3, page 19, 2012)
  - o Restrictive cardiomyopathy
  - o Stress-induced cardiomyopathy – "Takotsubo"
  - o Dilated cardiomyopathy: symptoms / signs of HF arrhythmias or sudden cardiac death, associated with
    - One or two ventricles
      - Dilated
      - ↓ function

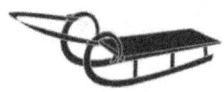

➢ Clinical

- Take a directed history and perform a focused physical examination for the three major types of cardiomyopathy.

  - Congestive failure
    - Often tricuspid regurgitation (TR)
    - Large flask-shaped heart
    - Low voltage ECG
    - Atrial fibrillation and LBBB common

  - Constrictive (often due to amyloidosis)

  - Hypertrophic cardiomyopathy
    - Angina
    - Syncope
    - Sudden cardiac death (SCD)
    - Dyspnea
    - Jerky arterial pulse
    - 3rd heart sound (S3)
    - Variable late systolic murmur down LSE (distinguish from AS)
    - Decreased by negative inotropic drugs

Source: Burton JL. *Churchill Livingstone* 1971, page 17.

Dilated Cardiomyopathy (DCM)

➢ Definition

  - A disease of heart muscle characterized by dilation of the cardiac chambers and reduction in ventricular contractile function.

➢ Demography

  - Incidence $30/10^5$ per year

➢ Pathophysiology

  - Diseased myocardium → neurohormonal activation → dilated cardiac chambers → tricuspid / mitral regurgitation (TR / MR) → Atrial / ventricular arrhythmias → SCD (sudden cardiac death)

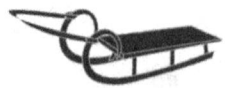

- Give the causes of **dilated cardiomyopathy**

    o Idiopathic
      - 50%

    o Reversible
      - Alcohol
        LV, or LV plus RV dilated, hypokinetic
      - Dugs (causing tachycardia)
        ▪ Cocaine
        ▪ Amphetamine

    o Caution: use labetalol rather than B-blockers ($\rightarrow$ coronary vasoconstriction)
      - Tachycardia, including takotsubo (stress-induced cardiomyopathy)

    o Others
      - Myocarditis
      - Arrhythmogenic RV dysplasia

➢ Diagnosis
    o Echocardiogram
      - 2 dimensional
      - Doppler
    o Radionucleotide ventriculorgraphy
    o Note
      - Endomyocardial biopsy not recommended

➢ Treatment
    o Treat symptomatic HF in the usual manner
    o Anticoagulation (INR 2-3) for history of
    o Corticosteroids / immune suppression
    o For EF ≤ 35% and NYHA II-III symptoms despite 3 mon of optimal medical therapy
      - ICD (implantation cardiac defibrillator)
      - Cardiac resynchronization (if QRS ≥ 120 ms [intraventricular conduction delay])
    o IABP (intraaortic balloon pump) or LVAD (left ventricular assist device) as bridge to cardiac transplantation
    o Mitral valve annuloplasty / replacement for symptomatic severe MR (mitral regurgitation)

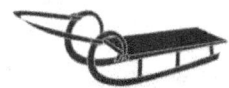

Hypertrophic Cardiomyopathy (HCM)

➢ Definition
- o Pathophysiology outflow tract obstruction leading to diastolic dysfunction
- o Asymmetric focal septal or diffuse hypertrophy of the LV (left ventricle) in the absence of known or identifiable ("idiopathic") conditions which cause ↑ afterload
- o May be autosomal dominant in half of patients
- o Common idiopathic disorders of the myocardium associated with
  - Hypertrophy of ventricles (especially asymmetric septal hypertrophy)
  - ↓ compliance of LV
  - ↓ size of LV
  - ↓ relaxation in diastolic
  - LV outflow tract obstruction +/- (↑ outflow obstruction with ↑ LV contractility / ↓ volume of ventricle)

➢ Demography
- o Prevalence
  - 1/500 persons (200 / 10^5)
- o Early onset often is
  - Inherited
  - Seen in athletes
  - Common cause of SCD (sudden cardiac death, especially age 10 to 35 yr)
- o Late onset in older persons with hypertension
- o Autosomal dominant in 50% → first degree relatives require echocardiogram to screen for HCM

➢ Genetics
- o Inherited from
  - Autosomal dominant
  - Variable penetrance / phenotype expression
  - Mutation in myosin heavy-chain gene

➢ Pathophysiology
- o ↑ LA
- o ↓ LV (from hypertrophy)
- o LVOT obstruction

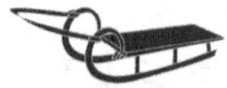

Mastering the Boards: Cardiology   A.B.R. Thomson

- ➢ Causes / associations
  - o Ischemia
  - o HF (heart failure)
  - o Arrhythmias
  - o CVA (cardiovascular accident ["stroke"]
  - o Mortality rate ~ 5% per year
    - - HF (heart failure)
    - - CVA
    - - SCD (sudden cardiac death)

- ➢ Clinical

SO YOU WANT TO BE A CARDIOLOGIST!

- • Give the mechanism for development of the murmur of MR (mitral regurgitation) in HCM.
  - o LVOT (left ventricular outflow tract) obstruction displaces MV (mitral valve) anteriorly during systole → MR murmur

---

CLINICAL SKILLS

  - o Virtually the only circumstance when ↓ preload (Valsalva maneuver, standing) → ↑ systolic murmur is HCM (hypertrophic cardiomyopathy)
  - o In the patient with HCM, give the significance of a double (bisferious) carotid pulse
    - Not all patients with HCM have obstruction of outflow, and the physical finding which suggests this double peak carotid pulse.

- ➢ Clinical

- • Perform a focused physical examination of the cardiovascular system for HCM (hypertrophic cardiomyopathy).

  - o Pulse
  - o Precordium
    - - Palpation
    - - Auscultation
      Systolic murmur
        - - LSB (left sternal border)
        - - ↑ by Valsalva, standing
        - - May be associated with murmur of mitral regurgitation

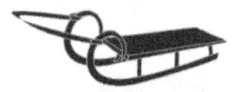

➤ Complications

  o Mid-systolic murmur caused by LVOT (LV [left ventricular] outflow tract) obstruction

  o Intensity of murmur of HCM and positioning

	Preload	HCM murmur intensity
- Valsalva, squatting	↓	↑ (unmasks, or ↑ LVOT obstruction)
- Raising legs	↑	↓

➤ Diagnosis

  o ECG
  - ↑ Q waves
  - T waves upright in leads with Q waves
  - Inverted if apex of LV is hypertrophic
  - Two-dimensional
  - Doppler flow
  - ECG not diagnostic, with abnormal ST-segment and T-waves, plus LV hypertrophy

  o Exercise echocardiogram
  - Early detection of gradient before hypertrophy

  o CMR (cardiovascular magnetic resonance)
  - Early detection of small areas of hypertrophy

CLINICAL ALERT

  o HCM plus ↑ risk of SCD suggested on Holter monitoring by NSVT (non-sustained ventricular tachycardia)

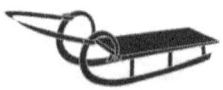

Mastering the Boards: Cardiology   A.B.R. Thomson

- Give the clinical features used to **distinguish** the murmur of **HCM** (hypertrophic cardiomyopathy) from AS (aortic stenosis)

Clinical	AS	HCM
o Apex beat	- Single	- "triple ripple"
	- Sustained	
o Carotid		
- Pulse	- Pulsus bisferiens (rise-fall-rise)	- Parvus (low volume rise)
		- Tardus (slow rise)
- Radiation	Yes	No
o Murmur		
- Associated AR	No	Sometimes
- Maneuvers (intensity)		
▪ Valsalva	↓	↑
▪ Squat → stand	↓	↑
▪ Stand → squat	↑	↓

xxxxxxxxxxxxxxxxxxxxxxxxxxxxxxxxxxxxxxxxxxxxxxxxxxxxxx

SO YOU WANT TO BE A CARDIOLOGIST!

A young man with a known midsystolic murmur since age 20 has successfully placed in his provincial track team, and is offered to try out for the national Olympic team.
- Give the changes on echocardiogram which help to distinguish HCM versus "athlete's heart".

Features on echocardiogram	HCM	Athlete's heart
Hypertrophy	Asymmetrical	Symmetrical (concentric)
Wall thickness	> 15 mm	≤ 15 mm
LV end-diastolic diameter	< 55 mm	> 55 mm
↑ LA	Yes	No
Abnormal diastolic function	Yes	No

Abbreviations: HCM, hypertrophic cardiomyopathy; LA, left atrium; LV, left ventricle

A patient with a diagnosis of HCM proven by echocardiogram moves to your practice area to attend the local university. His previous internist, who was a classmate at medical school and whose competence you trust, describe in her referral letter that the patient had a significant LVOT (left ventricular outflow tract) obstruction. You auscultate the young man's precordium, and there is no murmur.

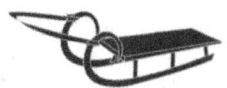

- Give the explanation for the loss of a previously auscultated murmur in HCM.
  - In about 5% of persons with HCM, the LV (left ventricular) hypertrophy and fibrosis may undergo remodeling which may lead to a dilated cardiomyopathy and loss of the original LVOT obstruction caused by the hypertrophy.
  - Note of caution
    - Assess this patient's EF and NYHA symptom class: if EF ≤ 35%, NND symptoms NYHA class II or III, patient still has ↑ risk of SCD (sudden cardiac death)

- ➢ Treatment
  - Perform risk stratification for SCD (sudden cardiac death)
  - Treatment options are complex depending upon
    - Risk for SCD
    - Symptoms
    - Genotype
    - Phenotype
    - Progressive HF (heart failure) refractory to medical treatment
    - Systolic function
    - LVOT obstruction
  - No strenuous exercise
  - EV ≥ 50% - BB → CCBs → diosopyamide
  - EV < 50% - ACEI
  - Outflow gradient > 50 mm Hg
    - Septal ablation
    - Surgery

  - Lifestyle
    - Holter monitoring (NSVT [non-sustained supraventricular tachycardia])
    - Stress testing
    - Avoid vigorous exercise
  - Genetic counseling and family screening of 1ˢᵗ degree relatives

  - Symptoms
    - B-blockers
    - Non-dihydropyridines
      Calcium channel blockers
      Diltiazem, verapamil
  - Arrhythmias
    - Treat, but preventative therapy not proven to be of benefit

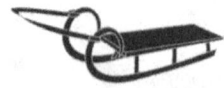

o Atrial fibrillation (AF)
   - Anticoagulation for chronic or paroxysmal AF
   - Chronic suppression of HF (if cardioversion contraindicated / fails)
     ▪ Amiodarone
     ▪ Disopyramide
     ▪ Procainamide
   - Cardioversion for acute HF
   - Control ventricular response before cardioversion with B-blockers, or CCB (diltiazem, verapamil)

o ICD (implantable cardiac defibrillator)
   - For high-risk HCM
o Dual-chamber pacing
   - ↓ symptoms, but not survival

o Pacemaker
   - Procedures ~25% ↓ LVOT (LV outflow tract) gradient
   - ↓ symptoms, but not survival

o Surgery
   - Septal myotomy-myectomy +/- mitral valve replacement (MVR)
   - Catheter-based ablation of septum with alcohol
   - Cardiac transplantation

SO YOU WANT TO BE A CARDIOLOGIST!

* In patients with HCM (hypertrophic cardiomyopathy), give the features which suggest the patient is high-risk and that placement of ICD (implantable cardiac defribrillator) may be appropriate.

o SCD (sudden cardiac death)
   - Genetic mutations in myosin heavy-chain gene
   - Prior SCD / sustained ventricular tachyarrhythmia (SVT)
   - Family history of SCD
o Clinical
   - Syncope (or near syncope)
     ▪ Recurrent, or with exertion
     ▪ Especially in young persons
   - Hypotension with exercise
o ECG / Holter
o Diagnostic imaging thickness of wall of myocardium > 30 mm

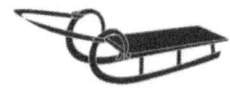

WATCH YOUR STEP IN TREATING HCM

DO **not** use
- o Digoxin
  - - Positive inotropic effect → ↑ ventricular outflow obstruction
- o Diuretics in HCM (especially if there is severe LV outflow obstruction)
  - - Diuretics → preload ↓ may ↑ obstruction and ↓ cardiac output
- o Dihydropyridines CCBs (e.g. Nicardipine, nisoldipine, israipine ↑ vasodilation
- o Nitrates   } ↑ LV outflow gradient
- o Vasodilators
- o Prophylactic antiarrhythmic drugs for NSVT
  - - May ↑ risk of arrhythmias when used prophylactically

Abbreviations: CCB, calcium channel blockers; NSVT, non-sustained ventricular tachycardia

---

Restrictive cardiomyopathy (RC)

➤ Definition
- o Stiffening of the right and left ventricles, with or without ↓ volume in the ventricles, resulting in ↑ intracavity pressures, ↓ filling volume and ↓ function of the ventricles
- o Normal EF (ejection fraction, normal thickening of wall of ventricles)
- o Rigid myocardium leading to ↓ filling of RV (right ventricle)

➤ Pathophysiology
- o Rigid ventricular wall leading to ↑ diastolic ventricular pressure ↑ preload pressure, ↓ filling of ventricles, diastolic dysfunction, pulmonary hypertension and R-sided HF (↑ end diastolic pressure in LV and RV).

- o Rigid, stiff myocardium (with or without infiltration) → ↓ diastolic filling of ventricles
  - - ↑ RV / LV filling pressures
  - - Systolic function N/↓ → ↑ intracardiac pressures

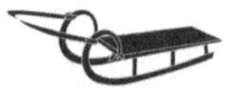

➢ Causes

    ○ Primary
        - Idiopathic
        - Inherited mutations
            ■ Genes encoding
                - Troponin I and T
                - β-myosin heavy chain
            ■ Proteins of sarcomeres
            ■ Some mutations that cause HCM may cause RC, or
            ■ A type of HCM with a restrictive phenotype
    ○ Secondary:

• Give the **causes** of restrictive cardiomyopathy.

○ Endomyocardial disease	- Fibrosis - Post-radiation damage - Carcinoid syndrome - Hypereosinophilic syndrome - Drug toxicity antracycline
○ Infiltration	- Amyloid - Hemochromatosis (restrictive or dilated cardiomyopathy) - Sarcoidosis - Globotriaosylceramide (Fabry disease) from X-linked deficiency of α-galactosidase - Glycogen storage disease
○ MSK disease	- Scleroderma
○ Endocrine	- Diabetes
○ Immune	- Systemic sclerosis (scleroderma) - Eosinophilic (Loffler endocarditis)
○ Iatrogenic (drugs)	- Anthracyclines - Radiation

➢ Clinical
    ○ Features of right- and left-sided ventricular failure
    ○ S3 gallop, force apex impulse (in S- [systolic] HH [heart failure] or constrictive pericarditis, there is a S3 gallop, but apex is hardly / not palpable)
    ○ 5-yr mortality rate ~ 35%

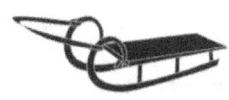

➢ Diagnosis
  o Note of caution
  o ↑↑ β-naturatic peptide (> 800 pg/mL)
  o ECG
    - ↓ QRS voltage precardial leads ≤ 10 mV
    - Limb leads ≤ 5 mV
    - Amyloid infiltration
      ▪ ↓ voltage
      ▪ ↓ progression of R-wave
    - Sarcoid infiltration
      ▪ Conduction abnormalities
  o Echocardiogram
    - ↑ Early diastolic filling rate
    - ↓ filling of RL and LV
    - EF normal
      ▪ ↑ RA and LA
      ▪ Wall thickness normal
      ▪ ↑ CVP (central venous pressure)

  o Echocardiogram with Doppler
    - ↑ thickness of myocardium
    - ↓ diastolic filling
    - ↓ / N systolic function
    - ↑ RV / LV filling pressures
    - ↑ intracardiac pressures

  o Cardiac CT, MRI, PET

  o Cardiac catheterization
    - ↑ filling pressures, RV and LV
    - Abnormal dip-and-plateau filling pattern on pressure tracing of RV and LV

  o Biopsy of endomyocardium only if diagnosis unclear

  o Note: RCM must be distinguished from constrictive pericarditis

- Give the features which help to **differentiate restrictive cardiomyopathy (RC)** from **constrictive cardiomyopathy (CC)**.

Features	RC	CC
o Pericardial knock (loud S3)	Rare	Common
o Friction rub	No	Yes
o BNP concentration	↑↑	N / ↑
o Chest X-ray, pericardial Ca^{2+}	No	Yes

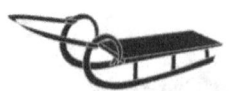

Features	RC	CC
○ MRI: ↑ pericardial thickness	Yes	No
○ Echocardiogram		
- Atrial enlargement	Yes	No
- LV hypertrophy	Yes	No
○ ↓ fall in LV filling during inspiration	No	Yes
○ Cardiac catheterization, R-side: diastolic pressure LV – RV	No	Yes
- Shifting of ventricular septum back-and-forth during diastole	No	Yes
- Effusion	No	Yes
- Early filling velocity across MV / TV, with rapid decrease in velocity	No	Yes
- ↑ filling with inspiration	No	Yes
- Abnormal motion of septum during diastole	No	Yes

Abbreviations: CC, constrictive cardiomyopathy; LV, left ventricle; MV, mitral valve; RC, restrictive cardiomyopathy; TV, tricuspid valve;

➢ Treatment

○ Treatment underlying conditions and complications

• Give the therapy of restrictive cardiomyopathy.

○ Treat underlying / associated disorders
- Hypertension
- Diabetes
- CAD

○ ACEI / ARBs
- ↓ diastolic dysfunction
- ↑ diastolic filling

○ Loop diuretics
- Diuretic, as needed (↑ diastolic filling), and used continuously so as not to ↓ fully pressure → ↓ SV (stroke volume)
- Caution: do **not** use high doses of loop diuretics, since the ventricular volumes are normal or ↓, and ↓ LV / RV volume → ↓ SV / ↓ CO → orthostatic hypotension, syncope

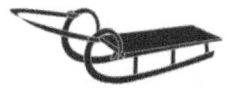

- o BB / CCBs (non-dihydropyridine) if
  - Symptoms persist despite loop diuretics, or
  - Atrial tachyarrhythmias
  - β-blockers and CCB (calcium channel blockers to ↑ diastolic filling, used cautiously so as not to ↓ CO (cardiac output)
  - Do **not** use BB / CCBs in the presence of conduction abnormalities (may precipitate third-degree heart block)
- o ICD for
  - Syncope
  - Ventricular arrhythmias
- o Pacemaker for
  - High-grade conduction defects

Abbreviations: BB, beta blocker; CAD, coronary artery disease; CCB, calcium channel blocker; CO, cardiac output; CT, computed tomography; ICD, implantable cardiac defibrillation; LV, left ventricle; MRI, magnetic resonance imaging; PET, positron emission tomography; RV, right ventricle; SV, stroke volume

---

SO YOU WANT TO BE A CARDIOLOGIST!

- Give the name of the medication sometimes used to treat heart failure (HR) or arrhythmias, which must not be used in restrictive cardiomyopathy caused by amyloidosis.

  - o Do **not** give digoxin in the patient with cardiac amyloidosis
  - o Amyloid fibrils in heart bind digoxin extracellularly → hypersensitivity / toxicity

---

CT/MRI will show pericardial thickening in both restrictive cardiomyopathy (RC) and constrictive cardiomyopathy (CC).

- In addition to treat the associated heart disease, give the treatment of restrictive cardiomyopathy caused by sarcoidosis and by hypereosinophilic syndrome (Loffler endocarditis).

- **Sarcoidosis**

  - o Corticosteroids

  - o Anti-malarials
    - Chloroquine
    - Hydroxychloroquine

  - o Immunosuppression
    - Cyclosporine
    - Methotrexate

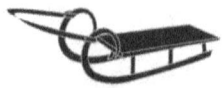

- **Loffler endocarditis**
  - Corticosteroids
  - TK (tyrosine kinase) inhibitor
  - Interferon
  - Cyclosporine
  - Chemotherapy
  - If cardiac thrombus present
    - Anti-coagulate with warfarin

- Give the difference seen on ECG of the cardiomyopathy seen with sarcoidosis vs. amyloidosis.

Condition	Nature of myocardial involvement	Low voltage on ECG
o Sarcoidosis	Patchy	No
o Amyloidosis	Diffuse	Yes

Tachycardia-mediated Cardiomyopathy

- Caused by sustained rapid atrial or ventricular arrhythmias
- Control rate of arrhythmia to improve cardiomyopathy
- Recurrence of tachyarrhythmia → rapid recurrent cardiomyopathy

Peripartum Cardiomyopathy

➤ Definition
  - LV dysfunction [newly] diagnosed in the last month of pregnancy up to 5 months postpartum

➤ Demography
  - Incidence ~ $30/10^5$ deliveries
  - ↑ incidence in
    - African American women
    - Older mother
    - Multiparty
    - Multiple pregnancy
    - Gestational hypertension

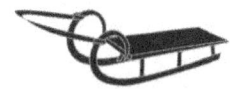

- ➢ Etiology / associations
  - ○ Viral triggers e.g.
    - – Coxsakie virus
    - – Parvovirus B19
    - – Adenovirus
    - – HSV
  - ○ Autoimmune myocarditis in mother
    - – Fetal cells pass into
    - – Mother (microchimerism)
  - ○ Abnormal prolactin cleavage product
  - ○ Clinically suspect in pregnant or recently post-partum mother with
    - – HF (heart failure, displaced PMI point of maximal impulse; aka apical impulse), or SCD (sudden cardiac death)

- ➢ Diagnosis
  - ○ Echocardiogram
    - – ↓ EF (ejection fraction)
    - – LV dilation
  - ○ ECG
    - – LVH (LV hypertrophy)
    - – Abnormal ST T waves

Clinical Alert

- • Give what is the main cause of pregnancy-related maternal death in North America.
  - ○ Even though about half of women who develop peripartum cardiomyopathy within 6 mon of delivery, the leading cause of pregnancy-related maternal death is pericardium cardiomyopathy, which leads to
    - – Heart failure
    - – Arrhythmias
    - – Thromboembolism

- • Give what is the profile of the woman who develops peripartum cardiomyopathy.
  - ○ > 30 yr
  - ○ African-Canadian
  - ○ Multiparous
  - ○ Multifetal pregnancy
  - ○ Preeclampsia
  - ○ Hypertension during pregnancy (gestational hypertension)

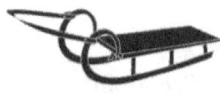

> Treatment
>> o B1-selective blockers
>>> - Metoprolol
>>> - Atenolol
>> o ACE inhibitors (hydralazine during pregnancy)
>> o Diuretics
>> o Digoxin
>> o Heparin for thromboembolism → Coumadin after delivering
>> o Counseling if LV function does not return to normal → avoid further pregnancies

- Give the reason why the selective B1-blockers are used for peripartum cardiomyopathy.

  o Avoid non-selective B blockers during pregnancy, since they may ↑ uterine relaxation

- Give the treatment of peripartum cardiomyopathy.

  o The usual treatment is used for complications, such as
    - Heart failure *do not use
      - ACE inhibitors
      - ARBs■ Aldosterone antagonists
      - Amiodarone
    - Arrhythmias
      - Warfarin when EF < 35%
      - See clinical alert below
  o IVIG (intravenous immune globulin)
  o Pentoifylline (to ↓ TNF-α)
  o Bromocriptine (↓prolactin)
  o Ventricular assist devise
  o Heart transplantation
  o If LV dysfunction persists, avoid further pregnancies

Sudden Cardiac Death (SCD)

> Risks

Persons with HCM are at risk of SCD (sudden cardiac death). Risk stratification is necessary, since a person with≥ 1 high (major) risk factor or ≥ 2 low (minor) risk factors benefit from prophylactic placement of an ICD (intracardiac defibrillator). Because of the importance of placing an ICD to prevent SCD, it is appropriate to expect that you know which patient with HCM to refer, and therefore to test you on these major and minor risk factors for SCD.

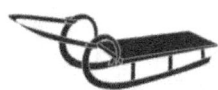

- Give risk factors for sudden cardiac death (SCD).

➢ Major
  - o VT (ventricular tachycardia; spontaneous and sustained)
  - o Previous cardiac arrest
  - o First-degree relative with SCD

➢ Minor
  - o VT (non-sustained)
  - o Syncope (with no explanation)
  - o Exercise response
    - Reduced, or
    - Hypotensive
  - o Perfusion study
    - Microvascular disease
  - o Echocardiogram
    - LV septal wall > 30 mm
    - LV outflow obstruction

SO YOU WANT TO BE AN HCM CARDIOLOGIST SPECIALIST!

Most episodes of sudden cardiac death (SCD) do not occur with vigorous physical exercise.

- Give 5 major factors predictive of **SCD in HCM** (hypertrophic cardiomyopathy).
  - o VT (ventricular tachycardia)
    - Causing previous cardiac arrest
    - Spontaneous sustained
    - Spontaneous non-sustained
  - o Syncope, unexplained
  - o Family history, SCD
  - o Exercise stress test
    - ↑ BP < 20 mm Hg
    - ↓ SBP
  - o Echocardiogram
    - LV wall ≥ 30 mm
  - o Note: If there are none of these major predictive factors for SCD, the NPA (negative predictive accuracy > 95%)

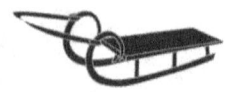

CONGENITAL HEART DISEASE

The following conditions will be considered
- PFO (patent foramen ovale)
- ASD (atrial septal defect)
- VSD (ventricular septal defect)
- PDA (patient ductus arteriosus)
- PVS (pulmonary valve stenosis)
- Aortic coarctation
- Tetralogy of Fallot
- Eisenmenger's syndrome

- Give the anatomic classification of congenital heart disease

    - Shunts (R → L or L → R)
        - R and L heart shunts

    - Valvular defects
        - Aortic or pulmonary stenosis
        - Bicuspid aortic valve (predisposes to later aortic stenosis)
        - Tricuspid atresia

    - Complex lesions
        - Fallot tetralogy
        - Transposition of the great vessels
        - Ebstein anomaly
        - Combinations of defects

Source: Davey P. *Wiley-Blackwell* 2006, page 174.

SO YOU WANT TO BE A PEDIATRIC CARDIOLOGIST!

- Give the four commonest causes of cyanotic heart diseases of infancy.

The Four T's:
- **T**etralogy of Fallot
- **T**ransposition of the great vessels
- **T**ricuspid regurgitation
- **T**otal anomalous pulmonary venous connection

Source: Baliga RR. *Saunders/Elsevier* 2007, page 89.

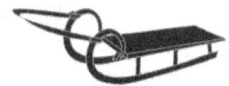

- Give the physiological classification of congenital heart disease based on the presence or absence of cyanosis.

- **Acyanotic**

  ➢ With L → R shunt
    o Ventricular septal defect (VSD)
    o Atrial septal defect (ASD)
    o Patent ductus arteriosus (PDA)

  ➢ With no shunt
    o Bicuspid aortic valve, congenital aortic stenosis
    o Coarctation of aorta
    o Dextrocardia
    o Pulmonary stenosis, tricuspid stenosis
    o Ebstein's anomaly

- **Cyanotic**
    o Ebstein anomaly (if an atrial septal defect (ASD) and R → L shunt are also present)
    o Truncus arteriosus
    o Transposition of the great vessels
    o Tricuspid atresia
    o Total anomalous pulmonary venous drainage
    o Eisenmenger syndrome (pulmonary hypertension and a right – to - left shunt)
    o Tetralogy of Fallot

Source: Talley NJ, et al. *Maclennan & Petty Pty Limited* 2003, page 85.

- Give the causes of cyanosis

  ➢ Central cyanosis
    o ↓ arterial oxygen saturation
      - ↓ concentration of inspired oxygen: high altitude
      - ↓ cardiac output: left ventricular failure or shock
      - Lung disease: chronic obstructive pulmonary disease with cor pulmonale, massive pulmonary embolism
      - Right-to-left cardiac shunt (cyanotic congenital heart disease)
    o Polycythemia
    o Hemoglobin abnormalities (rare): methemoglobinemia, sulphemoglobinemia

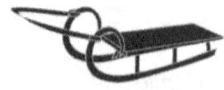

➢ Peripheral cyanosis
  o All causes of central cyanosis cause peripheral cyanosis
  o Exposure to cold
  o Arterial or venous obstruction

Source: Talley NJ, et al. *Maclennan & Petty Pty Limited* 2003, page 19.

- Give the chest X-ray findings seen in 3 common causes of congenital heart disease.

  o Causes
    - VSD
    - ASD (of the secundum type)
    - Patent ductus arteriosus (PDA)
    - Fallot's tetralogy (in order of frequency)

  o Chest X-Ray Findings
    - Boot-shaped heart
    - Enlarged right ventricle
    - Decreased pulmonary vasculature
    - Right-sided aortic arch (in 30% of cases)

SO YOU WANT TO BE A CARDIOLOGIST!

- Give the clinical circumstances should heart disease be suspected as being congenital in origin.

  o Young person
  o Murmur down left sternal edge
  o Presence of both cyanosis and clubbing
  o Presence of other congenital conditions:
    - Down syndrome : ASD (ostium primuim type of atrial septal defect)
    - Turner syndrome: coarctation of the aorta, pulmonary stenosis
    - Gargoylism: fibroelastosis
    - Marfan syndrome: ASA, dissecting aneurysm
  o Depending upon underlying history, presence of
    - Cyanosis
    - Clubbing
    - Polycythemia (secondary to low pO2)
    - Drawfism, or infantilism (retention in adult life of sexual characteristics of childhood)

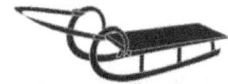

- Perform a focused physical examination to distinguish between dextrocardia, situs inversus, dextroversion, and levoversion.

		Dextro-cardia Side	Situs inversus	Dextro-version	Levo-version
o	Apex beat	R	R	R	L
o	Heart sounds	R	R	R	L
o	R. atrium	L	L		
o	Descending aorta	R	R	L	R
o	Lung		R, 2 lobes; L, 3 lobes		
o	Liver dullness		L		
o	Stomach	L	R	L	R
o	Associated				
	- Bronchiectasis and dysplasia of the frontal sinuses (Kartagener syndrome)	✓	✓	-	-
	- Cardiac malformation (CM)	✓	-	-	-
	- CM plus Turner syndrome*	✓	-	-	-
	- Asplenia	✓	-	-	-

*Turner syndrome: female, webbing of neck, ↑ carrying angle of elbow joint, gonadal dysgenesis

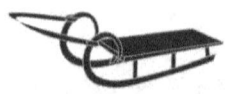

SO YOU WANT TO BE A PEDIATRIC CARDIOLOGIST!

- Give the complications of aortic coarctation.

    - Severe hypertension and resulting complications:
        - Stroke
        - Premature coronary artery disease

- Give the findings in Turner syndrome, Noonan syndrome and Bonnevie-Ullrich syndrome and give one clinical finding on inspection which all three have in common.

    - Webbed neck. Now let's consider differences in these three syndromes.

Turner syndrome

- Phenotypic females
- Ovarian dysgenesis
- Short stature
- Low-set ears
- "shield chest|
- Café-au-lait spots
- Freckles
- Heart congenital coarctation of aorta

Bonnevie- Ullrich syndrome

- Lymphedema of hands and feet
- Nail dystrophy
- Lax skin
- Short stature

Noonan syndrome

- Congenital pulmonary stenosis
- Pectus carinatum (forward projection of sternum)
- Short stature
- Mildly mentally challenged
- Hypertelevision
- Bleeding
- Skin changes

- Give 2 congenital disorders in which atrial fibrillation (AF) is common.

    - Atrial septal defect
    - Ebstein anomaly

Source: Baliga RR. *Saunders/Elsevier* 2007, pages 32 and 33.

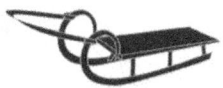

Patent Foramen Ovale (PFO)

- o Persistent valve-like opening covered by a membrane on the left side
- o May cause paradoxic embolus (peripheral vein or RA embolus goes to systolic circulation, e.g. brain, kidney rather than lung
- o With RAH and LAH, large
- o Defect produced like ASD
- o A PFO allows blood to pass directly from RA → LA (right-to-left shunt)
- o ↑ risk of CVA (cerebrovascular event, i.e. "stroke") from paradoxical embolism
- o Risk of orthodeoxia platypnea syndrome
- o Detection of PFO by echocardiogram (TTE or TEE) is increased with IV injection of bubbled (agitation) saline, followed by coughing or valsalva maneuver
- o If PFO causes CVA, begin anti-platelet therapy
- o If recurrent CVA, perform surgical closure of PFO

Atrial Septal Defect (ASD)

➢ Types

- o Primum
  - Persistal hole in ostium primum, with incompetence of the AV valves.

- o Secundum ASD
  - Persistent hole in ostium secundum (second hole in the septum premum in not blocked off in the normal manner by the septum secundum)

➢ Clinical
- o May be asymptomatic, or associated with
  - Atrial fibrillation (AF)
  - Pulmonary artery hypertension
  - Tricuspid regurgitation (TR)
  - Complete heart block
  - Anomalous pulmonary venous drainage
  - PDA (patent ductus arteriosus)

Adapted from: Mangione S. *Hanley & Belfus* 2000, page 251.

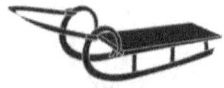

- Perform a focused physical examination for ASD.

o	Inspection	- No cyanosis unless PHT reverses shunt (RA → LA → LA → RA)
o	JVP	- Normal,, or - "a" and "v" waves become equal
o	Pulse	- May be associated with atrial fibrillation
o	Palpation	- PMI – normal, or diffuse - Heave – LSE (left sternal edge)

o	Heart sounds	. S_2
		  ▪ Wide
		  ▪ Split
		  ▪ Fixed

o	Murmur	- Large L → R shunt - Mid – diastolic - Tricuspid area - Murmur of TR, often with onset of AF - Murmur of mitral stenosis (MS)

MCQ Name Alert

ASD + MS murmur = Lutenbach syndrome

---

o	Signs of PHT	- Eisenmenger syndrome
o	Hand (Holt-oram syndrome)	- Hypoplastic thumb - Thumb is in line with other digits - Accessory phalanx

o	Associated syndromes	- Fallot trilogy
		  ▪ ASD
		  ▪ PS
		  ▪ RVH
		- Lutembacher syndrome
		  ▪ ASD
		  ▪ MS (rheumatic)

Abbreviation: PS, pulmonary stenosis; MS, mitral stenosis; RVH, right ventricular hypertrophy; PMI, apex impulse, point of maximum impulse; AF, atrial fibrillation; TR, tricuspid regurgitation.

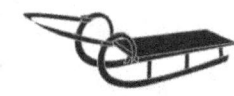

Atrial septal defect (ASD): ostium secundum (at the left sternal edge)

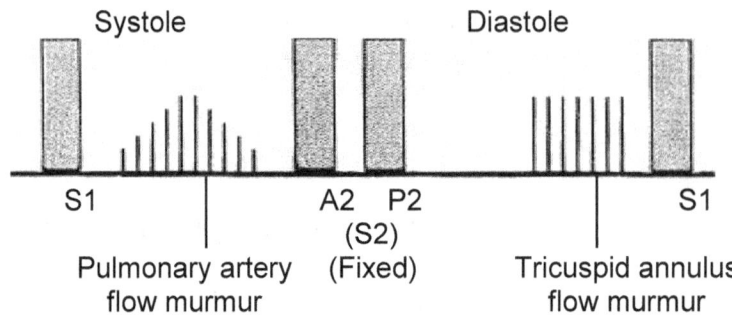

Adapted form: Talley NJ, et al. *Maclennan & Petty Pty Limited* 2003, page 84.

MCQ Alert

- Give what is the Murmur of ASD

  o ASD itself is not associatied with a murmur.

---

     o ECG   - RAD (right axis deviation)
                             - RBBB (right bundle branch block)

     o Note
        - These clinical and ECG findings may vary, depending upon whether the ASD is associated with
           ▪ MR (from a cleft in MV [mitral valve])
           ▪ TR (from cleft in TV [tricuspid valve])
           ▪ VSD (ventricular septal defect)

     o Another note:
        - Ostium primum – most commonly has associated MR, TR, VSD
        - Ostimum secundum – most frequent type

- Perform a focused physical examination to distinguish between a secundum and a primum ASD.

     o JVP
        - ↑ a wave
     o Murmur
        - Tricuspid diastolic murmur
        - Pulmonary systolic ejection murmur
        - Primum is also accompanied by pansystolic murmur (due to incompetent AV valves)
           ▪ RBBB plus left axis deviation

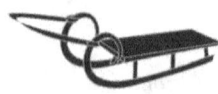

- o Sounds
  - ↑ P₂
  - P₂ widely split
- o ECG
  - RBBB plus right axis deviation

➤ Diagnosis
- o TTE (transthoracic echocardiogram)
- o Agitated saline contrast injection
- o Cardiac catheterization
  - Calculate pulmonary-to-systemic blood flow (Qp : Qs)

➤ Treatment
- o Indications
  - Symptoms
  - Associated pulmonary hypertension
  - When Qp : Qs > 1.5-2.0
  - ↑ RA, ↑ RV
  - Large L → R shunt
- o Ostium primum ASD defect → surgical closure
- o Ostium secundum ASD defect → percutaneous closure
- o Before placement of pacemaker (↓ risk of systemic thromboembolism)

➤ Contraindications
- o Normal pulse
- o Do not close an ASD if there is shunt reversal (L → R → L)

➤ Pregnancy planning
- o 10% of offspring children will have ASD
- o Higher risk of ASD is associated with genetic syndromes

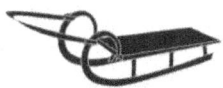

Dextrocardia

➢ Terms

➢ Clinical

- Perform a focused physical examination for dextrocardia.
  - Apex beat is on the right side.
  - Heart sounds heard on the right side of the chest
  - Liver dullness on the left side
  - Possible bronchiectasis
  - Mazinkonski's sign – not named after this person!
    - Dextrocardia without evidence of situs inversus, usually associated with cardiac malformation
    - May occur with cardiac malformation in Turner's syndrome

Source: Baliga RR. *Saunders/Elsevier*, 2007, page 83.

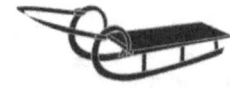

> Differential

- Perform a focused physical examination to distinguish between acquired versus congenital dextrocardia.

  o Congenital dextrocardia may be associated with
    - Basal bronchiectasis
    - Malformed frontal sinuses
    - Situs inversus (transposition of viscera, with dullness over left ribs anteriorly, and tympany over right ribs anteriorly

  o Acquired right lung disease
    - Collapse
    - Effusion (large)
    - Pneumothorax (large)

Ventricular Septal Defect (VSD)

Ventricular septal defect (VSD) (at the left sternal edge)

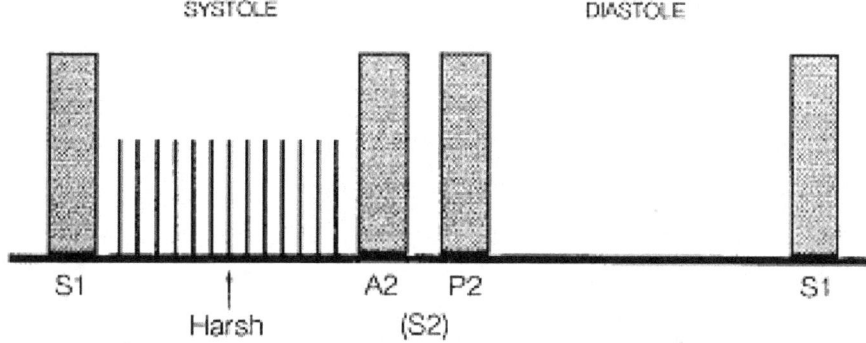

Source: Talley NJ, et al. *Maclennan & Petty Pty Limited* 2003, page 83.

  o LV → RV → development of PHT (pulmonary hypertension)

  o 4 types

  o May be close spontaneously

> Causes
  o Congenital
  o Rupture of the interventricular septum (e.g. complication of myocardial infarction)

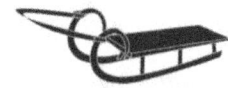

➤ Types

• Give the types of VSD.

   ○ The supracristal type (above the crista supraventricularis):
     - A high defect just below the pulmonary valve and the right coronary cusp of the aortic valve
     - The latter may not be adequately supported, resulting in aortic regurgitation
     - In Fallot tetralogy this defect is associated with the rightward shift of the interventricular septum
     - In double-outlet left ventricle with subaortic stenosis the supracristal defects associated with a leftward shift of the septum

   ○ The infracristal defect, which may be in either the upper membranous portion of the interventricular septum, or the lower muscular part
     - Small defects (maladie de Roger; curiously, a very loud murmur)
     - Swiss cheese appearance (multiple small defects)
     - Large defects
     - Gerbode defect (defect opening into the right atrium

Source: Baliga RR. *Saunders/Elsevier* 2007, page 169.

➤ Clinical

   ○ History of endocarditis

   ○ Day 3-7 post STEMI

   ○ New pansytolic murmur (left sternal edge)

   ○ Thrill, from high L→R flow

   ○ ~50% of VSDs occur with anterior wall MI (myocardial infarction)

   ○ Findings which suggest that the VSD is **hemodynamically important**

     - Apex, displaced LV impulse

     - Diastolic murmur (murmur)

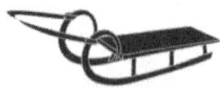

- Perform a focused physical examination for a ventricular septal defect.
    - ○ Pulse   – Usually normal
    - ○ Palpation   – PMI
        - ▪ Dynamic
        - ▪ Displaced - laterally
        - – Pulsation over pulmonary trunk and RV heave
        - – Thrill
            - ▪ L-LSE (left lower sterna edge)
    - ○ Heart sounds   – S_2 normal – with small defects
        - – S_2 split
        - – $A_2 \downarrow$ - with large defects
        - – P_2 only – RV = LV pressure
        - – $\uparrow P_2$ – PHT (pulmonary hypertension)
        - – The murmur of a VSD is usually
            - ▪ Pansystolic Q loudest in the L- ICS 3,4 (left third and fourth left intercostals spaces)
            - ▪ Radiates over the precordium
            - ▪ Associated thrill
            - ▪ Radiates to the axilla
            - ▪ Associated with a S_3
    - ○ Murmurs
        - – Small defect (muscular VSD)
            - ▪ Ejection murmur
            - ▪ High frequency
        - – Moderate defect
            - ▪ Systolic
                - -Pansystolic
                - -L-LSE
                - -Diminishes with development of PHT
            - ▪ Diastole
                - - Mid-diastole
                - - Rumple
                - - Apex
                - - Decrescendo if VSD associated with AR
        - – Continuous in systole and diastole, with no interval of a silent pause
        - – May cover entire systole, or be decrescendo, crescendo, or mixed crescendo/decrescendo
        - – Best heard L. LSB
        - – If there is a crescendo pattern, it starts after S_1
        - – Usually due to PDA (patent ductus arteriosus)
        - – When pulmonary hypertension (PHT) develops, diastolic component disappears.
        - – With further worser PHT, the continuous murmur completely disappears.

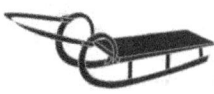

➢ Complications
  o Heart failure (HF)
  o RV outflow obstruction (muscular infundibular obstruction)
  o Aortic regurgitation
  o Infective endocarditis
  o Pulmonary hypertension and reversal of shunt L → R → R → L (Eisenmenger complex)
  o Pulmonary hypertension (PHT)
  o Bacterial endocarditis
  o Myocardial infarction (VSD from rupture of interventricular septum)

➢ Signs of associated conditions

  o VSD as part of a syndrome
    – Fallot tetralogy
    – TA (truncus arteriosus)
    – Double – outlet RV
    – AV canal defects
  o VSD as an association
    – Down syndrome
    – Transposition of the great arteries
    – PDA (patent ductus arteriosus)
    – ASD, secundum (arterial septal defect)
    – Coarctation of the aorta
    – Valvular defects
      ▪ Pulmonary stenosis
      ▪ Pulmonary atresia
      ▪ Tricuspid atresia

- In the context of VSD, give the meaning of Graham Steell murmur, and the Eisenmenger complex.

  o Graham Steell murmur   - Murmur of PR (pulmonary regurgitation) in person with VSD in which the flow through the defect decreases from the development of PHT, (the usual left - to- right shunting falls)

  o Eisenmenger complex   - The left - to – right flow in the VSD reverses with the development of pulmonary hypertension

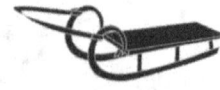

> Treatment

- Give the treatment of VSD.
  - Before development of pulmonary hypertension (PHT)
    - Percutaneous device closure
    - Surgical closure indicated for worsening
      - AR or TR
      - ↑ LV overload
      - Endocarditis, recurrent
  - After PHT develops (VSD RV → LV plus PHT = Eisenmenger syndrome)
    - Vasodilators for symptoms
    - Remember – closure is not done at this stage
    - Pregnancy planning
      - VSD + PHT
      - Recommended against pregnancy
    - High mortality
      - Medical therapy
        - > 90%
      - Surgical
        - > 50%

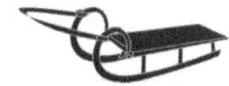

Mastering the Boards: Cardiology A.B.R. Thomson

~~~~~~

Cautionary Points about ASD and VSD

- o Do not close ASD if there is shunt reversal
- o Do not close VSD if there is large R → L shunt and pulmonary hypertension (Eisenmenger syndrome)

~~~~~~

Patent Ductus Arterosus (PDA)

➢ Definition

- o "Machinery" murmur heard best below the left clavicle in patient with persistent fistula between aorta and pulmonary artery
  - Clubbing
  - Small PDA plus history of endocarditis transcatheter closure large PDA + PHT
    - ▪ Do **not** close
- o Persistance of fetal connection between pulmonary artery into aorta

➢ Clinical

- Perform a focused physical examination for patent ductus arteriosus (PDA).

  - o Inspection
    - Cyanosis
    - Clubbing
      - "Differential cyanosis" in feet and not in hands

  - o Pulse
    - Collapsing
    - Differentiate from
      - AR (aortic regurgitation)
      - CHB (complete heart block)
      - Anemia
      - Hyperthyroidism
      - Paget's disease
    - ↑ PP due to ↓ DBP (PP = SBP-DBP)
    - Corrigan pulse (also seen in AR)

  - o Palpation
    - Heaving apex beat
    - Thrill, 2nd L-ICS
    - LA, ↑ LV (unless PHT develop
    - LVH, RVH; late, RV → LV shunt, with cyanosis

  - o Heart sounds
    - S_2 absent or widely split
    - ↑ P_2 with development of PHT

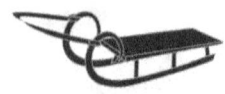

- o Murmur
  - Pansystolic (continuous "machinery") murmur, L-ICS-2
  - Continuous (systolic and diastolic) all over precordium, or medial to left midscapula
  - Systolic murmur begins after S_1, peaks with S_2, and may extend into early diastole (Gibson murmur)
  - Rarely only a systolic murmur
  - Differentiate from
    - Venous
      - Venous hum
      - AV anastomosis – intercostals vesssels, post rib fracture
      - AV fistula – coronary, pulmonary
    - Rupture sinus of valsalva
    - Murmur
      - MR plus AR
      - VSD plus AR

- o Associations
  - VSD (ventricular septal defect)
  - PS (pulmonary stenosis)
  - Coarctation of aorta
  - Hypoplastic left heart syndrome
  - Critical congenital aortic stenosis

- o Complications
  - Development of PHT
  - Signs of PHT
    - ↑ P_2
    - Clubbing and cyanosis of toes
  - Diastolic and then systolic murmur disappear
  - HF
  - Septic emboli
  - Bacterial endocarditis
  - Pulmonary artery endarteritis
  - Pulmonary emboli
  - Intraventricular bleeding
  - Broncho-pulmonary dysplasia
  - NEC (necrotizing enterocolitis)
  - Rupture of aneurysmal and calcified ductus

Abbreviation: L-ICS-2, second left intercostals space; PHT, pulmonary hypertension; LSE, left sterna edge; AR, aortic regurgitation; VSD, ventricular septal defect.

Adapted from: Baliga RR. *Saunders/Elsevier* 2007, pages 78 and 79.

 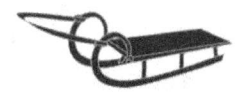

➢ Chest x-ray
- Large right atrium
- Right ventricular hypertrophy (RVH)
- Prominent, pulsating pulmonary arteries
- Hilar dance (prominent, pulsating hilar shadows)
- Small aorta

 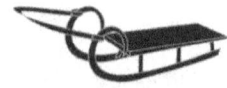

Tetralogy of Fallot

➢ Definition
  o VSD, subarterial
  o Pulmonary stenosis (PS), valvular or infundibular
  o Aortic override
  o RV hypertrophy

➢ Inheritance
  o Offspring of parents with TofF 5%
    - With chromosome 22q11.2 microdeletion, ~ 50%
  o Associated with Down syndrome
  o Dysmorphic facial characteristics not always present

➢ Clinical

• Perform a focused physical examination for tetralogy of Fallot.

  o Necessary findings
    - VSD with R → L shunt
    - PS (infundibular or valvular)
    - RVH
    - Dextroposition of the aorta, with overriding of the VSD

  o General
    - ↓ growth
    - Polycythemia

  o Skin/ hands
    - Clubbing
    - Central cyanosis

  o Precordium
    - Palpation
      ▪ Left parasternal heave with normal left ventricular impulse
    - Auscultation
      ▪ A2 > P2
      ▪ Ejection systolic murmur heard in the pulmonary area

• Give the physical findings after Blalock-Taussing shunt for tetratology of Fallot.

  o Radial pulse L < R
  o The arm on the side of the anastomosis (usually the left) may be smaller than the other arm
  o Blood pressure difficult to obtain (narrow pulse pressure in the arm supplied by the collateral vessels)
  o Thoracotomy scar

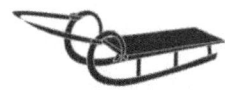

➢ Complications
  o Cyanotic and syncopal spells
  o Cerebral abscess
  o Endocarditis

➢ Associations - Conditions associated with Fallot (Stenson) tetralogy
  o Right-sided aortic arch
  o Double aortic arch
  o Left-sided superior vena cava (SVC)
  o Hypoplasia of the pulmonary arteries
  o Atrial septal defect (ASD)

Abbreviation: PS, pulmonary stenosis; RVH, right ventricular hypertrophy

Adapted from: Baliga RR. *Saunders/Elsevier* 2007, page 91.

SO YOU WANT TO BE A CARDIOLOGIST!

Fallot tetralogy is comprised of VSD with R → L shunt, pulmonary stenosis (PS), right ventricular hypertrophy (RVH), and dextroposition of the aorta.

• Give the extra feature which makes up Fallot pentology.

  o ASD
    - PHT plus reversed or bidirectional shunt from one of many cardiac defects (ASD, VSD, PDA)
  o Eisenmenger complex
    - VSD plus R → L shunt, without, or common associated PS

Source: Baliga RR. *Saunders/Elsevier* 2007, page 92.

SO YOU WANT TO BE A PEDIATRIC CARDIOLOGIST!

• Give the pathognomic "Coeur de sabot" finding on chest X-ray which suggest tetralogy of Fallot?

  o Aortic knuckle - normal
  o Pulmonary conus – concavity
  o Lower left heart border – upturned (due to RVH)
  o Hilum – enlarged right atrium and pulmonary artery
  o Lung fields – poorly seen

Abbreviation: RVH, right ventricular hypertrophy

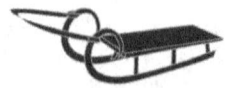

- Give the major extracardiac complications of cyanotic congenital heart disease.

  - CNS   - Cerebral emboli
    - Abscesses
  - Lung   - Hemorrhage
    - Thrombosis
  - Bone   - Scoliosis
    - Arthritis
    - Arthropathy
  - Kidney   - Dysfunction
  - GI   - Gallstones

➤ Treatment
  - Surgical repair
    - VSD
      ▪ Patch
    - PS
      ▪ Transannular patch → PR (pulmonary regurgitation) → TR (tricuspid regurgitation)
      ▪ Later replacement of pulmonary valve (percutaneous or surgical)
  - Control of atrial fibrillation
  - Consider maze procedure
  - Ambulation
  - Pneumatic compression devices
  - Filters on IV lines (↓ risk of paradoxical air embolism)
  - Phlebotomy for hyperviscosity syndrome
  - Treatment of iron deficiency
  - Operative correction before pregnancy

➤ Post-surgical follow-up (with TTE [transthoracic echocardiography]. CMR, catheterization)
  - PR (pulmonary valve regurgitation) → RV (right ventricular) dilation → TR (tricuspid regurgitation)
    - Requires reoperation
  - RVH (right ventricular hypertrophy)
    - ↑ risk of SCD (sudden cardiac death)
      ▪ Non-sustained VT (ventricular tachycardia)
      ▪ QRS > 180 msec

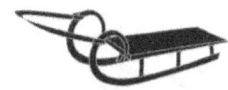

Eisenmenger Syndrome and Complex

➢ Definition
  o Pulmonary hypertension with a reverse or bidirectional shunt
  o Shunt (VSD, ASD, patent ductus arteriosus, persistent truncus arteriosus, single ventricle or common artrioventricular canal
  o Intracardiac L→ R shunt (from VSD, PAA, ASD) that reverses to R → L shunt and the development of cyanosis and pulmonary hypertension

➢ Clinical

SO YOU WANT TO BE A CARDIOLOGIST!

• Give the difference between Eisenmenger syndrome and complex.
  o Eisenmenger syndrome
    - PHT plus reversed or bidirectional shunt from one of many cardiac defects (ASD, VSD, PDA)
  o Eisenmenger complex
    - VSD plus R → L shunt, without, or common associated PS

• Give the findings on physical examination of the heart which suggest that the Eisenmenger complex is progressing to the Eisenmenger syndrome.
    o ↑ P2
    o Murmur becomes softer
    o L-side of heart becomes smaller

• In the context of Eisenmenger syndrome, give which type of associated shunt is the right ventricle enlarged?

  o With ASD causing Eisenmenger syndrome, the RV is enlarged.

  o Eisenmenger complex
    - Dextraposed aorta (partially arising from RV)
    - Large high VSD
    - Systolic murmur with a thrill; may have associated AR
    - Distinguish from tetrology of Fallot

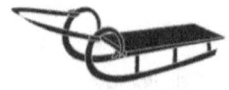

- Take a directed history and perform a focused physical examination for Eisenmenger syndrome.

- History
  - CNS
    - Cerebrovascular accidents (as a result of paradoxical embolization, venous thrombosis of cerebral vessels, or intracranial haemorrhage)
    - Sudden death
    - Brain abscess
  - Lung
    - Pulmonary embolization
    - Hemoptysis
  - Heart
    - Right ventricular failure
    - Paradoxical embolization
    - Infective endocarditis
  - Kidney
    - Hyperuricemia

- Physical examination
  - S2
    - VSD: single second sound
    - ASD: fixed, wide split second sound

Adapted from: Baliga RR. *Saunders/Elsevier* 2007, pages 88 and 89.

SO YOU WANT TO BE A PEDIATRIC CARDIOLOGIST!

- Give an example of a cyanotic cardiac condition where the cyanosis is more pronounced in the feet than in the hands.

  - Eisenmenger syndrome

HAVE YOU DECIDED NOT TO BE A PEDIATRIC BUT RATHER AN ADULT CARDIOLOGIST? NO WONDER!

- In the context of a systolic murmur, give the meaning of the 'Gallavardin phenomenon'.

  - The high-frequency components of the ejection systolic murmur may radiate to the apex, falsely suggesting mitral regurgitation (MR)

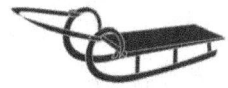

Mastering the Boards: Cardiology

A.B.R. Thomson

- Perform a focused physical examination of the cardiovascular system for Eisenmenger syndrome (ES).

  o General appearance
    - Central cyanosis (when R → L shunting occurs)
    - Cyanosis of lower torso > upper torso
    - Clubbing of fingers

  o JVP
    - 'a' waves
    - 'v' waves ES is associated with TR

  o Pulse
    - 'v' waves if AS is associated with TR
    - Atrial arrhythmias

  o Heart palpation
    - L. parasternal heave
    - Palpable P2

  o Heart sounds
    - ↑ P2
    - S2
      - Single VSD
      - Wide, fixed splitting of S2 – ASD
      - Reversed S2 splitting (A2 P2 → P2A2)
      - PDA: reverse split of second sound, and lower-limb cyanosis
    - Pulmonary ejection click

  o Murmurs
    - PR - early diastolic murmur (aka Graham Steell murmur)
    - TR - loud pansystolic murmur

  o Complications
    - HF
    - CVA
    - Brain abscess
    - SBE
    - Hemoptysis
    - Bleeding, thrombosis

Abbreviation: ASD, atrial septal defect; L, left side; PDA, patent ductus arteriosus; PHT, pulmonary hypertension; PR, pulmonary regurgitations; PTA, persistent truncus arteriosus; R, right side; RV, right ventricle; SBE, subacute bacterial endocarditis; SOL, space-occupying lesion; TR, tricuspid regurgitation; VSD, ventricular septal defect

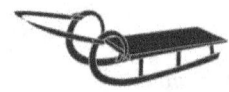

```
┌──────────────────────────────────────────────────────────────┐
│ SO YOU WANT TO BE A PEDIATRIC CARDIOLOGIST!                    │
│                                                                │
│ • Give when the hemodynamic severity of a VSD does not reflect │
│   its size.                                                    │
│ The hemodynamic severity is reflected by the L → R shunt. The  │
│ magnitude of this shunt may be reduced by                      │
│     ○ ↑ pulmonary arteriolar resistance                        │
│     ○ Hypertrophy of pulmonary outflow tract, leading to       │
│       pulmonary stenosis (from functional muscular             │
│       hypertrophic subvalvular pulmonary stenosis)             │
│                                                                │
│ • When does the typical pansystolic murmur of VSD occur only   │
│   in early systole.                                            │
│     ○ The VSD is usually in the membranous portion of the      │
│       ventricular septum. If the muscular part of the septum   │
│       contracts, the murmur occurs only in early systole.      │
└──────────────────────────────────────────────────────────────┘
```

➤ Treatment
- ○ Moderate exercise
- ○ Avoid high altitudes
- ○ Avoid long airplane rides
- ○ Prevent dehydration, iron deficiency
- ○ Avoid pregnancy (≥ 30% mortality rate)
- ○ Use IV lines with filters
- ○ Vasodilators

Hyperviscosity Syndrome

➤ Shunt

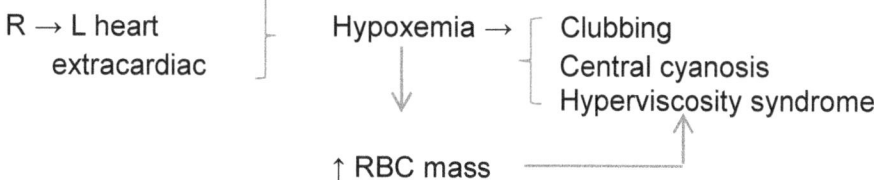

R → L heart extracardiac → Hypoxemia → Clubbing / Central cyanosis / Hyperviscosity syndrome; ↑ RBC mass

➤ Treatment
- ○ Phlebotomy plus fluid hydration ≤ 3 / yr when
  - - Hemoglobin > 20 g/dL
  - - Hematocrit > 65%
  - - Symptoms (no dehydration present)
- ○ Iron po for ~ 2 mon to replace iron lost by phlebotomy

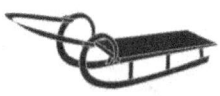

CARDIAC TUMORS

- Primary   -   Usually left atrial myxoma

- Secondary   -   Direct spread or metastasis
    - Lung, breast
    - Kidney, hepatocellular, adrenal (grow into IVC [inferior venacava] → right atrium)

- In all patients with LA myxoma, resect to ↓ risk of embolization

Ne'er walked the earth a greater man than he.

Micheal Angelo

 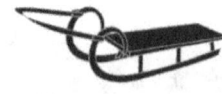

DISORDERS OF NON-CARDIAC VESSELS

Lower Leg Pain and Ulcers

➢ Clinical

- Perform a focused physical examination to determine the cause of leg pain.

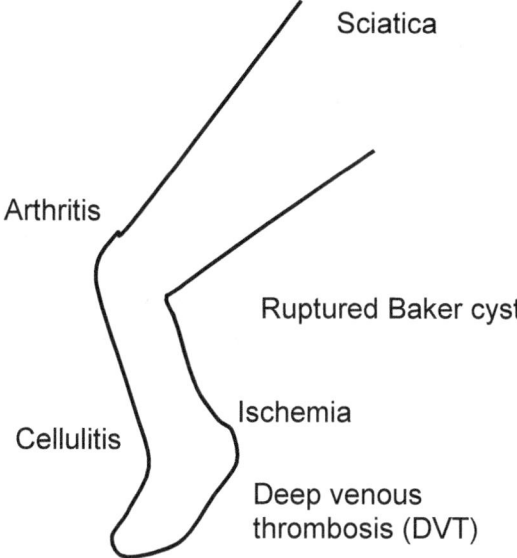

Adapted from: Davey P. *Wiley-Blackwell* 2006, page 17.

- Take a directed history for lower leg ulcers.

    - o Vein
        - Stasis, with pigmentation and stasis eczema around lateral malleoli

    - o Artery
        - Large vessel: artherosclerosis, thrombangitis obliterans
        - Small vessel: vasculitis (diabetes mellitus [DM], rheumatoid arthritis [RA], sickle cell disease)
        - Nerve: Peripheral neuropathy: DM, syphilis

    - o Skin
        - Benign
            - Pyoderma gangrenosum
            - S. Aureus
            - Tuberculosis (TB)
            - Fungus

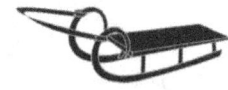

- Malignant
  - Basal cell cancer
  - Squamous cancer
  - Lymphoma
  - Melanoma
  - Kaposi sarcoma
- o Grading (pressure sores)
  - Grade I: erythema, skin intact.
  - Grade II: skin loss, epidermis or dermis (abrasion, blister, shallow crater).
  - Grade III: full thickness loss and damage to subcutaneous tissues.
  - Grade IV: extensive destruction, tissue necrosis or damage to the underlying muscle or bone.

Abbreviations: DM, diabetes mellitus; RA, rheumatoid arthritis; TB, tuberculosis

Adapted from: Talley NJ, et al. *Maclennan & Petty Pty Limited* 2003, Table 3.12, page 66; Ghosh AK. *Mayo Clinic Scientific Press* 2008, page 1053; Baliga RR. *Saunders/Elsevier* 2007, page 621.

- o Interpretation of findings

		Possible pathology	Finding
• Arterial	o	Raynaud disease	- Sharply demarcated pallor in fingers that changes over several minutes - Normal wrist pulses

	o	Arterial insufficiency	- Ulcers:
			  • Distal aspects of foot
			  • Painful
			  • Rapidly developing
			  • Often erythematous when infected

	o	Chronic arterial insufficiency	- Cool, pale extremity with hair loss
	o	Vasculitis	- Headache, temple soreness - Changes in skin colour and temperature - Swelling

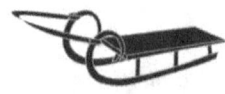

	Possible pathology	Finding
• Venous	○ Superficial phlebitis	- Warmth, painful to touch - Erythema due to inflammation of tissue around the vein
	○ Acute DVT	- Pain secondary to inflammation in the absence of superficial changes - Swelling of distal part of the extremity
	○ Venous obstruction	- Prominent veins in an edematous limb
	○ Chronic venous insufficiency	- Skin: - Warm and erythematous - Thickened skin (woody) - Increased pigmentation - May have brownish ulcers around the ankles

Abbreviation: DVT, deep vein thrombosis

Permission granted: McGee SR. *Saunders/Elsevier* 2007, Table 1, page 249.

- Take a directed history and perform a focused physical examination of the most common types of lower leg ulcer.

	Type of ulcer			
	Venous	Arterial	Arteriolar	Neurotrophic
• History				
○ Onset	Trauma +/-	Trauma	Spontaneous	Trauma
○ Course	Chronic	Progressive	Progressive	Progressive
○ Pain	No (unless infected)	Yes	Yes	No
• Physical (ulcer)				
○ Location	Medial aspects of leg	Toe, heel, foot	Lateral, posterior aspect of foot	Plantar
○ Surrounding skin	Stasis changes	Atrophic	Normal	Callous
○ Ulcer edges	Shaggy	Discrete	Serpiginous	Discrete
○ Ulcer base	Healthy	Eschar, pale	Eschar, pale	Healthy or pale

Source: Ghosh AK. *Mayo Clinic Scientific Press* 2008, page 1053.

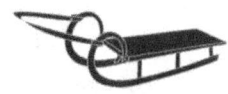

494

- Take a directed history to differentiate between intermittent claudication (from atherosclerosis and peripheral vascular disease) and pseudoclaudication (from spinal stenosis).

	Claudication	Pseudoclaudication
o Character	Cramp, ache	"Parasthetic" pins and needles
o Bilateral	+/-	+
o Onset	Walking	Walking & Standing
o Walking distance	Constant	Variable
o Relief	Standing still	Sitting down, leaning forward

Adapted from: Ghosh AK. *Mayo Clinic Scientific Press* 2008, page 1044.

Peripheral Vascular Disease (PVD)

➢ Definition
   - Arterial and venous insufficiency in the lower leg
   - Atherosclerosis of the aortic bifurcation or arteries of the legs, leading to ↓ ABI (ankle-brachial index, leg SBP / ARM ABP [systolic blood pressure] of ≤ 0.90
   - Each ↓ ABI by 0.1 is associated with a 10% ↑ risk of a major CV (cardiovascular) event

- Give the main diseases affecting arteries of varying sizes.

Size of artery	Main lesions
o Large	– Arteriosclerosis – Syphilis – Embolism (due to clots, or rarely tumour or fungus emboli) – Takayasu disease
o Medium	– Polyarteritis nodosa – Monckeberg sclerosis – Giant cell arteritis – Buerger's disease – Arteritis of severe infection and malignancy – Embolism – Arteriosclerosis

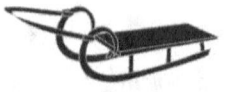

Size of artery	Main lesions
o Small arteries and arterioles	– Hypertension – Dermatomyositis – Scleroderma – Raynaud's phenomena – Rheumatoid arthritis – Ergotism

Source: Davey P. *Wiley-Blackwell* 2006, page 233.

- Give 3 common effects of diabetes on blood vessels.

  - o Atheroma
  - o Hypertensive arterial sclerosis
  - o Small vessel disease
    - Retina
      - Microaneurysm
      - Retinitis
    - Kidney
      - Intercapillary glomerulosclerosis

- Give the differences in the signs & causes of peripheral vascular disease (PVD).

  - o Obstructive
    - Claudication
    - Absent pulses
    - Colour changes
      - Leg elevation – foot blanching
      - Leg depression – slow venous filling
    - Common causes
      - Atherosclerosis

    - Atrial tachycardia
      - Polyarteritis
      - Embolism
  - o Non – obstructive
    - Raynaud's phenomenon (white, blue, red)
    - Pain
    - Paresthesia
    - Coldness
    - Common causes (AT-complete)

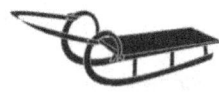

Clinical Tip

From the location of exercise-associated leg pain, or a bruit / murmur, give the approximate location of the narrowing on the artery in the person with PAD (peripheral arterial disease).

Site	Artery
Buttock, thigh	Aortoiliac area
Calf, upper leg	Superficial femoral
Lower leg, foot	Popliteal area

- Take a directed history for and perform a focused physical examination for peripheral vascular disease (arterial and venous insufficiency) in the lower extremities.

- History

  - Claudication
    - Leg claudication
    - Location and severity of pain at rest, on exertion, at night
    - Onset/offset
    - Distance to develop claudication
    - Aching in lower legs, especially when dependent
    - Parathesia
    - Pallor
    - Paralysis
  - Impotence
  - Associated conditions/risk factors
    - Hypertension
    - Hyperlipidemia
    - Hyperhomocysteinemia
    - Obesity
    - Diabetes
    - Physical inactivity
    - Smoking
    - Causes of L/R- HF
    - Family history
  - Personal past history of CAD, PVD, rheumatic fever, cardiac murmur, cardiac surgery, cardiac events, medications

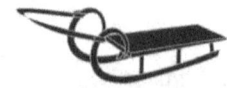

- Physical examination

- Inspection
  - Pulses
    - Compare femoral, popliteal, tibial, dorsalis, pedis pulses; carotid, radial, brachial, abdominal aorta and renal arteries
    - Asymmetrical foot coolness
    - Pallor on leg elevation
    - Redness on leg dependency (positive Buerger test)
    - Muscle atrophy
    - Bruits, thrills of abdominal aorta and femoral arteries

  - ↓ pulse femoral, popliteal arteries
  - ABI and/or symptoms of
    - ≤ 0.90, compatible with PVD
    - ≤ 0.40, usually accompanied by ischemic rest pain

  - Signs and /or symptoms of
    - Diabetes
    - Hyperlipidemia
  - Limbs
    - Size
    - Symmetry
    - Edema
    - Muscle atrophy

  - Skin
    - Colour/pigmentation
    - Texture
    - Loss of hair on toes
    - Ulcers/scars
    - Gangrene
    - Nails (colour, texture)
    - Venous distribution (engorgement, varicosities)

- Palpation
  - Temperature (compares both limbs)
  - Capillary refill (compares both limbs)
  - Edema (compares both limbs)
  - Pulses (rate, rhythm, amplitude, waveform)
  - Palpation: carotid, radial, brachial, abdominal aorta; renal, femoral, popliteal, dorsalis pedis, tibial arteries
  - Pitting edema

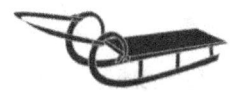

- Auscultation
  - o Bruits (carotid, abdominal aorta, renal, iliac, femoral)

- Special manoeuvres
  - o Leg elevation test for pallor
  - o Dependency test for dusky rubor

Trendelenburg	Perthe
o Raise leg from supine position to drain the veins	- While patient stands, apply tourniquet to mid thigh
o Apply tourniquet to mid thigh	- Instruct patient to walk for 5 minutes and watch what happens to the engorged veins while the tourniquet is in place.
o Have patient stand and watch the refilling of the collapsed veins with and without the tourniquet	

  - o Interpretation
    - - Tourniquet in place, with standing the initially collapsed;
      - ▪ veins below the tourniquet become more engorged with walking (and pain develops in the leg) → the valves of the communicating veins are incompetent and the DVS is blocked;
      - ▪ veins below tourniquet empty with walking → valves of communicating veins are competent, and deep venous system (DVS) is competent;
    - - saphenous vein (SV) refills → the valves of the communicating veins are incompetent (backfilling)

  - o Tourniquet removed; with standing
    - - Veins below the tourniquet are still engorged with walking, the valves of both the communication and the saphenous vein are incompetent; the initially collapsed SV refills → the valves of the SV are incompetent (backfilling)

What is" the best"?

  - o The "best tests" for diagnosing PVD from physical examination are
    - - Wounds or sores on foot
    - - Abnormal foot colour or coolness
    - - Absent pulses
    - - Limb bruit
    - - Venous filling time > 20 seconds

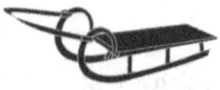

Mastering the Boards: Cardiology   A.B.R. Thomson

SO YOU WANT TO BE A CARDIOLOGIST!

- In the context of peripheral vascular disease, give what is the Buerger test.

  o Blanching" upon raising legs and "rubor" on dependency

- In the context of peripheral vascular disease, give what is the De Weese test.

  o Disappearance of palpable distal pulses after exercise

- Tests of arterial insufficiency

➢ Clinical
   o Ankle/brachial index – compare palpated systolic BP values in brachial and either dorsalis pedis or posterior tibial arteries (normal A/B >1)
   o Capillary refill time
   o Venous filling time
   o Ausculatory bruit

➢ Diagnostic imaging

   o Doppler ultrasound, CTA, MRA (CT or MR angiography), invasive angiography

SO YOU WANT TO BE A CARDIOLOGIST!

When ratio of the ipsilateral blood pressure in the ankle to the brachial artery (ABI) is ≤ 0.90, then PVD (peripheral vascular disease) is suggested. However, diabetes is associated with PVD, and in diabetes the arteries may be calcified, leading to an increase in ABI, perhaps into the normal range. Thus, in diabetes the ABI may be falsely normal (> 0.90), even if these truly is PVD.

- Give the clinical test for PVD which should be performed in the patient with a non-compressible artery and ABI > 90

   o Determine the TBI, the toe-brachial index

Abbreviations: BP, blood pressure; CAD, coronary artery disease; L/R-CHF, left-/right-sided congestive cardiac failure; PVD, peripheral vascular disease

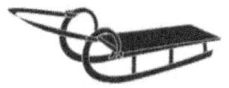

➤ Differential

- o Arteries   - Popliteal entrapment syndrome
-    - Chronic compartment syndrome

- o Vein

- o PNS   - Sensory neuropathy
-    - Lumbar radiculopathy
-    - Lumbar spinal stenosis

- o Muscle   - Tenderness
-    - Wasting

Abbreviation: PNS, peripheral nervous system

Adapted from: Jugovic PJ, et al. *Saunders/ Elsevier* 2004, page 143.

- Within the context of PVD (peripheral vascular disease), give the meaning of the Leriche syndrome.

- o The Leriche syndrome is atherosclerotic obstruction within the aortoiliac system resulting in
  - ↓ femoral pulses
  - Claudication in the hip and buttocks
  - ED (erectile dysfunction)

➤ Grading system for lower extremity arterial occlusive disease

| | ABI | |
Grade	Supine Resting	Post exercise
o Normal	1.0-1.4	No change or increase
o Mild disease	0.8-0.9	> 0.5
o Moderate disease	0.5-0.8	> 0.2
o Severe disease	< 0.5	< 0.2

Abbreviation: ABI, ankle to brachial systolic pressure index

Source: Ghosh AK. *Mayo Clinic Scientific Press* 2008, Table 25-3, page 1044.

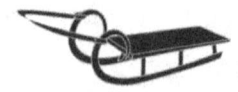

- Give the grading system for lower extremity arterial occlusive disease (AOD), using ankle – to – brachial systolic pressure index

Grade of AOD	Supine Resting	Post exercise
o Normal	1.0-1.4	No change or increase
o Mild	0.8-0.9	> 0.5
o Moderate	0.5-0.8	> 0.2
o Severe	< 0.5	< 0.2

Source: Ghosh AK. *Scientific Press*, 2008, Table 25-3, page 1044.

- Take a focused history and perform a directed physical examination to distinguish between chronic vs acute (critical) ischemia.

		Acute	Chronic
o Pain	- At rest	+	-
	- With exercise	-	+
	- Predictable distance	-	+
	- Relief with rest	-	+
o Examination	- Ulcers	+	-
	- Gangrene	+	-
	- Bruits	+	-

Adapted from Jugovic PJ, et al. *Saunders/ Elsevier* 2004, pages 143-5.

- Give the performance characteristics of physical examination for peripheral vascular disease (PVD).
  - o While the previously taught physical findings of atrophic skin, absent lower limb hair and capillary refill time ≥ 5 seconds all have positive likelihood ratios of < 2, other traditional signs have considerable merit.

Finding	PLR
o Inspection	
- Wounds or sores on foot	7.0
- Foot colour abnormally pale, red, or blue	2.8
- Atrophic skin	1.7
- Absent lower limb hair	1.7

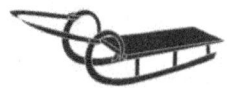

Finding	PLR
o Palpation	
- Foot asymmetrically cooler	6.1
- Absent femoral pulse	6.1
- Absent posterior tibial and dorsalis pedis pulses	14.9
- At least one pedal pulse present	
o Auscultation	
- Limb bruit present	7.3
o Ancillary tests	
- Capillary refill time ≥5 seconds	1.9
- Venous filling time > 20 seconds	3.6

Abbreviations: PLR, positive likelihood ratio; NLR, negative likelihood ratio; NS, not significant; PVD, peripheral vascular disease

Adapted from: McGee SR. *Saunders/Elsevier* 2007, Box 50-1, page 600.

> Differential

- Take a directed history and perform a focused physical examination to differentiate between arterial vs venous insufficiency.

	Arterial insufficiency	Venous insufficiency
History of pain		
o Location	- Toes, points of previous trauma, lateral malleolus	- Medial and lateral malleoli
o Pain	- Intermittent claudication (exercise pain), rest pain	- None, or ache in lower legs on dependency
o Paraesthesia	- Yes	- No
o Paralysis	- Yes	- No
Physical examination		
o Skin		
- Colour	Pale, pigmented, Shiny atropic	Brown red
- Thickness	↑	N
- Ulcers	Yes (medial malleolus)	Yes (lateral malleolus)
- Temperature	Cold	Warm
- Tenderness	Yes	Yes
- Swelling	Yes	Yes
- Prominent veins	No	Yes
- Loss of hair	Yes	No

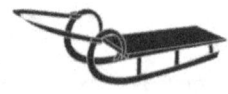

	Arterial insufficiency	Venous insufficiency
o Skin	- Gangrene - Thick, ridged nails	- Skinny leg
o Palor	- White (leg up), red (leg down)	- Normal, or blue (leg down)
o Palor (cold)	- Yes	- No
o Pitting edema	- Yes	- Yes
o Pulses	- ↓	- Normal
o Bruit	- Yes	- No

Adapted from: Filate W, et al. *The Medical Society, Faculty of Medicine, University of Toronto*, 2005, page 249; Jugovic PJ, et al. *Saunders/ Elsevier* 2004, page 144.

General Reminder

    o Aortoiliac disease is associated with ↑↑ risk of distal embolization

---

- Perform a focused physical examination to **distinguish between peripheral vascular disease** (PVD) **and Spinal Stenosis** (SpSt).

	PVD	SpSt
↓ / absent pulses	+	-
↑ pain		
- With exercise	+	-
↓ pain		
- Standing	-	+
- With rest	+	-
- When sitting / lying	-	+
- Bend forward	-	+

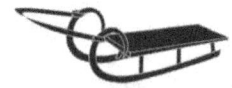

➤ Treatment

- o Screening
  - ≥ 65 yr
  - ≥ 55 yr plus smoking, or diabetes
  - Leg symptoms with exertion
  - Non-healing leg ulcers

- o Risk management
  - Smoking cessation program
  - Treat associated
    - Hypertension
      - Targets < 140 / 90 mm Hg
      - Diabetes, CKD < 130 / 80 mm Hg
    - > 24 h poor prognosis
      Hyperlipidemia (target cholesterol < 100 mg/dL) (statins)
    - Diabetes
    - Weight management
    - Ramipril (to ↓ risk of MI, CVA, vascular death)
    - B-blocker if indicated for other reasons

- o Anti-platelet agents
  - ASA
  - Clopidogrel

- o Pain control
  - Exercise
  - Cilostazol
  - Pentoxifylline for non-tolerance of cilostazol

- o Revascularization
  - Aortioliac artery
    - Endovascular stenting
  - Common femoral artery
    - End arterectomy, with possible surgical repair
  - Superficial femoral artery
    - < 3 cm length endovascular
    - > 5 cm open surgery

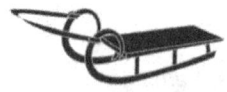

Cilostazol is a phosphodiesterase inhibitor used to ↑ pain-free walking distance in persons who have PAD (peripheral artery disease).

- Give the properties which contribute to the usefulness of cilostazol in persons with PAD (peripheral arterial disease), and give its major contraindication.
  - o Cilostazol has properties which contribute to its usefulness to treat peripheral vascular disease, including
    - Anti-platelet aggregation
    - Arterial vasodilation
    - Must not be used in presence of HF (heart failure)
  - o Clinical caution: do not use ciclitazol for PVD when there is
    - A history of HF
    - Current ↓ LVEF

Internittent claudication may be caused by PVD (peripheral arterial disease) or by spinal stenosis (SpSt)

Acute Limb Ischemia (ALI)

➢ Pathogenesis
  - o Acute and marked reduction in blood flow to limb resulting from
    - Severe atherosclerosis
    - Associated
      - ▪ Thrombosis
      - ▪ Embolization

➢ Clinical
  - o Limb pain at rest
  - o ↓ muscle power
  - o ↓ sensation
  - o ↓ pulse (including on Doppler ultrasound)
  - o Pale, cool limb

➢ Treatment
  - o Risk stratification for medical or surgical therapy (please see below)
  - o Suggested general approach to urging and treatment choice for ALI (acute limb ischemia)
  - o Anti-platelet and heparin therapy
  - o Intra-arterial thrombosis

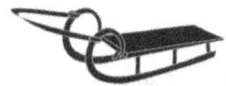

- o Surgery
  - - Expected survival
    - • > 2 yr, bypass surgery
      < 2 yr, balloon angioplasty
  - - Below the knee implant
    - • Drug-eluting stent

	Doppler study arterial blood flow	Muscle weak	Sensation loss	Treatment
o Action needed now	Yes	No	No	Anti-platelet and anti-thrombotic therapy
	No	No	Toes	
o Urgent	No	Mild-moderate	>toes	Revascularization bypass angioplasty stent
o Too late	No	Severe	Marker	Amputation

Peripheral Pulses

"Keeping your finger on the pulse"

Mangione Pearls

- o "The greater amplitude of distal arteries makes them better suited for the evaluation of salable findings, such as pulsus paradoxus and pulsus alternans"

- o "The analysis of the arterial pulse for the evaluation of left ventricular outflow obstruction is less reliable in older patients with hypertension or atherosclerosis"

Adapted from: Mangione S. *Hanley & Belfus* 2000, page 180.

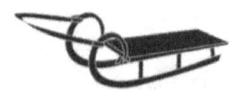

Arterial Pulse

- o The primary upstroke wave occurs in systole, and is palpable

- o The percussion wave is the early part of the primary wave, which is caused by the ejection of blood from the LV into the central aorta

- o The interface between the percussion wave and the tidal wave is the anacrotic notch (not palpable, only seen on tracings)

- o The tidal wave is the mid – to – late systolic part of the primary wave, (forward flow) which is caused by the passage of blood from the central to the peripheral portions of the aorta (reverse flow).

Adapted from: Mangione S. *Hanley & Belfus*, 2000, page 182.

Shape / Contour

There are three types of double – peak pulses, pulsus bisferiens, bifid pulse, and dicrotic pulse.

- • Pulse contours

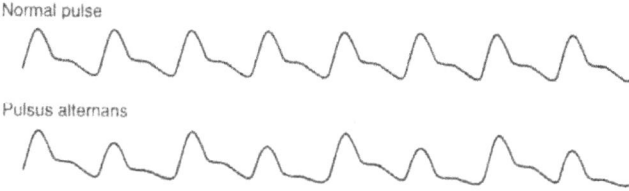

Normal pulse

Pulsus alternans

- o **Pulsus alternans** is a regular pulse that has alternating strong and weak beats.

Pulsus bisferiens

- o **Pulsus bisferiens** and the dicrotic pulse have two beats per cardiac cycle; and both beats are systolic.

  - o A double – peaked arterial pulse, with both peaks in systole, and both peaks usually the same height (strength)
  - o Characterized by   - Rapid upstroke
    - ↑ amplitude
    - Rapid downstroke

  - o Caused by   - Aortic regurgitation
    - High output states
  - o The pulsus bisferiens may be heard as a
    - "pistol shot" femoral bruit
    - Duroziez' double murmur

Adapted from: Mangione S. *Hanley & Belfus* 2000, page 185.

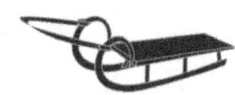

    o   In persons with combined AR plus AS, what is the typical pulse?

         Biferiens

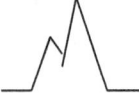

- Bifid pulse

➢ The "spike and dome" double pulse is palpated at the bedside only when there is severe HOCM.
  - The initial "spike" is caused by early and rapid emptying of the LV.
  - The second "dome" wave of the bifid pulse is caused by the emptying which occurs after the HOCM-associated obstruction.

Source: Mangione S. *Hanley & Belfus*, 2000, page 185.

- Dicrotic pulse

Dicrotic pulse

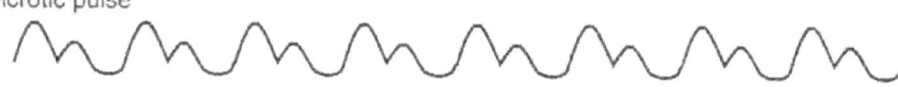

- In the dicrotic pulse one is systolic and the other beat is diastolic.
- The first peak is from emptying of the LV during systole
- The second peak is from emptying in diastole
- Longer interval between first and second peak than the shorter interval in the bisferiens or bifid pulse.
- The dicrotic pulse requires elastic arteries to be palpated (not palpated in older persons)
- Causes: low-output states
  - Pericardial tamponade (during inspiration
  - Severe congestive cardiomyopathy

Pulsus paradoxus   Inspiration

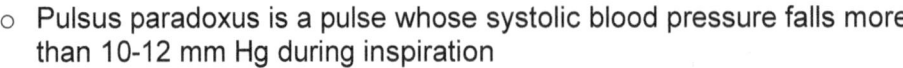

- Pulsus paradoxus is a pulse whose systolic blood pressure falls more than 10-12 mm Hg during inspiration

Pulsus Paradoxus

➢ Definition

  o ↓ SBP ≥ 20 mmHg on inspiration

• Perform a focused physical examination for pulsus paradoxus (exaggeration of normal fall.

➢ Heart
  o L-/R- HF
  o Pericarditis ± tamponade
  o AR
  o ASD

➢ Lung
  o COPD

Abbreviation HF, heart failure; AR, Aortic regurgitation; ASD, atrial septal defect

Adapted from: Mangione S. *Hanley & Belfus* 2000, pages 30-31and 63-66 .

  o What is the effect of inspiration on pulse rate and volume?
    – ↑ pulse rate and volume
  o When pulse rate and volume decrease on inspiration, this is called "pulses paradoxicus"
    – Pulsus paradoxicus is commonly caused by
      ▪ Reactive airway disease (asthma)
      ▪ Constrictive pericarditis pericardial effusion
      ▪ Obstruction of the SVC (superior vena cava)

xxxxxxxxxxxxxxxxxxxxxxxxxxxxxxxxxxxxxxxxxxxxxxxxxxxx

SO YOU WANT TO BE A CARDIOLOGIST!

• What is "**reversed** pulsus paradoxus"?

  o Pulsus paradoxus: inspiratory fall in systolic blood pressure (SBP) > 12 mm Hg (some authors say >10 mm Hg)
  o Reversed pulsus paradoxus:
    – Expiratory fall in SBP>10 mm Hg
    – Caused by
      ▪ HOCM
      ▪ inspiration
      ▪ acceleration of the sinus heart rate
      ▪ intermittent inspiratory positive pressure breathing in L-CHF.

Source: Mangione S. *Hanley & Belfus* 2000, page 31.

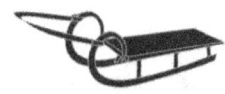

Mastering the Boards: Cardiology   A.B.R. Thomson

SO YOU WANT TO BE A CARDIOLOGIST!

- About 98% of persons with pulsus paradoxus have cardiac tamponade. Give the other causes.

- Lung
    - Mechanical ventilation, the amount of pulsus paradoxus, correlates with the degree of the patient's auto-positive end-expiratory pressure (auto-PEEP) (a measure of expiratory difficulty in ventilated patients).
    - Hyperventilation
    - Valsalva maneuver
    - HF
    - Asthma
    - Emphysema
    - Obesity

- Heart
    - Atrial septal defect (ASD)
    - Severe left ventricular dysfunction (especially with uremic pericarditis)
    - Regional tamponade (tamponade affecting only one or two heart chambers, a complication of cardiac surgery)
    - Severe hypotension
    - Aortic regurgitation (AR) - **BEWARE**: with AR from type A aortic dissection, the hemopericardium may eliminate the pulsus paradoxus (PP), so the lack of PP in a person with dissection does not exclude tamponade.

Source: McGee SR. *Saunders/Elsevier* 2007, page 130.

SO YOU WANT TO BE A CARDIOLOGIST!

- Give causes a rapid arterial upstroke when input and cardiac pulse pressure are normal.
    - VSD, mitrial regurgitation
    - HOCM (hypertropic obstructive cardiomyopathy

A rapid arterial upstroke occurs with high output states (e.g. anemia, exercise, thyrotoxicosis, pregnancy, beriberi, Paget disease; AV fistulas
- Give the meaning of "spike and dome bifid pulse"?
    - First peak from rapid early-systolic emptying of ventricle, then an obstruction, followed by another emptying (second peak).
    - Association with severe HOCM

Source: Mangione S*Hanley & Belfus* 2000, page 185.

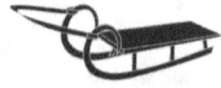

Pulsus Parvus et Tardus

➢ Definition

- A pulse that has a small volume and rises slowly (slow upstroke amplitude)

Pulsus parvus et tardus

➢ Pathophysiology
- ↓ LV outflow, e.g. aortic stenosis
- ↓ LV contraction, e.g. cardiomyopathy
- ↓ LV filling, e.g. mitral stenosis

SO YOU WANT TO BE A CARDIOLOGIST!

- Give the difference in the cause of pulsus parvus by itself versus pulsus parvus et pulsus tardus.

  - Pulsus parvus, ↓ amplitude of upstroke
    - ↓ LV contraction
    - ↓ LV filling
  - Pulsus parvus and pulsus tardus
    - Amplitude plus slow upstroke
    - Aortic stenosis (AS)
    - Mitral stenosis (MS)
    - Cardiomyopathy
    - ↓ LV filling or contraction

SO YOU WANT TO BE A CARDIOLOGIST!

- Give the difference between pulsus parvus plus tardis, versus hyperkinetic pulse.

  - Pulsus parvus plus pulsus tardis (low amplitude plus slow upstroke) usually means presence of aortic stenosis
  - Hyperkinetic pulse (rapid upstroke, high amplitude): wide pulse pressure, aortic regurgitation. Normal pulse pressure, mitral regurgitation

---

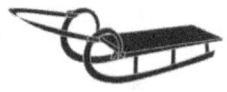

- Description of characteristic pulses

Pulse	Description	Causes
o Pulsus parvus (Hypokinetic pulse)	– Small volume, weak pulse from ↓ LVSV	▪ Hypovolemia ▪ LV failure ▪ Shock ▪ MI ▪ Restrictive pericardial disease ▪ Arrhythmia
o Pulsus tardus	– Small volume, slowly rising pulse – Delayed with respect to heart sounds	▪ Aortic stenosis
o Hyperkinetic pulse	– Strong, bounding pulse	▪ SV - Heart block - Hyperdynamic circulation - Fever - Anemia - Exercise - Anxiety ▪ Reduced peripheral resistance - Patent ductus arteriosus - Arteriovenous fistula
o Collapsing	– Quick rise, quick fall	▪ ↑ CO
o Waterhammer	– Quick rise, full expansion, quick fall	▪ AR
o Bisferiens	– Double peaked pulse, mid systolic dip	▪ AR, AS ▪ Hypertrophic cardiomyopathy
o Alternans	– Alternating amplitude of pulses (More easily detected in conjunction with blood pressure measurement)	▪ HF

Abbreviations : LVSV, left ventricular stroke volume; LV, left ventricle; MI, myocardial infarction; SV, stroke volume CHF, congestive heart failure ; CO, cardiac output ; AR, Aortic regurgitation ; AS, Aortic stenosis

Source: Filate W, et al. *The Medical Society, Faculty of Medicine, University of Toronto* 2005, Table 3, page 251 and Table 4, page 252.

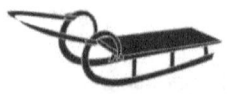

SO YOU WANT TO BE A CARDIOLOGIST!

- Palpation of the peripheral arterial pulse is a time-honoured part of the physical examination. Under what circumstances should you palpate the peripheral arteries on both sides of the body, the peripheral arteries in the upper and lower portions of the body, and the carotid or brachial arteries?

  o Right and left sides, considering possible asymmetry
  - Thrombosis
  - Atherosclerosis
  - Embolism
  - Dissection
  - External compression/ occlusion

  o Upper and lower peripheral arteries
  - In hypertension patient who may have coarctation of the aorta, or supravalvular aortic stenosis

  o Central arteries
  - When trying to characterize the form of the arterial wave

Hyperkinetic pulse

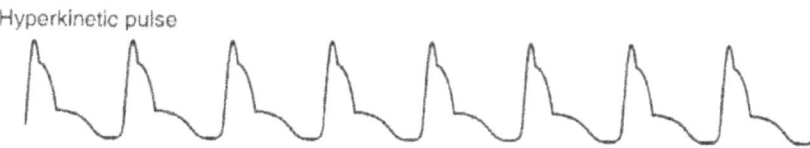

- Perform a focused physical examination for causes of rapid ventricular contraction and low peripheral vascular resistance.

  o AV fistula
  o Thyrotoxicosis
  o Exercise
  o Anemia
  o Paget's disease
  o Beriberi
  o Pregnancy

- Perform a focused physical examination of the pulse to distinguish between the hyperkinetic pulse of AR versus MR.
  o Definition of hyperkinetic pulse
  - Rapid upstroke ($\uparrow$ speed of contraction)
  - $\uparrow$ amplitude ($\uparrow$ SV [stroke volume])
  o AR - $\uparrow$ PP (pulse pressure)
  o MR – PP is normal

Permission granted: McGee SR. *Saunders/Elsevier* 2007, page 125.

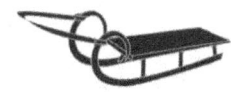

- Take a focused history and perform a directed physical examination for causes of **hyperkinetic heart syndrome** causing an abnormally wide pulse pressure (PP) (PP > 50% of systolic BP).

➢ Increased pulse pressure
  o Heart
    - Aortic regurgitation
    - Patent ductus arteriosus (PDA)
    - AV fistula
  o Lung
    - Hypercapnia
  o Metabolic
    - Fever
    - Anemia
    - Beriberi
    - Hyperthyroidism
  o Bone
    - Paget disease
  o Liver
    - Cirrhosis
  o Skin
    - Severe exfoliative dermatitis
  o Pregnancy

➢ Reduced pulse pressure (PP; PP < 25% of SBP).
  o Aortic stenois
  o Constrict percarditis
  o Cardiac tamponade
  o Tachycardia
  o Hypotension

➢ Differences in blood pressure between arms or between arms or between the arms and legs.
  o Occlusion or stenosis of the artery of any cuase
  o Coarctation of the aorta
  o Dissecting aortic aneurysm
  o Patent ductus arteriosus
  o Supravalvular aortic stenosis
  o Thoracic outlet syndrome

 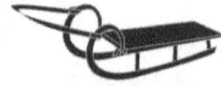

- Give the causes of differences in blood pressure between arms or between arms or between the arms and legs.

    o Heart
      - Patent ductus arteriosus (PDA)
      - Supravalvular

    o Aorta
      - Coarctation of the aorta
      - Dissecting aortic aneurysm
      - Aortic stenosis (AS)

    o Artery
      - Occlusion or stenosis of the artery of any cuase
      - Thoracic outlet syndrome

Adapted from: Baliga RR. *Saunders/Elsevier* 2007, page 94.

Abnormal arterial pulse patterns

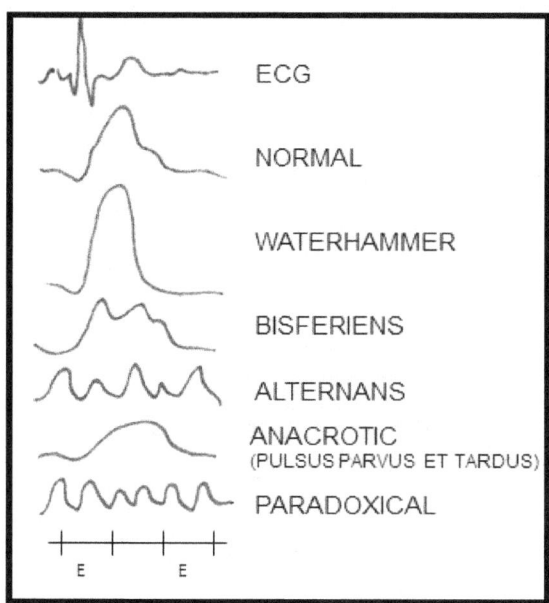

Source: Filate W, et al. *The Medical Society, Faculty of Medicine, University of Toronto* 2005, page 252.

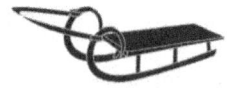

Pulse Pressure

- Perform a focused physical examination for an abnormally **widened pulse pressure**.

➤ Definition: pulse pressure > 50% of systolic blood pressure

➤ Causes
  - Hyperdynamic heart syndrome ($\uparrow$SV, $\downarrow$PVR)
  - Aortic regurgitation
  - Patent ductus arteriosus (PDA)
  - Exercise
  - Anemia
  - Arteriovenous fistulas
  - Beriberi
  - Paget's disease
  - Cirrhosis
  - Pregnancy
  - Thyrotoxicosis
  - Severe exfoliative dermatitis

Abbreviations: PVR, peripheral vascular resistance; SV, stroke volume.

SO YOU WANT TO BE A CARDIOLOGIST!

- Give the influence of the pulse pressure (PP) on the interpretation of the palpation of a rapid arterial upstroke.

  ➤ $\uparrow$ PP, rapid upstroke
    - Normal collapse
      - Mitral regurgitation
      - VSD
      - HOCM
    - Rapid collapse – aortic regurgitation
    - Hyperkinetic heart syndromes (high – output states)
  ➤ PP, rapid upstroke
    - Emptying into a low pressure area[1]
      - VSD
      - MR
    - Emptying into a high pressure area[2] - HOCM

1 rapid emptying of LV
2 LVH, delayed LV obstruction

Adapted from: Mangione S. *Hanley & Belfus* 2000, page 184.

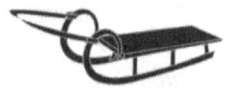

Mastering the Boards: Cardiology   A.B.R. Thomson

Carotid Bruits in an asymptomatic patient

- Auscultated in 16% of normal adults, and in 15% of children (<15 yrs)
- Increases the risk of TIAs/CVAs and the need for coronary artery bypass by 3-fold
- Seen in 10% of the surgical population
- Not predictive of perioperative CVA
- Are predictive of transient post operative dysfunction and behavioural problems

Source: Simel DL, et al. *JAMA* 2009, pages 107 to 110.

> **Quiz yourself**

- Give what does the peripheral pulse tells you about blood pressure (BP).

  - Systolic BP   -   Pressure on peripheral artery needed to obliterate the pulse

  - Diastolic BP   -   Volume of pulse

- Give causes of unequal radial pulses, yet equal brachial pulses.
  - Abnormal position of radial artery
  - What causes unequal radial and brachial pulses?
    - Obstruction of artery: thrombus, embolus, aneurysm, mediastinal compression

- Give the maneuver to perform on physical examination to be certain in that of the peripheral pulse volume seems to be abnormal.

  - Suspicion of pulse volume being
    - Large: rise arm
    - Small: lower arm

- Give why the patient with systemic hypertension does not necessarily develop a collapsing pulse.
  - A collapsing pulse is the result of an increase in the pulse pressure
  - The pulse pressure is the difference between the systolic and the diastolic blood pressures [SBP & DBP, respectively]).
  - In systemic hypertension, there is an increase in both SBP & DBP, so the pulse pressure (SBP minus DBP) may not be sufficient to cause a collapsing pulse.

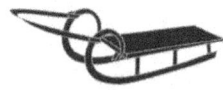

- Give causes of a **collapsing pulse**.
  - Aortic regurgitation (AR)
  - AV shunts
  - 3rd – degree heart block
  - Fever (may be associated with "dicrotic" pulse)
  - Anemia
  - Chronic liver disease

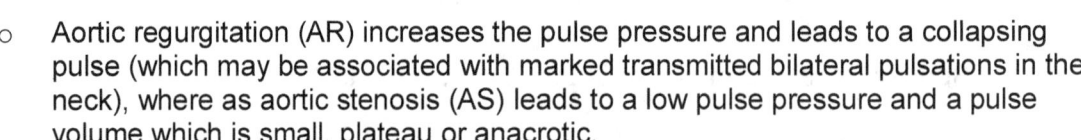

  - Aortic regurgitation (AR) increases the pulse pressure and leads to a collapsing pulse (which may be associated with marked transmitted bilateral pulsations in the neck), where as aortic stenosis (AS) leads to a low pulse pressure and a pulse volume which is small, plateau or anacrotic.
  - Jugular venous distention (JVP) is associated with a, c and v waves. What are the causes of ↑ JVP and the absence of pulsations?
    - The pressure in the jugular veins is increased because of obstruction in the superior vena cava (SVC) or in the jugular veins themselves.
  - Under what circumstance will the hepato-jugular reflex be absent in the person with ↑ JVP?
    - ↑ JVP due to venous obstruction

SO YOU WANT TO BE A CARDIOLOGIST!

- Give what is Friedrich ataxia (FA), and what are the associated cardiac abnormalities.

  - CNS degeneration
    - Spinocerebellar tracts
    - Posterior columns
    - Pyramidal tracts
  - MSK abnormalities
    - Kyphoscoliosis
    - Pes cavis
  - Cardiac abnormalities in FA
    - Cardiomegaly
    - Arrhythmias
    - Conduction defects

- In the context of increased pulse pressure in one limb (due to AV fistula), what is the area of the Branham sign? (compressing the area of suspected AV fistula causes ↓ HR).

  - Branham sign is bradycardia caused by inhibiting the ↑ RA pressure caused by the fistula, thereby inhibiting vagal and stimulating the sympathic pathway [Bainbridge reflex]).

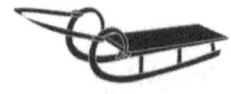

Mastering the Boards: Cardiology   A.B.R. Thomson

- Multiple tests are available for the diagnosis of structural heart disease. Give the diagnostic test(s) recommended for 7 of the following types of cardiac disease.

Cardiac condition	TTE	TEE	3 DE	RA	CATH	CMR	CT
○ HF (heart failure)	+						
○ Cardiomyopathy	+					+(ARVC)	
○ Valve disease	+	+ (AV)	+ (MV)			+ (AV)	+ (AV)
○ Prosthetic valve		+					
○ ASD / VSD			+				
○ Endocarditis		+					
○ Congenital heart disease	+				+	+	
○ Pulmonary hypertension	+						
○ Pericardial disease	+						
○ LA thrombus		+					
○ LV function	+		+	+		+	
○ RV function						+	
○ Coronary arteries					+		+
○ Myocardial disease / viability						+	

Abbreviation: ARVC, arrhythmogenic RV [right ventricular] cardiomyopathy; ASD, atrial septal defect; CATH, cardiac catheterization; CMR, cardiovascular magnetic resonance; LA, left atrium LV, left ventricle; RV, right ventricle

---

SO YOU WANT TO BE A CARDIOLOGIST!

- In which conditions may the pulse rate in one arm differ from that in the other.

  ○ Usually, slowing of the pulse on one side occurs distal to the aneurymal sac. Thus, an aneurysm of the transverse or descending aortic arch causes a retardation of the left radial pulse. Also, the artery feels smaller and is more easily compresses than usual An aneurysm of the ascending aorta or common carotid artery may result in similar changes in the right radial pulse.

Source: Baliga RR. *Saunders/Elsevier* 2007, page 94.

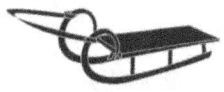

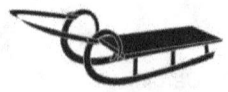

INDEX

Note: Page number followed by "f" or "t" indicates figure and table respectively.

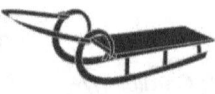

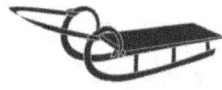

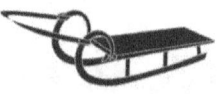

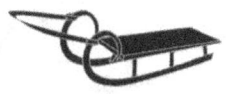

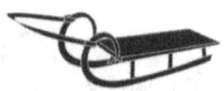

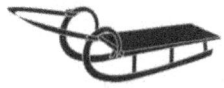

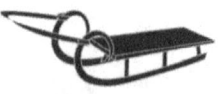

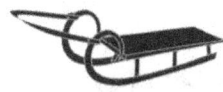

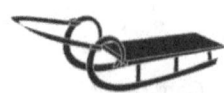

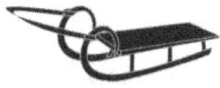

Mastering the Boards: Cardiology   A.B.R. Thomson

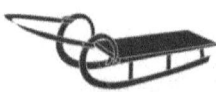

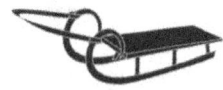

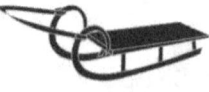

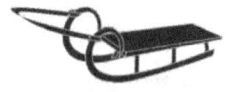

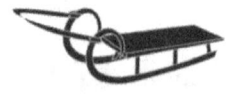

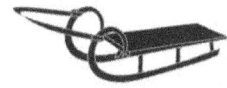

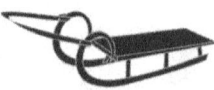

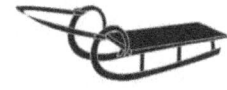

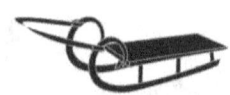

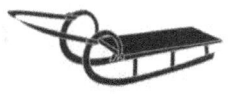

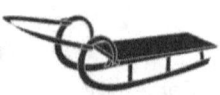

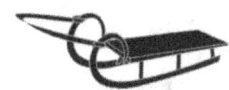

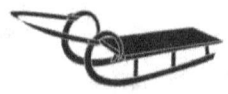

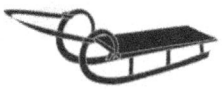

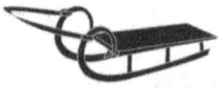

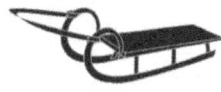

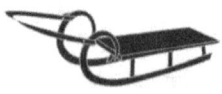

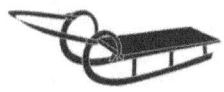

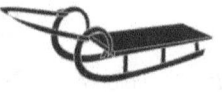

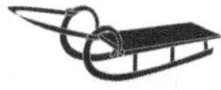

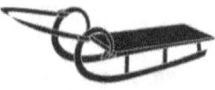

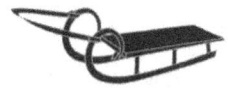

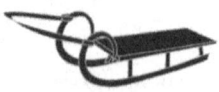

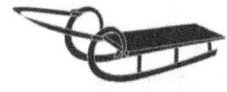

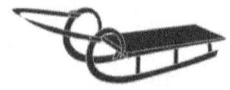

www.ingramcontent.com/pod-product-compliance
Lightning Source LLC
Chambersburg PA
CBHW080755180526
45168CB00006B/2216